D0523173

allergy & asthma
RELIEF

allergy & asthma
RELIEF

Featuring **the Breathe Easy Plan**
Seven Steps to Allergen Resistance

WILLIAM E. BERGER, M.D.
AND DEBRA L. GORDON

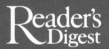

The Reader's Digest Association
Pleasantville, New York/Montreal

Project Staff

Editor
Neil Wertheimer

Designer
Rich Kershner

Photo Researcher
Leslie Caraballo

Copy Editor
Jane Sherman

Indexer
Nanette Bendyna

Illustrator
Rod Little,
Information Illustration

Reader's Digest Health Publishing

Editor in Chief and Publishing Director
Neil Wertheimer

Managing Editor
Suzanne G. Beason

Art Director
Michele Laseau

Production Technology Manager
Douglas A. Croll

Manufacturing Manager
John L. Cassidy

Marketing Director
Dawn Nelson

Vice President and General Manager
Keira Krausz

Reader's Digest Association, Inc.

President, North America Global Editor-in-Chief
Eric W. Schrier

Notice to our readers

The information in this book should not be substituted for, or used to alter, medical therapy without your doctor's advice. For a specific health problem, consult your physician for guidance. The mention of any products, retail businesses, or websites in this book does not imply or constitute an endorsement by the authors or by the Reader's Digest Association.

Copyright © 2004 by The Reader's Digest Association, Inc.
Copyright © 2004 by The Reader's Digest Association (Canada) Ltd.
Copyright © 2004 by The Reader's Digest Association Far East Ltd.
Philippine Copyright © 2004 by The Reader's Digest Association Far East Ltd.
All rights reserved. Unauthorized reproduction, in any manner, is prohibited.

Reader's Digest is a registered trademark of The Reader's Digest Association, Inc.

Library of Congress Cataloging-in-Publication Data
Berger, William E.
  Allergy and asthma relief : the breakthrough approach to ending the attacks and feeling great--all the time! / by William E. Berger and Debra L. Gordon.
      p. cm.
  Includes index.
  ISBN 0-7621-0507-0 (hardcover) -- ISBN 0-7621-0604-2 (paperback)
  1. Asthma--Popular works. 2. Allergy--Popular works. I. Gordon, Debra L.
II. Title.
  RC591.G675 2004
  616.2'38--dc22
                                    2004000707
0-7621-0507-0 hb
0-7621-0604-2 pb

Address any comments about *Allergy and Asthma Relief* to:
Editor in Chief
Reader's Digest Home and Health Books
Reader's Digest Road
Pleasantville, NY 10570-7000

To order additional copies of *Allergy and Asthma Relief*, call 1-800-846-2100.

For more Reader's Digest products and information, visit our website **rd.com**

Printed in the United States of America.
1 3 5 7 9 10 8 6 4 2 (hb)
1 3 5 7 9 10 8 6 4 2 (pb)
US 4422H/G

acknowledgments

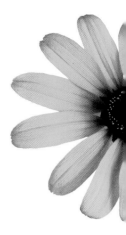

I wish to thank my coauthor, Debra Gordon, for her extraordinary efforts in helping to put this important and often complex information into a highly readable and interesting format. Our professional collaboration has been one of the most enjoyable and productive experiences of my career as a physician and educator. I am sure that Debra will not miss our cell phone discussions at all hours of the day and night to get the wording of a sentence in this book just right to best describe a particular condition or treatment regimen.

I feel particularly privileged to work with a superb clinical and research staff, including my associates in practice, Mark Sugar, M.D., Janis Davidson, R.N., C.P.N.P, and Ellen Schonfeld, R.N., C.P.N.P., who are truly dedicated to providing the highest-quality medical care to our patients with asthma and allergic disorders. A very special thanks to our administrator, Georgia Beams, who helped me start Allergy and Asthma Associates of Southern California in Mission Viejo over 25 years ago and is still the glue that holds everything together. Thanks to my son, Michael, and my daughter, Johanna, for their encouragement and confidence that their dad would get this project done on time and to the best of his abilities. Last, I especially want to thank my wife, Charlette, for her loving support and understanding during the entire process of making this book a reality. I know that it isn't easy to be married to a physician who spends his whole workday caring for allergy and asthma patients, then comes home and spends his free time writing a book about taking care of allergy and asthma patients. Now maybe we'll have more time for golf??!!

—William E. Berger, M.D.

After years of interviewing and working with physicians on a variety of health-related topics, I can spot the good ones pretty quickly. From our very first correspondence, I knew William E. Berger, M.D., was one of them. Despite having a hectic practice that includes significant clinical research, as well as holding the position of president of the American College of Allergy, Asthma, and Immunology during the time we worked on this book, Dr. Berger was never more than a phone call away. He never lost his patience, read every draft carefully, provided extremely well thought out and well-crafted revisions, and never made me feel foolish when I stumbled over the difference between nasal steroids and nasal antihistamines. He's just been a joy to work with.

I also want to thank the other experts who helped craft this book, most notably the fine physicians at the National Jewish Medical and Research Center in Denver. Harold Nelson, M.D., was a great help in walking me through the future of allergy and asthma treatment, while Esther L. Langmack, M.D., contributed immeasurably to the chapter on alternative approaches. Additionally, Joe Spahn, M.D., was fabulous when it came time to talk about allergies and asthma in children. Out in front, though, was Bill Allstetter, the public relations guru at the center, who always found the perfect expert for me to interview.

In addition, I want to thank the women who shared their experiences with asthma and allergies (and those of their families) in response to my panicked request on the bulletin board of the Freelance Success network.

Agreeing to write a book is always a relatively easy proposition; actually creating a final product is quite another thing. The fact that you are holding said product in your hands is due in no small part to the incredible work of the editorial staff at Reader's Digest Books. To Neil Wertheimer, who kept me going with his wit and laid-back attitude and who did what every writer prays her editor will do by making me seem like a better writer than I really am. To Rich Kershner, who designed the book you're holding so that you really want to read through it all. And to Jane Sherman and Suzanne Beason, whose copyediting and proofreading skills saved me from several embarrassing faux pas and you from any inconsistencies or inaccuracies. **—Debra Gordon**

contents

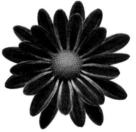

PART THREE

the **breathe easy** plan

PART FOUR

special **situations**

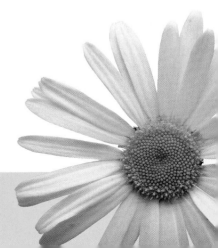

taking
control
of allergies & asthma

Controlling your condition: It sounds so simple doesn't it? In fact, it's something that, for most people with allergies and asthma, often seems nearly impossible to achieve.

A stunning 94 percent of people with allergies say the condition reduces their quality of life, affecting their productivity, sleep, concentration, and even sex, according to a survey by the American College of Allergy, Asthma, and Immunology. And if you thought that asthma was just a sometime annoyance, think again: Asthma is a chronic condition that often permanently scars the lungs, severely impacting your respiratory health throughout your life.

Yet most people treat their asthma and allergies as mild inconveniences, something an over-the-counter pill or nasal spray can resolve. Hard to believe? Consider that only half of the people with allergies who were questioned in one survey considered the disease to be a serious medical condition, and nearly two-thirds didn't see an allergist or other doctor the last time their symptoms acted up.

With allergies and asthma reaching epidemic proportions among the American population today, this laissez-faire attitude cannot continue. Far too many people have simply resigned themselves to a life of being miserable, of seeing the everyday joys that most people experience simply pass them by.

And so we bring you *Allergy & Asthma Relief*, featuring the Breathe Easy Plan. It's a program I'm proud to attach my name to, and one I'm convinced will work. Why? Well, after 25 years of treating patients who have these chronic conditions, of developing plans to help them live fuller, healthier lives, I am convinced that it takes more than a prescription to "breathe easy." Instead, it takes a comprehensive plan, one that incorporates everything from where you work and where you sleep to the doctor who treats your condition.

That's just what we've tried to provide for you in this book. As you work your way through *Allergy & Asthma Relief*, and, most important, as you implement the Breathe Easy Plan that forms the heart of the book, I guarantee that you will find yourself feeling the kind of relief you have sought for years.

That doesn't mean it will be easy, though, for it's never easy to change. Indeed, we'll ask you to change your eating habits, your home environment, your reactions to stress, and even your workplace environment. But as you launch the Breathe Easy Plan, remember:

- The plan is based not only on decades of scientific research but also on the best clinical practices in use today. The steps in the Breathe Easy Plan aren't theoretical; they work, and work well.
- Many of the changes you will be asked to make go far beyond just controlling allergies or asthma. The dietary changes, environmental improvements, supplement program, and stress-relief techniques you will be doing will also help your weight, your heart, your energy, your immunity from diseases, and even your outlook on life.

To make the Breathe Easy Plan as easy as possible to do, we've made the steps extremely specific. At no point should you have any trouble knowing what to do or why. We've also removed the element of time. This is not a 2-week or 12-week program; while it is best done sequentially, you can do it at your own pace, with the knowledge that it has the power to provide a lifetime of allergy and asthma relief if implemented correctly.

Through it all, we provide you with the motivation to make the necessary changes and, most important, to stick with them for the long term. We teach you how to evaluate your own progress, how to talk with your physician about your medications and overall care, and how to incorporate other approaches into your comprehensive program.

So take a deep breath (you can do it!), sit back, and relax. You've just taken the most important first step toward a lifetime of allergy and asthma relief.

William E. Berger, M.D.

William E. Berger, M.D

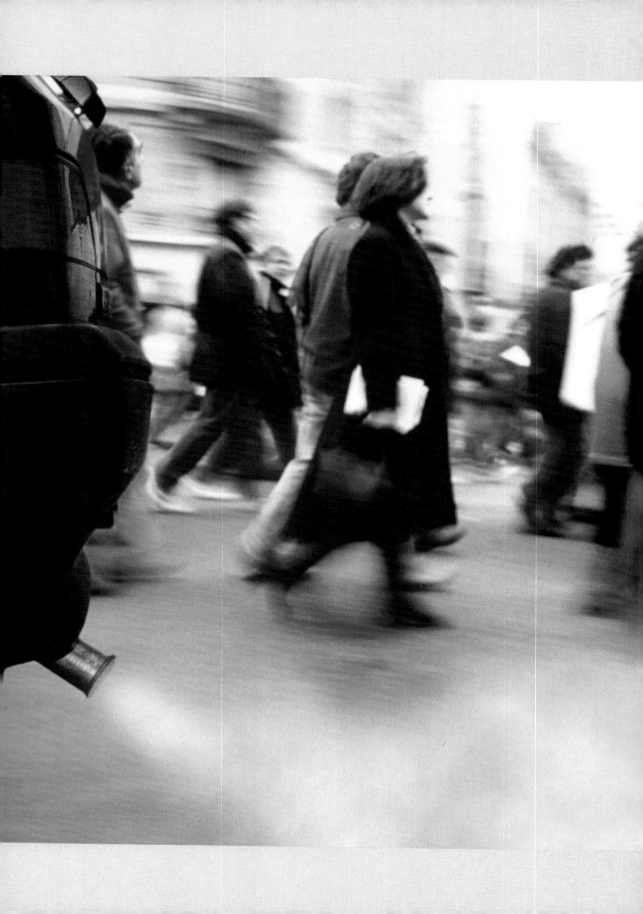

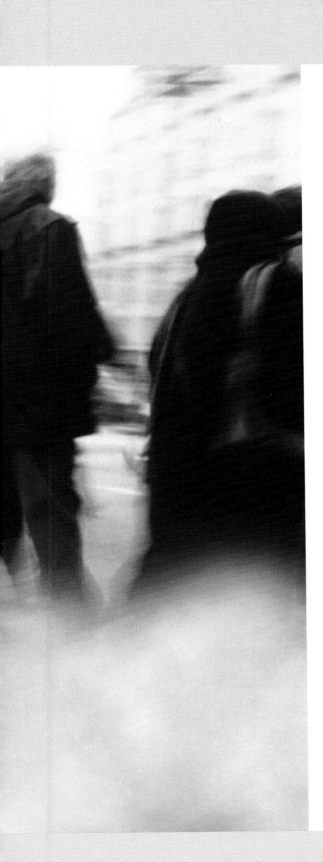

PART ONE

the problem

Is *epidemic* too strong a word
to describe the rise of allergies
and asthma in our modern world?
Probably not. An astounding
number of people today struggle
with the sneezing, wheezing,
and discomfort of allergies and
asthma. The reasons are complex
and conflicting, but also fascinating.

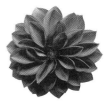

chapter one

an epidemic in the air

Augustus Caesar. Peter the Great. Ludwig von Beethoven. Charles Dickens. Teddy Roosevelt. John F. Kennedy. Leonard Bernstein. Liza Minnelli. Kenny G. Jackie Joyner-Kersee. All famous people—and all afflicted with asthma, allergies, or both.

Of course, you don't have to be President of the United States, a torch singer, or an Olympic gold medalist to have these diseases; you just need to be human. These days, asthma and allergies are reaching epidemic proportions in the United States and other countries, pressuring already overloaded health care systems, putting children's long-term health at risk, and costing employers billions in lost workdays and productivity.

The diseases themselves aren't new. More than 1,000 years ago, Persian physician Ali Razi wrote "An Article on the Reason Why Abou Zayd Balkhi Suffers from Rhinitis When Smelling Roses in Spring." In it, he reported on his philosophy teacher, who complained annually of sinus pain and inflammation "when the smell of flowers amplifies the illness." The recommended treatment might make today's allergy shots seem benign by comparison: In cases of severe nasal pressure, Ali Razi wrote, the patient's hair should be cut and his head covered with mustard.

In the early 1800s, London physician John Bostock, who studied his own affliction, provided the first detailed account of seasonal allergies. He coined the phrase "hay fever" because his condition typically worsened during haying season. The condition was so rare back then, however, that Bostock wrote, "I have not heard of a single unequivocal case among the poor."

Today, of course, the condition is the opposite of rare. While accurate statistics are hard to come by, professional estimates maintain that allergies and asthma together affect roughly 50 million adults, making them the most common chronic health problems in the United States (high blood pressure is number two). Likewise, asthma and other respiratory diseases (including allergic rhinitis) are the most common chronic conditions among children.

Given those statistics, chances are good that you or someone you know suffers from the itchy eyes, sneezing, wheezing, runny nose, and general misery of allergies or from the choking, can't-get-a-breath suffocation of asthma. That's why you're reading this book. You know how miserable it is to live your life stuck in an air-conditioned house on beautiful spring days, tethered to an inhaler like a dog to a tree, with your only pet a goldfish or turtle.

What you probably don't know is how simple it is to live a complete and active life—dog and all—even if you have allergies or asthma. That's what this book and our Breathe Easy Plan will show you.

a pervasive problem

Look around you. One out of four Americans has some kind of allergic disease, and the numbers have been rising exponentially in the past 20 years. Gail Shapiro, M.D., of the Northwest Allergy and Asthma Center in Seattle, recalls that when she finished training 30 years ago, a famous professor of pediatrics told her he didn't think they needed an allergist on staff. "We never hospitalize anyone for asthma," he said. Today, asthma is the leading cause of hospitalization for children and one of the top reasons young adults wind up in the hospital. It is also the primary reason for about 14 million doctor's visits and 2 million emergency room visits a year.

Dr. Shapiro also rarely saw a case of food anaphylaxis as a resident, and she recalls that back then, she and

by the numbers

- Americans make 9 million visits to office-based physicians each year because of hay fever, a.k.a. allergic rhinitis.

- Asthma-related conditions are responsible for 14 million doctors' visits and 2 million emergency room visits a year in the United States.

- Allergic rhinitis costs the country about $6 billion a year in direct medical costs and lost productivity.

- Thirty-four Americans die each day—more than 12,000 a year—from asthma-related causes.

her fellow doctors thought the condition—a severe, life-threatening allergic reaction—was "some kind of mental thing." Today, she says, it's a rare pediatric resident who hasn't seen someone come into the emergency room near death from anaphylaxis, and more than 600 people die each year from anaphylaxis related to food, latex, medication, or insect allergies.

"Allergies are definitely more prevalent today," says Marc E. Rothenberg, M.D., Ph.D., section chief of allergy and clinical immunology at Children's Hospital Medical Center of Cincinnati. In fact, the past five decades have seen tremendous growth in the incidence of all immune-based diseases, with allergies and asthma very much "the tip of the iceberg," he says.

For instance, atopic dermatitis (itchy rash, or eczema) is the most common skin condition in children under age 11, with 10 percent of children diagnosed with it in the 1990s, compared with just 3 percent in the 1960s. About 8 percent of American children have food allergies today, compared with about 2 percent of adults, suggesting that the incidence has increased since we adults were kids (contrary to popular wisdom, children *don't* usually outgrow allergies).

And allergic rhinitis—the run-of-the-mill, hay fever kind of allergy—affects up to 40 percent of children in the United States and a total of 35 million people overall. As for asthma . . . well, those rates have been growing faster than corn in July. The number of Americans with asthma more than doubled

Top 5 Myths of Allergies and Asthma

1 **Some dog breeds, such as Chihuahuas, are better for people with asthma and allergies.** REALITY: It's the protein in the pet's saliva, dander, and urine that causes allergies in some individuals, not the hair. Since all dogs have dander, saliva, and urine, there are no particular breeds that are better for people with asthma and allergies.

2 **Asthma can be cured.** REALITY: There is no cure for asthma. However, with the proper diagnosis and treatment, people with asthma can lead normal, active lives with little disturbance to quality of life.

3 **Moving to Southwestern states will cure asthma and allergies.** REALITY: Moving to Southwestern states may relieve allergies for a few months, but new allergies to local plants in the new area can develop within a short period of time. There is no place you can move to escape from allergies and asthma.

4 **Children outgrow asthma.** REALITY: Asthma is a chronic state of hyperresponsiveness. Some children have asthma symptoms that clear up during adolescence, while others worsen, but the tendency toward oversensitive airways remains. Unfortunately, there is no way to predict a child's clinical progress.

5 **Allergies are a harmless problem.** REALITY: Allergies are a serious problem and should be treated effectively. If left untreated, they can lead to decreased quality of life, including impaired sleep and learning ability as well as absences from school and work. Untreated allergies can also result in other chronic respiratory problems, such as asthma and sinusitis, and skin disorders such as eczema and urticaria (hives). Some allergies, such as those to foods, drugs, and insect stings, can even lead to life-threatening anaphylaxis—a systemic allergic reaction that can sometimes be fatal.

between 1980 and 1999, from 6.8 million to 17.3 million reported cases, according to the Centers for Disease Control and Prevention in Atlanta, and the number of deaths from asthma tripled between 1977 and 1998— from 1,674 to 5,438—despite new medications and better understanding of the disease.

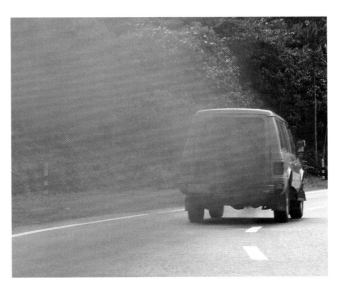

The weird thing about this boom in allergies and asthma? No one really knows why it's happening.

Oh, there are lots of theories. Some blame it on genetics, but while genetics certainly play a role in asthma and allergies, our genetic traits change far too slowly to account for such a sudden increase. And some allergic reactions, such as those produced by many plants, dyes, metals, and chemicals, have no genetic basis.

Other theories include:

Japanese research suggests the airborne waste from car exhaust could be affecting the mucous membranes in the lungs and nose, boosting allergic responses.

■ **We're spending more time indoors** and are thus exposed to more indoor allergens and air pollutants.

■ **Our world is** *too* **clean,** preventing our immune systems from doing their jobs properly (see "Are We Too Clean?" on page 18).

■ **An epidemic increase in obesity rates,** coupled with a dramatic drop in fruit and vegetable consumption, is playing havoc with our immune systems.

■ **Airborne waste materials from fossil fuel** combustion (for example, exhaust from cars and power plants) could be affecting the mucous membranes in the lungs and nose, boosting allergic responses, Japanese research suggests.

■ **Complications during pregnancy,** particularly those related to the uterus, such as preeclampsia, hemorrhage after birth, or preterm contractions, could be resulting in a higher risk of allergies and asthma for the children born of those pregnancies.

■ **Immune system defects** resulting in allergies and asthma are set early in life, probably in the fetal stage, and are locked into one's "immunological memory," researchers say. In recent years, scientists have mapped several allergy-asthma genes, finding that genes not only reflect a risk of developing asthma but also determine how severe the disease will be once it develops.

Yet despite decades of research and data, a report issued in March 2002 found that researchers were no closer to understanding the roots of the asthma epidemic than they were when it first began 20 years earlier. They're hampered by the absence of a standardized system for monitoring trends, as well as flawed and inconclusive data.

The very complexity of diseases like asthma and allergies also makes identifying a cause or causes difficult. In fact, it's quite likely that there is no single disease called "asthma" but rather multiple diseases that fall within the realm of asthma, just as there are multiple forms of headaches. Also, as with any complex chronic disease, such as heart disease, diabetes, or arthritis, there will never be just one cause or just one treatment. Instead, as we learn more about the genetics of individuals, it's likely that treatments will become more individualized.

defining allergies and asthma

Whether it's a plain-Jane pollen/dust mite/cat dander allergy, a life-threatening food allergy, disfiguring and endlessly itching eczema, or chest-tightening asthma, allergies and asthma are real diseases, not simply irritating annoyances that will go away if you just stop thinking about them. Yet that's how they were once viewed—as conditions of the mind. As recently as 20 years ago, even doctors believed that allergies and asthma were caused by anxiety, hysteria, and an overall "weak constitution." Today we know they're the result of a complex biochemical confluence among the immune system, the environment, and your own genes. We'll cover that in more detail in later chapters.

Although they seem to go together like bacon and eggs, allergies and asthma are actually two different diseases—albeit ones that exist on the same continuum, with asthma at the far end and allergies somewhere in the middle. There's even a name for the close connection between the two: allergic airway syndrome, or rhinobronchitis. Although allergies may contribute to asthma (about 80 percent of people with asthma also have allergies, and people with allergies are three times more likely than those without to develop asthma), asthma doesn't cause, or even contribute to, allergies. Often, people with allergies have no symptoms of asthma, but when they're exposed to cold air, exercise, or infection, they show significant bronchial "hyperresponsiveness," or asthma-like symptoms. They don't have asthma per se, but their lungs do have a greater tendency to react to these situations in an asthma-like manner than those of someone who doesn't have allergies.

Researchers suspect several reasons for the conjunction between allergies and asthma.

■ **Similar anatomy.** The microscopic anatomy of the tissues in the nose and lungs are almost identical, with very similar cells. Both are exposed to the same allergens and irritants, and they respond similarly.

How the Respiratory System Works

While it sounds simple—provide your body with oxygen, rid your body of carbon dioxide—the process of respiration is decidedly complex. Here are the key parts of the respiratory system and what they do.

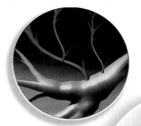

TERMINAL BRONCHIOLES: Like the tiny twigs that provide nourishment to the leaves of a giant tree, these ultrathin branches are the last in a line of bronchial tubes that transport gases to and from the alveoli.

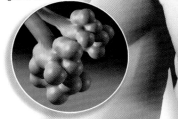

ALVEOLI: These clusters of hollow sacs are where gases are exchanged between the lungs and the bloodstream.

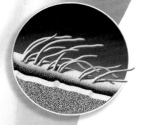

CILIA: Millions of these tiny hairs line the respiratory tract, beating at 12 to 16 strokes per second and creating waves that move germ-catching mucus up and out of the lungs.

NASAL CAVITY

TRACHEA: Similar to the trunk of a tree, this large tube is the passageway for all the gases entering and leaving the lungs.

INTERCOSTAL MUSCLES: These muscles connect rib to rib and help open and close the rib cage when you breathe.

TRACHEA

TERMINAL BRONCHIOLES

ALVEOLI

STERNUM

INTERCOSTAL MUSCLES

RIGHT LUNG

LEFT LUNG

DIAPHRAGM

DIAPHRAGM: This key muscle for breathing forms a curved sheath below your lungs. When you breathe in, your diaphragm drops, increasing the size of your lungs.

STERNUM: This plate of bone down the center of your chest holds in place the lung-protecting rib bones in the front of your body.

Are We Too Clean?

Although no one knows why the incidence of allergies and asthma is skyrocketing in this country, a leading theory holds that our world (at least the United States and other Western countries) is simply too clean. Some researchers call this the hygiene theory. One researcher, Marc E. Rothenberg, M.D., Ph.D., section chief of allergy and clinical immunology at Children's Hospital Medical Center of Cincinnati, calls it the delinquency theory, as in the immune system has so little to do that it turns into a kind of physiological "juvenile delinquent," just itching to get into trouble. It's a much-studied theory: Since 1997, scientists have published more than 6,000 research reports examining the apparent links between civilized living and allergies and asthma.

The problem stems from the tremendous advances we've made in the past 50 years in combating infectious diseases, parasites, and other pathogens. With vaccines eliminating many previously common childhood diseases, antibiotics van-

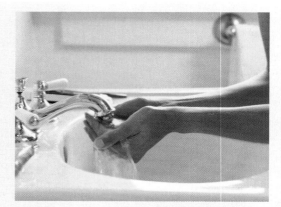

quishing others, and the American penchant for cleanliness (just think about the tremendous explosion in sales of antibacterial wipes, soaps, and lotions), a germ doesn't stand a chance.

This means the immune system is left sitting around, twiddling its virtual thumbs. Its entire function is to recognize the difference between "self" and foreign bodies. Self is fine, and some foreign bodies are bad (think about HIV and E. coli). Yet many foreign bodies you come in contact with (such as the hundreds of food proteins you eat and

■ **The nasal-bronchial reflex.** Nerve fibers originating in the upper airway connect to the lungs, allowing allergic reactions in the nose to cause a reflex in the lungs.

■ **Nasal blockage resulting in increased mouth breathing.** This, in turn, means the air that's taken in isn't warmed or filtered as it is when it's breathed through the nose, possibly triggering spasms as it moves into the lungs.

■ **Postnasal drip of inflammatory material.** Inflammatory chemicals commonly found in the noses of people with allergic rhinitis drip into the lungs while they sleep, causing asthma to worsen.

As we said, however, allergies and asthma *are* two different conditions. So let's start with allergies.

Simply put, if you have allergies, you have a hypersensitive immune system, one that responds entirely inappropriately to things such as plant pollen, other grasses and weeds, certain foods, latex, insect bites, or certain drugs, all of which are known as allergens.

The most common allergy is allergic rhinitis. It's an inflammation of mucous membranes that occurs when allergens touch the lining of the nose. Allergic the thousands of molecules you breathe in daily) are also fine. The immune system has to learn at an early age how to tell the good foreign bodies from the bad, just as a toddler has to learn what "hot" means. One way it does this is through encounters with endotoxins, molecules that occur naturally in every bacterium's outer envelope and are released into the environment any time bacteria die.

The fewer endotoxins your immune system encounters in childhood, the less likely it will learn that important difference. Instead, it may just start attacking *all* foreign bodies—as well as your own body. The result: diseases ranging from allergies and asthma to autoimmune conditions such as multiple sclerosis and rheumatoid arthritis.

Some evidence supporting this theory can be found in the disparate rates of allergy and asthma within a country. Studies in both Europe and the United States show that people living in rural and farm homes had far less atopy (genetic risk of allergies) and asthma, even though they had much higher exposure to endotoxins from living near animals. For instance, a study in Basel, Switzerland, showed that children of part-time farmers had a 76 percent higher risk of hay fever and other allergies than those of full-time farmers, suggesting that greater exposure to the farm environment can be more protective. Another study of asthma prevalence in children living on the Pacific atolls of Tokelau and in Tokelauan children living in New Zealand, a more modern environment, found that just 11 percent of the children living on the atolls had asthma, compared with 25 percent of Tokelauan children in New Zealand.

The fact that a spate of recent studies shows that children who have pets when they're young are less likely to develop allergies when they're older also lends credence to the theory.

Obviously, this doesn't mean you should send your children out to the woods to fend for themselves, but maybe you can relax the hypervigilance many parents have and consider getting them a dog. The bottom line: A little dirt won't kill 'em—and it may even help.

rhinitis is characterized by sneezing; congestion; itching and dripping of the nose; and itchy, watery eyes. It can be seasonal—affecting about 36 million Americans—or perennial, meaning it never goes away.

Not sure if you have allergies? Well, if you're constantly sneezing, sniffling, and clearing your throat; if your head feels like it contains more stuffing than a down comforter; if just the sight of peanuts can make your skin break out in hives; or if the skin under your eyes looks as if you've been in a brawl, chances are good that you do. Allergies are rarely fatal, and the handful of deaths that occur each year are from food, medication, or insect allergies, not the most common allergic rhinitis. You'll learn much more about rhinitis, and even be able to take a quiz that can tell you if you may have it, in chapter 3.

Asthma, on the other hand, can make you pretty darn sick, pretty darn quick. A chronic—meaning it doesn't go away—disease of the pulmonary system, or lungs, it's made worse by that overactive immune system. Symptoms include coughing, wheezing, and shortness of breath. During an asthma attack, the airways (bronchial tubes) in your lungs react to some stimulus, or trigger. They become inflamed and make more mucus than usual. At the same time, the muscles around the airways tighten, making it hard to breathe.

Blame It on Mom

Wondering whether you have allergies? Ask your mom when she started menstruating. Researchers in Finland reviewed a study of 5,000 pregnant women who had been asked when they began menstruating. They then gave the women's now-30-something children allergy tests for various types of grasses and house dust mites. They found that mothers whose periods started when they were younger than 12 were almost 1.5 times more likely to have children who later developed allergies than those who started menstruating at 16. Why? Well, the researchers don't really know, but they do have their theories. One is that differences in the maternal estrogen environment, which manifested itself in the varying ages of menstruation, somehow programmed the immune systems of the fetuses.

People with asthma describe an attack as feeling as if they're "breathing through a straw" or are drowning. In a way, they *are* drowning as their airways squeeze shut and their lungs become starved for air. Although there's no cure for asthma, it can be treated and controlled. You'll learn more about asthma in chapter 4.

Both allergies and asthma attack indiscriminately, regardless of race, age, socioeconomic status, and overall health. They don't care if you're a 98-pound weakling or a pro football player. You can develop allergies and asthma in childhood or in your sixties; in Phoenix, Arizona, or Portland, Oregon. Your age, sex, race, and socioeconomic status may, however, play a role in your *risk* of developing these diseases and in their severity.

For instance, although African-Americans have only a slightly higher prevalence rate of asthma than whites, they're three times more likely to die or be hospitalized because of it. Much of the reason probably relates to poverty, since people living in poverty have less access to quality medical care and often have no choice about where they live or work. Thus, their exposure to asthma triggers, such as insect droppings, diesel emissions from trucks and buses, and other toxic chemicals, is much greater. But researchers from Johns Hopkins University in Baltimore recently discovered that some African-Americans may have a particular gene that predisposes them to asthma.

Women are about one-third more likely than men to have asthma, and they're twice as likely to die from it. One study of female high school students found that girls reported significantly more frequent and severe symptoms of asthma and other allergic diseases than boys did. One possible reason could be the use of birth control pills, but researchers really don't know how to account for the difference. An October 2002 study also found that women with endometriosis are more likely than other women to have autoimmune disorders, including asthma, allergies, and eczema.

Now that you know *what* asthma and allergies are, it's time to turn your attention to the *whys*. Just what's going on in your body that can make something as simple as a grain of pollen wreak so much havoc? You'll find out in chapter 2.

chapter two

why your
immune
system
falters

When it comes to the causes of allergies and asthma, you can forget the usual suspects. They're not infectious diseases, so viruses and bacteria can't be blamed. Nor can you blame working too hard, standing in the rain, eating too much fat, or being attractive to mosquitoes.

Instead, blame yourself—or more specifically, your immune system, the same one that's designed to protect you from harm. When you have allergies or asthma, it acts like a cat on speed: hyperalert to any potential invader, seeing enemies where it should see friends, and ready to fly into action at the slightest provocation or even a peaceful interaction.

To understand why your immune system sometimes goes haywire, you first need to understand how things are *supposed* to work, so come with us on an intimate tour.

the guardian of health

If you've read anything about the immune system, you've undoubtedly seen it portrayed as a miniature army that's constantly on the defense against attack,

What's the Difference between Atopic and Allergic?

If your doctor says you're atopic, it doesn't mean you're losing your hair or your train of thought. It just means you have a genetic predisposition to allergies, certain skin conditions, or food or drug hypersensitivities. If a condition is known as atopic, it means that genetics play a role in who's likely to get it. Allergic rhinitis and, as has been recently discovered, latex allergies are atopic; allergies to insects and drugs are not usually hereditary, so they wouldn't be called atopic.

To put it another way, someone who is allergic reacts adversely to exposure to allergens; someone who is atopic is genetically predisposed to developing allergies. Thus, you can be atopic without being allergic, and you can be allergic without being atopic. If you're atopic without being allergic, though, don't get too comfortable—you're at a much higher risk of developing allergies than someone without atopy.

How do you know if you're atopic? Well, call your mom—or your dad, brother or sister, aunts, uncles, and cousins. If they had allergies—any kind of allergies, not just rhinitis—you're probably atopic. If so, you should follow the Breathe Easy Plan in part 3 even if you haven't developed full-blown allergies yet; it may reduce your exposure enough to prevent your immune system from becoming hypersensitive.

equipping its "soldiers" with the weapons necessary to fight evil, uh, germs, and always girding itself for battle. You can almost feel tiny spears being thrown around inside your body.

The reality is far less warlike. If we had to come up with a better analogy, it would be the security operation at a busy airport. Here's why: With every breath you take, with every bite of food you eat, with every touch on your skin, your body encounters and processes millions of foreign cells and molecules. As with the tens of thousands of people passing through airport corridors each day, the vast majority of substances passing through your body are welcome and harmless. But every now and then, something harmful slips through—an airborne virus, a splinter in your finger, an unseen bit of mold on a piece of bread. A well-functioning immune system, using a broad array of covert tactics and screens, identifies and disposes of unwelcome substances, usually unnoticed by the rest of your body.

Just as for airport security, the greatest challenge for the immune system is distinguishing the good from the bad. That balance is crucial. A weak immune system can allow viruses and bacteria to proliferate in your body or make healing from injury difficult and slow. That's why diseases that suppress immunity, such as AIDS, are so dangerous.

The other side of the pendulum is also problematic. An overactive immune system can attack the very thing it's supposed to protect—you. For example, rheumatoid arthritis is a disease in which your immune system attacks one or more of your joints. An overactive immune system can also view foreign bodies that are generally safe, such as the proteins in food, as potential terrorists that need to be eliminated. It's this latter state you have to worry about with allergies and, to a lesser extent, asthma.

Understanding how the immune system differentiates between welcome and unwelcome cells is the key to understanding the causes of allergies and asthma. That's what we'll explain next.

telling self from non-self

The immune system operates on one fundamental truth: There is "self," and there is "non-self." Ideally, immune system cells go after only non-self molecules, such as bacteria, viruses, fungi, parasites, and even tumors, and leave self cells, such as nerve, muscle, and brain cells, alone. In most cases, that's just what happens.

The immune system knows which are "good" cells and which are "bad" cells because the surface of every cell in your body sports special proteins called human leukocyte antigens, or HLAs. Immune cells also identify intruders by characteristic shapes, called epitopes, that protrude from them. Think of HLAs and epitopes as a cell's ID badge, proclaiming its right to be in your body. As immune cells circulate, looking for foreign bodies to eliminate, they're constantly scanning the landscape for any HLAs they don't recognize. If they see a cell without the appropriate identification, a complex series of events begins, eventually ending with the destruction of the invader.

These intruders run the gamut, from the bacteria and viruses mentioned above to pollen grains or molecules of the oil in poison ivy. Even chemicals, drugs, and particles (such as latex powder) count as foreign. They're all called antigens, and they're the alarm bells that startle the immune cells into action.

The cells doing the detect-and-destroy work are white blood cells. Millions of them circulate in blood and tissues, helping to defend your body from infection. There are five main types.

1. Lymphocytes. Think of these cells as the surveillance team, constantly circulating throughout your body on the lookout for antigens. When they find any, they develop plans for attacking the invaders and convey those plans to other members of the immune system team. They also form the institutional memory of the immune system, storing those plans of attack on what amounts to a cellular hard drive, then calling it up again if the antigens reappear. There are two types of lymphocytes:

T lymphocytes, or T cells, secrete potent substances to attract the immune system cells that do the actual destruction work. Then they serve as a kind of cheerleading squad to keep the defense team at its job. Certain T cells do more than simply mark the antigens: They also attack and destroy diseased cells.

B lymphocytes, or B cells, are immune cells that actually produce antibodies, specialized fighter proteins that help your immune cells do their job. B cells have long memories for their enemies and may remain in your body for years, ready at any time to turn into little antibody factories whenever an antigen they recognize appears. This is how vaccination works: A tiny bit of a (usually) killed virus, or antigen, such as polio, measles, or flu, is injected into your bloodstream, provoking your B cells to create antibodies. Then, if you ever encounter the fully functional form of the virus, your body can quickly marshal its defenses and produce millions of the required antibodies without delay. If your B cells had never met up with that particular antigen before, the antibody response would be much slower, and the intruder could gain the upper hand.

2. Macrophages. These large cells engulf and destroy large particles such as bacteria or yeast.

3. Neutrophils. The most numerous white blood cells, neutrophils are the first to arrive on the scene after an injury occurs. Their favorite food is bacteria, and one neutrophil can eat about a dozen bacteria, destroying them with a substance that's similar to household bleach. The cells don't live long—about 12 hours—and if they eat their fill before then, they die sooner. Even in death, however, they have a mission to fulfill: releasing little chemical "SOSs" that alert and attract more neutrophils.

4. Eosinophils. These white blood cells secrete chemicals that trigger the inflammatory process (described on page 26) and help destroy foreign cells. They work together with lymphocytes and neutrophils, both of which release

The White Blood Cells

Circulating in your blood and scattered through all the tissues of your body is an army of defensive cells collectively known as white blood cells, or leukocytes. Their name is derived from their appearance under a microscope, which is colorless compared with the red blood cells with which they circulate in the bloodstream. Here are the five main types.

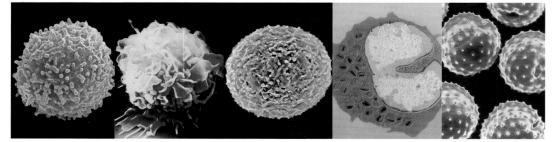

LYMPHOCYTES Found mostly in the lymphatic system, these search your body for cells that don't belong there and alert other cells to their presence.

MACROPHAGES These engulf and destroy large cells, such as bacteria or yeast, as well as the debris from natural cell formation in a growing body.

NEUTROPHILS The most common type of white blood cells in the bloodstream, they are first to appear at the site of an injury. Their job is to consume unwelcome cells.

EOSINOPHILS These make up 4 percent or less of active white blood cells. They attack larger cells, in part by secreting toxins that trigger inflammation.

BASOPHILS When they encounter damaged tissue, these cells release granules of germ-killing toxins and histamine, a substance that triggers inflammation.

certain substances that attract eosinophils to a particular site so they can release parasite-killing toxins. Eosinophils can play a big role in asthma. When they're called to a site during an allergic or asthmatic attack, they release toxins inappropriately, damaging the lining of air passages. Thus, one focus of asthma treatment is to stop eosinophils from accumulating in the lungs and prevent those already there from causing damage. That's the goal of steroid inhalers.

5. Basophils. Also called granular leukocytes, these white blood cells are filled with granules of toxic chemicals that can digest microorganisms. Basophils are also implicated in allergy attacks because, like eosinophils, they release a host of chemicals that contribute to the inflammatory response, including histamine (hence the use of *anti*histamines to treat allergies).

the lymphatic system

The immune system is much more than a mishmash of cells, however; it's a true system, with its own transportation network and rest stops, known as the lymphatic system. This pipeline of veins and capillaries similar to blood vessels runs throughout your body. It collects lymph fluid from the spaces around cells and returns it to the bloodstream. Throughout this transportation network are way stations called lymph nodes—small, bean-shaped masses found in places such as your neck, groin, and armpits. They're filled with lymphocytes and act as filters for the lymph fluid, removing microorganisms and other pathogens so the lymphatic cells can destroy them on the spot. That's why your neck and underarms feel tender when you're sick; the lymph nodes there are working overtime, filtering and destroying the antigens responsible for your illness.

The spleen is part of this system, functioning like a super-size lymph node. Lying in the upper left side of your abdominal cavity just under your diaphragm, it serves as a truck stop for immune cells, which wait there until they're needed. It also filters blood, which is why, although you can get along just fine without a spleen (it's often injured in traumatic accidents and subsequently removed), you may be more prone to infections if your super-size filter is gone.

Your tonsils and adenoids, small organs found at the back of your throat, also play a role. They're the birthplace of phagocytes, immune cells that target bacteria that enter the mouth.

The third and final major player in the immune system is the thymus gland. Located just over your heart in the upper right part of your chest, it acts like a boarding school for T lymphocytes, secreting a hormone that helps the T cells mature into their various types.

inflammation

Remember the two types of white blood cells called basophils and eosinophils? They're the immune cells that trigger the inflammatory reaction. Inflammation is a cornerstone of the immune system, but it can be a double-edged sword, especially when it comes to allergies and asthma.

Inflammation, in simplest terms, is what happens when a part of your body swells and heats up. It's your body's response to a host of insults: invasion by bacteria or viruses, injury, or reaction to your own tissues. When tissues are injured, they and the cells that flock to the injury release a barrage of chemicals, including histamine, bradykinin, serotonin, and others. These chemicals cause blood vessels to leak fluid into the tissues, leading to swelling, redness, and heat. This in turn throws a kind of barrier around the foreign substance,

How Inflammation Works

To most of us, "inflammation" means that a body part has become red, hot, and swollen. That's true, but the fascinating story lies in the "how" and "why." In fact, inflammation is your body's quick response mechanism for repairing tissue that is injured or infected.

1. A foreign body (germ, splinter, or allergen) is detected by white blood cells, which release several chemicals to launch a healing response.

2. Small blood vessels near the site leak fluid (causing swelling) and other white blood cells (which attack the foreign body). In addition, blood flow to the area increases, causing it to redden and heat up.

3. Tissue damage and signals from white blood cells trigger nerve pain receptors, increasing the pain of the injury. The goal: to make it difficult for you to use the hurt body part until it heals.

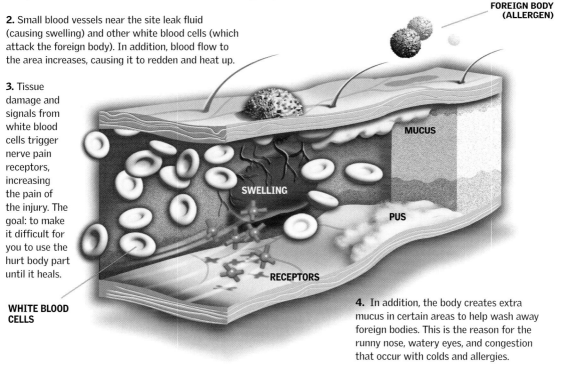

FOREIGN BODY (ALLERGEN)

MUCUS

SWELLING

PUS

RECEPTORS

WHITE BLOOD CELLS

4. In addition, the body creates extra mucus in certain areas to help wash away foreign bodies. This is the reason for the runny nose, watery eyes, and congestion that occur with colds and allergies.

5. Dead tissues, dead bacteria, and spent white blood cells accumulate to form pus.

preventing it from escaping into the body and infecting other tissues. The chemicals also attract white blood cells that "eat" the foreign substance as well as dead or damaged cells. The pus that often forms after an injury, then, is a mixture of dead tissue, dead bacteria, and live and dead macrophages.

Inflammation also increases mucus secretions, resulting in the runny nose, watery eyes, and congestion associated with allergic reactions. It can also cause the smooth muscles of your airways to constrict, resulting in the tightening sensation and gasping for air so common during an asthma attack. Inflammation is usually a beneficial healing process, but when it continues unabated, problems develop because it can harm tissues.

understanding antibodies

Now on to the antibodies, bringing us closer to how this whole system fits with allergies and asthma. As we noted earlier, the white blood cells known as B lymphocytes secrete proteins called antibodies. Your blood contains more than 1 *trillion* antibodies, and with every new threat—even previously unseen viruses like the one responsible for severe acute respiratory syndrome (SARS) in the winter of 2003—the B cells spew out new forms of antibodies. Most antibodies don't actually destroy the foreign invaders; they just latch onto them and mark them in some way so other immune system cells can do the dirty work, or they send out chemical signals calling other white blood cells to action.

Antibodies are made up of chains of molecules that form a Y shape. The sections that make up the tips of the Y's arms vary greatly from one antibody to another; this is called the variable region. It develops a unique shape based on the antigen it was created to react to, so it can "lock" onto that antigen just like a key fitting into a lock. Sometimes this locking neutralizes the antigen on its own, rendering it harmless; sometimes it ruptures the cells of the foreign body; and sometimes it forces antigens to clump together, creating a sitting-duck target for other immune cells to attack.

Your blood contains 1 trillion Y-shaded chains of molecules called antibodies and with every new threat— such as the SARS virus—your immune system creates new antibodies.

The stem of the Y links the antibody to the white blood cells that may be required to destroy the pathogen. This stem is identical in all antibodies of the same class and is called the constant region.

There are five classes of antibodies, each with a slightly different function and operating method. Scientists call them immunoglobulins, or Igs for short.

Of the five, IgE is the one we could call the "allergy antibody," since IgE antibodies are the main culprits contributing to allergies. Normally, they are present in tiny quantities in the body and are produced in response to relatively large invaders, such as parasites like ringworm and fluke. That's one reason allergies are far less prevalent in less developed parts of the world and why some researchers think our predilection for cleanliness has gone too far. They theorize that when people come into contact with these parasites, IgE goes out and does its job. If it never gets a chance to do its job, it begins to act out like a bored teenager. Instead of attacking parasites as it's supposed to do, it begins attacking proteins and molecules it *should* recognize as perfectly harmless, such as dust and peanuts and pollen.

When that happens, the IgE binds the allergen molecule either to basophils, the white blood cells described earlier, or to cells called mast cells, found in the mucous linings of tissues throughout the body, such as the throat, nose, lungs, skin, or stomach lining. This binding triggers the mast cells or basophils to release inflammatory chemicals, such as histamine, prostaglandins, and leukotrienes.

Recapping Our Story

Getting confused? Here's a cheat sheet on the science of allergies, as described in this chapter.

A. White blood cells are a major component of the immune system. These cells float freely in the bloodstream, seeking out and destroying viruses, bacteria, and other things that shouldn't be there.

B. There are five types of white blood cells.
- Lymphocytes
- Macrophages
- Neutrophils
- Eosinophils
- Basophils

C. There are two main types of lymphocytes: T cells and B cells.

D. B-lymphocytes create antibodies, which are proteins that latch onto pathogens, marking them for destruction by the other white blood cells.

E. There are five types of antibodies: IgA, IgD, IgG, IgM, and IgE.

F. IgE is the antibody involved in allergic reactions. It binds to mast cells in moist tissues in the body, sensitizing them to an allergen. When the allergen comes along, it interacts with the IgE antibody, which then signals the mast cell to release chemicals that cause the allergic reaction.

G. Basophils and eosinophils are also involved in allergic reactions. These white blood cells, like the mast cells, release chemicals that also contribute to the inflammatory reaction.

H. The result is an allergy attack: coughing, runny nose, itchy eyes, and so on.

It's these chemicals—not the actual dust mites, cat dander, or peanut proteins—that are responsible for the miserable coughing, wheezing, runny nose, itchy eyes, and itchy skin of an allergy attack. Because the mast cells are constantly calling up new recruits in the form of additional basophils and eosinophils, the attack can continue long after the allergen has been removed. In fact, one way that doctors screen for allergies is to measure the levels of IgE and eosinophils in your blood; if they're high and you haven't just returned from Africa or some other place where you could have been infected with parasites, chances are you've got allergies.

how allergies happen

The immune system can fail—and fail quite spectacularly, at that—in three main ways.

First, there's the failure most people are familiar with: weakened immunity. This is what happens as a result of chronic, or long-term, illness. For example, cancer—as well as cancer treatments—can greatly weaken your immune system.

Stress also weakens immunity. It turns out that the very chemicals released when you're under stress, such as adrenaline, are the same chemicals that keep your immune system in check so it doesn't get out of control. If you're under the kind of chronic, grinding stress that comes with a job you hate, money issues, too many deadlines, problems with your kids, an overcommitted life, or concerns about relationships, your body releases these chemicals nonstop. They in turn suppress your immune system, leading to a whole host of problems, ranging from colds and other viruses to cancer and heart disease.

HIV, which causes AIDS, also suppresses the immune system. The virus does this by deliberately attacking certain T cells, causing vulnerablity to numerous infections from very basic pathogens we live with all the time. People with AIDS eventually die not from the virus itself but from some ancillary disease that has taken advantage of their weakened immune systems.

The second category of immune system failure is overactivity. Autoimmune diseases such as multiple sclerosis, Crohn's disease, lupus, and type 1 diabetes fall into this category. These diseases occur because the immune system fails to recognize "self" cells as safe and begins attacking them as invaders. In Crohn's disease, for instance, it attacks cells in the gut; in diabetes, it kills off insulin-producing cells in the pancreas; and in multiple sclerosis, it attacks the surface of brain cells.

The third category of immune system breakdown is the one that results in allergies and asthma. It has some characteristics of overactive immunity in that the immune system reacts to the wrong thing. Instead of attacking your own cells, though, it attacks normally harmless molecules such as food proteins and

Inside an Allergic Reaction

Allergens are foreign substances that are not harmful to your body but which your immune system has learned to attack anyhow. Once an allergen is detected by your immune system, a fast but complicated process begins that leads to the sneezing, congestion, and other symptoms of allergies.

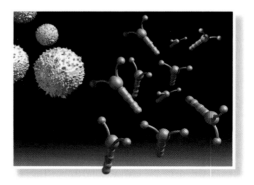

1. Initial exposure to an allergen causes your body to create Y-shaped antibodies unique to that allergen. These antibodies then stay in your body, ready to pounce if the allergen shows up again.

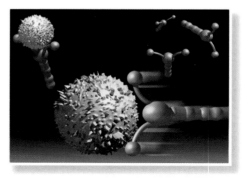

2. On the next exposure to the allergen (which could occur years or even decades later), the antibodies discover it and immediately lock onto it.

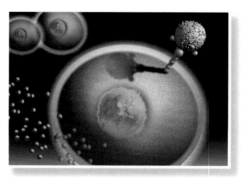

3. The antibody then attaches to a mast cell lining your nose, throat, lungs, or elsewhere, which in turn triggers the release of inflammatory chemicals. The inflammatory process begins, with swelling, creation of mucus, reddening, heat, and vessel constriction. Voilá—an allergic reaction.

pollens in an overreaction that is tantamount to using a fire hose to put out a match.

Most people with allergies have some genetic predisposition to them, a code deep within their ancestral material that presents the *possibility* of allergies or asthma. But just because you have a genetic recipe for a condition doesn't always mean you're going to develop that condition, and with allergies and asthma, it takes the right environment to provide the final ingredient. Plus, you can wind up with an allergy even with no genetic predisposition if you're exposed to the substance frequently enough. For instance, latex allergies were nearly unheard of until the 1980s, when the AIDS epidemic resulted in health care providers and emergency personnel using dozens of latex gloves a week.

Beyond the Usual Allergies

Although the majority of allergies are provoked through the IgE-mediated response, called Type I response, there are three other hypersensitivity immune responses.

Cytotoxic reactions (Type II). This type of hypersensitivity involves the destruction of cells, particularly red blood cells and platelets, which can affect the ability of your blood to clot. These reactions typically occur with mismatched blood transfusions.

Immune complex reactions (Type III). This type of reaction often occurs three weeks or so after you've taken the final dose of a drug like penicillin, and it plays a role in the development of autoimmune diseases. With a Type III reaction, you usually feel as if you have the flu, with fever, skin rashes, hives, and swollen, tender lymph nodes. It can result in lung or kidney damage.

Cell-mediated reactions (Type IV). This type of reaction results in allergic contact dermatitis, a skin rash that occurs when you touch something to which you're allergic. More on that in chapter 14.

The allergic response works like this: An initial exposure to an allergen—such as pollen, dust mites, pet dander, or shrimp protein—causes your body to increase production of IgE. Each IgE is specific to an allergen; therefore, a person with multiple allergies will have different IgEs for each allergen. The IgEs stick to mast cells or basophils, thus sensitizing you to a particular allergen.

This initial exposure could happen years before an allergy actually occurs, even in the womb. That's why some researchers suspect that peanut consumption by pregnant or breastfeeding women could be a major reason for the growing number of peanut allergies in children in the United States. When the children start eating peanut butter at age 2 or 3, the reaction is triggered. Or say your child is stung by a bee when she's 10. She doesn't have an allergic reaction then, but when she's stung again a year later, boom! Or maybe you've been exposed to penicillin again and again, not through pills but through hormones in the hamburgers you ate. One day, you get strep throat, and your doctor prescribes penicillin. The drug is the final straw, tipping your sensitivity into a full-blown allergy.

When this happens, the IgE molecules go wild. Now they recognize the allergen as a foreign substance, lock onto it in that lock-and-key manner, and tie it to a mast cell or basophil, which in turn triggers the release of inflammatory chemicals such as histamine, prostaglandins, and leukotrienes and leads to symptoms such as bronchial constriction, coughing, and wheezing.

That initial reaction is called the early phase reaction. It can be followed several hours later by another reaction in which chemicals released by the mast cells send out another call for inflammatory cells (basophils and eosinophils). In some people with perennial allergies, the tissue never returns to normal and can be inflamed and sensitized even by a nonallergic trigger such as cigarette smoke or perfume (to which you don't have an actual *allergy*.)

Allergic reactions are usually localized—that is, they happen right at the spot in which the allergen is detected. Get an allergen on your skin, and your skin reacts. Get an allergen such as pollen in your nose, and your sinuses become inflamed. However, if an allergic reaction is severe enough to occur throughout your body, you get anaphylaxis, in which your entire body goes into shock. This is a deadly situation that can be stopped only with emergency doses of epinephrine, which puts the brakes on the immune reaction.

putting it all together

So what does all this have to do with asthma? A lot, as it turns out. Although asthma is defined more as a respiratory condition than an immune system disorder, it has its roots in the immune system. For instance, an initial "trigger" in asthma may be the release of inflammatory chemicals from the immune system. These cells lead to the production of too much mucus and increase the responsiveness of the smooth muscles in the airways, making them more likely to close up.

Asthma is a chronic condition, as you'll see in chapter 4. Asthma attacks are just the acute phase of the disease. For all that we know today about the role of the immune system in asthma and allergies, there is still more that we *don't* know about these diseases, particularly asthma. Ironically, the devastating AIDS epidemic has had one silver lining: It has resulted in an explosion of knowledge and understanding about the immune system. That understanding is leading to new treatments for everything from cancer to allergies and may well change the very nature of how we diagnose and treat these diseases.

In the next three chapters, we'll go more deeply into the most common form of allergies, allergic rhinitis; asthma; and one of the most dangerous forms of allergies, food allergies. As you read those chapters, you'll find that your mini-course in the immune system will stand you in good stead.

all about
allergies

You're sneezing, your throat is scratchy, and your eyes itch. Or you have this strange rash on your arms that just won't go away. Or raised red wheals have appeared on your chest and back. Or every time you eat shrimp, your lips and mouth swell, and you begin wheezing.

All of these are symptoms of allergies. In fact, as you'll learn throughout this book, there are numerous forms and types of allergies—nearly as many as there are allergy triggers. Later, we'll talk more about some of the less common types, such as food, insect, medication, and skin allergies. In this chapter, however, we're going to tackle the granddaddy of them all, the form of allergy responsible for the greatest misery in the most people: allergic rhinitis, or hay fever.

Allergic rhinitis usually shows up before age 20, but it can develop at any age. In fact, it may be diagnosed as early as the first year of life. Today, allergic rhinitis affects 40 percent of children and 20 to 30 percent of adults.

In years past, hay fever was viewed as nothing more than an annoyance, not really worth treating seriously and certainly not capable of inflicting the kind of economic and physical toll that we now know it does. Indeed, today we know that allergic rhinitis is associated with several other respiratory illnesses, including asthma, and that it can significantly affect your ability to work or study. In fact, studies find that people with allergic rhinitis miss 3.8 million days of work and school each year. Children miss more than 2 million days of school, and more than one-third of adults with hay fever say it decreases their work effectiveness. Overall, this allergy costs the United States about $2 billion in direct costs, with indirect costs estimated to be much higher.

Unfortunately, most Americans, even those who have allergies, underestimate the consequences. A national survey conducted by the American College of Allergy, Asthma, and Immunology in August 2002 found that while 94 percent of allergy sufferers reported that allergies affected their quality of life—including work productivity, sleep, concentration, and even sex—just 50 percent considered the disease to be a serious medical condition. Nearly two-thirds, or 64 percent, hadn't seen an allergist or other doctor the last time their symptoms flared up.

the allergy ripple effect

The primary symptom of allergic rhinitis is a stuffed and/or runny nose. When your nose behaves like this, doctors say it's chronically inflamed. This constant inflammation provides the perfect breeding ground for viruses and bacteria,

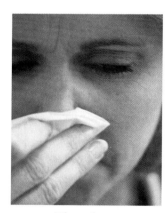

If you're prone to sinus infections ask your doctor to check you for allergies.

which can lead to numerous other problems, such as ear infections, sinus infections (sinusitis), and asthma. In fact, if you are prone to sinus infections, ask your doctor to check you for allergies.

Sinusitis affects about 31 million Americans a year. It's defined as an inflammation of the lining of the nasal sinuses, the hollow cavities within the cheekbones around your eyes and behind your nose. It can make an allergy attack feel like the sniffles. If you have sinusitis, chances are you also have a pounding headache, pressure behind your eyes and cheeks, toothache, green or gray nasal drainage, and postnasal drip. You may also lose your sense of smell and taste and have bad breath, along with chronic congestion.

About half of all people with sinusitis have allergies, and the theory is that the allergies lead to the sinus infections. It works like this: Normally, mucus and liquids drain from the sinuses through tiny openings about the size of a tip of a pen. Swelling due to an allergy can block that drainage, resulting in a buildup of mucus and providing a lovely spot for bacteria or viruses to thrive.

If allergies aren't treated, they can also lead to nasal polyps (pale, round outgrowths of the nasal lining) or swollen nasal turbinates (protruding tissues that

The Top 50 Allergy Capitals

Each year, the Asthma and Allergy Foundation of America (AAFA) ranks the top 50 U.S. cities for allergies. Researchers consider the average recorded pollen levels over the previous seven years, the length of the peak season for the most offensive pollen types, the number of antihistamine prescriptions written per capita in the previous year, and the number of board-certified allergists per capita. In 2003, the AAFA ranked the allergy capitals as follows:

1. Louisville, Ky.
2. Austin, Tex.
3. St. Louis, Mo.
4. Atlanta, Ga.
5. Charlotte, N.C.
6. Hartford/ New Haven, Conn.
7. Nashville, Tenn.
8. Raleigh-Durham/ Fayetteville, N.C.
9. Harrisburg/ Lancaster/ Lebanon/York, Pa.
10. Grand Rapids/ Kalamazoo/ Battle Creek, Mich.
11. Albuquerque/ Santa Fe, N. Mex.
12. Dallas/Ft. Worth, Tex.
13. Greenville/ Spartanburg/ Anderson, S.C.
14. Orlando/Daytona/ Melbourne, Fla.
15. Greensboro/ High Point/ Winston Salem, N.C.
16. Birmingham/ Tuscaloosa, Ala.
17. Indianapolis, Ind.
18. San Antonio, Tex.
19. Jacksonville/ Brunswick, Fla.
20. Houston, Tex.
21. Oklahoma City, Okla.
22. Memphis, Tenn.
23. Kansas City, Mo.
24. Phoenix, Ariz.
25. Las Vegas, Nev.
26. Baltimore, Md.
27. Boston, Mass.
28. Minneapolis/ St. Paul, Minn.
29. New York, N.Y.
30. Providence, R.I.
31. New Orleans, La.
32. Salt Lake City, Utah
33. Philadelphia, Pa.
34. Tampa/ St. Petersburg/ Sarasota, Fla.
35. Pittsburgh, Pa.
36. Columbus, Ohio
37. Cleveland/Akron/ Canton, Ohio
38. Albany/Schenectady/Troy, N.Y.
39. Detroit, Mich.
40. Seattle/ Tacoma, Wash.
41. Chicago, Ill.
42. Cincinnati, Ohio
43. Sacramento/ Stockton/ Modesto, Calif.
44. Washington, D.C.
45. Portland, Ore.
46. Milwaukee, Wis.
47. Norfolk/ Portsmouth/ Newport News, Va.
48. Denver, Colo.
49. San Francisco/ Oakland/ San Jose, Calif.
50. Los Angeles, Calif.

line the inside of your nose). Sometimes surgery is required to correct these problems. Untreated allergies can also cause dental and facial abnormalities, as described later, and can affect speech development in children.

In addition to the most common symptoms associated with allergic rhinitis—sneezing, runny nose, and watery eyes—it often disturbs sleep, so people spend their days in a fog of fatigue. Consequently, their ability to think, study, and process information is affected. They may also have difficulty remembering things, impaired hand-eye coordination, and decreased capacity to make decisions. Some of these symptoms may be caused by over-the-counter allergy remedies and others by a lack of sleep.

If congestion blocks your ear canals, it can interfere with hearing and affect learning and comprehension. Meanwhile, constantly blowing your nose and coughing can interrupt your concentration and ability to learn. But if you feel like you're moving in slow motion and your brain has turned to cotton candy, don't worry. Once you get your allergies fixed up with our Breathe Easy Plan in part 2, your alertness should come roaring back.

Allergies can also affect appearance. For instance, the dark under-eye circles called allergic shiners can make allergy sufferers look as if they've been pulling a string of all-nighters, although they're actually caused by swollen blood vessels under the eyes. Because many people with allergies breathe through their mouths, they're more likely to develop a high, arched palate (the roof of the mouth), an elevated upper lip, and an overbite, which may require orthodontic work. Then there's the nasal crease, a line across the lower part of the nose that forms from constantly rubbing it (known as the allergic salute). Finally, allergy sufferers may look as if they're constantly tired, in part, because of swollen adenoids, the lymph tissue that lines the back of the throat and extends behind your nose.

The Trouble With Allergies

When you think allergies, you usually think sneezing and wheezing. But allergies can affect your body in so many ways. Here are many of the possible affects, both short- and long-term:

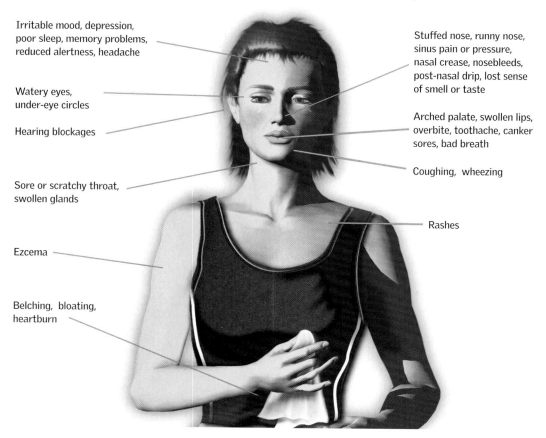

Irritable mood, depression, poor sleep, memory problems, reduced alertness, headache

Watery eyes, under-eye circles

Hearing blockages

Sore or scratchy throat, swollen glands

Ezcema

Belching, bloating, heartburn

Stuffed nose, runny nose, sinus pain or pressure, nasal crease, nosebleeds, post-nasal drip, lost sense of smell or taste

Arched palate, swollen lips, overbite, toothache, canker sores, bad breath

Coughing, wheezing

Rashes

Other common symptoms are chronic coughing; wheezing or shortness of breath; conjunctivitis, or pinkeye (red, swollen eyes); sore throat; frequent nosebleeds; post-nasal drip; bad breath; canker sores; an itchy palate; stomach problems, such as bloating, belching, and heart-burn; and irritability and depression. Just lovely, isn't it?

allergy or irritation?

Just because your nose is running and you're sneezing, that doesn't mean you have allergies. You could have a cold, sinusitis, or the plain-Jane form of rhinitis that's not associated with allergies. *Rhinitis* is just a term doctors use to describe the symptoms that result from nasal irritation, such as congestion or runniness. These symptoms can mimic allergic reactions but are not the result of the IgE immune response that occurs in allergies.

This is an important distinction. While your body may be irritated by

What's Your Rhinitis Type?

All allergic rhinitis is not created equal. Here are the three main types.

1 **Seasonal rhinitis.** This is what we think of when we think of rhinitis—occurring at certain times of the year, primarily in the spring and fall, when pollens (potent allergens) are at their peak. Although the timing of allergy season for you depends on where you live, the climate, and the season, that doesn't mean that moving will improve things. If you're prone to allergies, you'll probably just become allergic to something else in your new environment.

2 **Perennial rhinitis.** If you have perennial rhinitis, you have the dubious honor of being miserable year-round. It's likely that you're allergic to pet dander, dust mite and cockroach droppings, and mold, all allergy triggers that know no seasonality. You'll learn more about them later.

3 **Occupational rhinitis.** Blame it on your job; that's what your doctor will do. Occupational rhinitis results from a sensitivity to something at work, be it a chemical, the plants in the lobby, or the fibers in the carpet (but no, it's probably not the boss). If your symptoms occur only at work, improve or disappear on weekends and on vacation, and are shared by your col-leagues, ask your doctor to consider that something at work is literally getting under your skin.

any number of substances, an allergic response involves an immune system breakdown of a particular nature (which we described at length in chapter 2). Some doctors believe that what many people consider to be allergies are just irritations caused by, well, irritating things, such as dust or smoke.

Rhinitis that lasts less than six weeks is called acute, while persistent symptoms are called chronic. There's also infectious rhinitis, caused by viruses or bacteria, as with a cold or sinusitis, and vasomotor rhinitis, a run-of-the-mill drippy nose.

It works like this: Your nose normally produces mucus, which traps substances such as dust, pollen, pollution, and germs. Mucus flows back from the front of your nose and drains down your throat. If there's too much mucus, it drains down the front of your nose, too, and you get a runny nose. The more irritation, the more mucus your body produces to collect and dispose of the irritants. Numerous other things can also cause rhinitis, including temperature changes (think about how your nose runs when it's cold out), spicy food, some medications (including blood pressure drugs, birth control pills, and aspirin and other nonsteroidal anti-inflammatory drugs, such as ibuprofen and naproxen), cigarette smoke, perfume, alcoholic beverages such as beer and wine, cleaning solutions, and chlorine in swimming pools. You may even find yourself getting congested when you're sexually aroused.

pinning the blame

You're pretty sure you're allergic to *something*. The question is, *what?* Well, the only sure way to find out is with a skin or blood test, described in more detail in chapter 6. Here, we're going to outline the list of suspects, focusing, as we noted earlier, on those responsible for allergic rhinitis. Keep in mind that you can be allergic to several of these triggers at the same time and that one allergy may disappear while another comes to take its place.

What's Making My Nose Run?

You could have a cold. You could be encountering an irritant, such as smoke. Or maybe, just maybe, you could be having an allergic reaction. Here are questions to ask to see if your dripping nose is caused by nonallergic or allergic rhinitis.

1. Do you have a history of sneezing spells, itching of the nose and throat, and a large amount of watery nasal discharge?   yes ☐   no ☐

2. Do you have a family history of allergies?   yes ☐   no ☐

3. Do your symptoms respond favorably to treatment with antihistamines?   yes ☐   no ☐

4. Do your symptoms get worse during certain times of the year, such as spring or fall?   yes ☐   no ☐

5. Does exposure to animals such as cats or dogs cause nasal symptoms?   yes ☐   no ☐

Yes *answers to these questions are strongly suggestive of allergic rhinitis.*

1. Do you have fever and muscle or joint aches associated with your nasal symptoms?   yes ☐   no ☐

2. Do you have pain behind your eyes or above your upper teeth?   yes ☐   no ☐

3. Is your nasal drainage thick and/or discolored (green or yellow)?   yes ☐   no ☐

4. Are any other members of your household sick at the present time?   yes ☐   no ☐

Yes *answers to these questions usually suggest infectious rhinitis.*

1. Are your nasal symptoms brought on by changes in temperature or humidity?   yes ☐   no ☐

2. Are you very sensitive to scents in the air, such as perfume and cologne?   yes ☐   no ☐

3. Do cigarette smoke, cooking odors, and emotional stress cause nasal symptoms?   yes ☐   no ☐

4. Are antihistamines usually not helpful in alleviating symptoms?   yes ☐   no ☐

Yes *answers to these questions usually indicate vasomotor (nonallergic) rhinitis.*

something in the air

Airborne allergens, ranging from pollen and dust to mold spores, dander, and fibers, are the most common reason for rhinitis, with an estimated 35 million Americans allergic to these substances.

Let's start with pollen.

Even as many of us celebrate the demise of winter and the glory of spring, millions of allergy sufferers head to their TV rooms, eschewing the golf course, forgoing walks in the park, and considering investing in gas masks, all because the very same thing that's responsible for spring's beauty is also responsible for their misery. That would be pollen, the microscopic round or oval grains that plants use in lieu of sex to reproduce. Some use the grains to pollinate themselves, while others rely on insects, the wind, or even your clothes to carry the tiny particles around so they can do their business—namely, fertilizing other plants.

It's not the roses, daisies, and irises of spring and summer, however, that are to blame for your agony (unless you're a florist). Instead, look to the plain-Jane plants—trees, grasses, and weeds—without the showy flowers. That's because flowering plants depend on insects to carry their heavier pollen around, while run-of-the-mill plants produce particularly small, light, dry pollen granules that are custom-made for wind transport. And can they travel! Scientists have found ragweed pollen 400 miles out at sea and 2 miles high in the air. That's why simply clearing the area around you of offending plants isn't going to do any good. Plus, there's the sheer quantity of pollen: A single ragweed plant can generate a million grains a day.

Pollen occurs everywhere, in every state and country on every continent (even Antarctica). Even living in a high-rise apartment building in the midst of a city is no protection. Scientists in northern Spain found that residents of tower blocks in the city of Valladolid actually had a *higher* risk of pollen allergies than people who lived in villages in the local countryside. In fact, wrote one of the scientists, "Natural pollen sensitization appears to increase with the height of where the patient lived." The reason? Pollen rises as the air warms, then begins falling as it cools in the evening. The message: Keep your windows shut if you live in a high-rise.

Among North American plants, weeds are the most prolific producers

allergy sufferers ask

Am I Allergic to Cigarettes?

The short answer: No. Nor can you be allergic to perfume. You can, however, have a *sensitivity* to such substances, which can make your eyes water and your nose run and have you sneezing to beat the band—and if you have allergic rhinitis, you're more likely to have such sensitivities. But all those times you told the hotel clerk you were allergic to cigarette smoke and needed the only remaining nonsmoking room (which just happened to be a suite)? Well, it just isn't so. Next time, say "greatly irritated." It may not get you the upgrade, but it will be the truth.

The Usual Suspects

Allergens come from lots of seemingly unrelated sources, as this rogue's gallery shows. But they do have something key in common: They all are generated from living things. Your immune system is trained to attack viruses, bacteria and parasites, so it makes some sense that it might be hypersensitive to similar-size foreign proteins, organic chemicals, and molds.

Tree Pollen

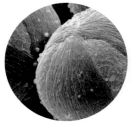

SYCAMORE This common tree puts off lots of pollen; a fuzz on its twigs and leaves can also trigger allergies.

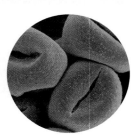

ASH Considered the No. 1 allergy plant in Mexico, this tree is found throughout North America.

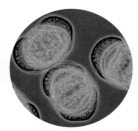

CEDAR Along with its juniper cousins, this cone-bearing evergreen is a major cause of hay fever.

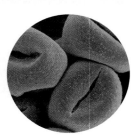

OAK This popular, common tree is mostly wind-polli-nated, and generates lots of microscopic pollen.

Grass Pollen

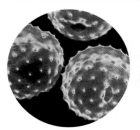

RAGWEED Among the worst allergy offenders, this weed thrives in areas where mankind has upset the ecosystem.

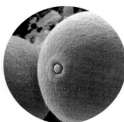

TIMOTHY GRASS One of many common grasses that trigger allergies. Others include Kentucky bluegrass and Bermuda grass.

Cockroaches

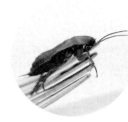

The saliva, feces, and bodies of these hardy urban bugs all generate allergens that can trigger attacks.

Pet Dander

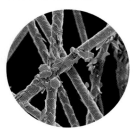

Cats and dogs constantly shed old skin cells, or dander, that carry all sorts of allergenic proteins.

Molds

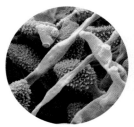

CLADOSPORIUM There are more than 30 types of molds in this genus. They often grow best in water-damaged environments.

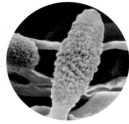

ALTERNARIA This unusu-ally shaped mold grows mostly on dead plants, par-ticularly grasses and cereals.

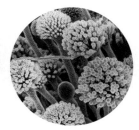

ASPERGILLUS This grows on decaying vegetation, such as compost heaps and fallen leaves, and often in air-conditioning systems.

Dust Mites

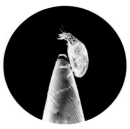

Half the size of a pen dot, these non-biting insects live just three months. They love beds for the warmth and food.

of allergenic pollen, with ragweed the major culprit; others include sagebrush, redroot pigweed, lamb's-quarters, Russian thistle (tumbleweed), and English plantain.

Grasses and trees, too, are important sources of allergenic pollens. Although more than 1,000 species of grasses grow in North America, only a few produce highly allergenic pollen. They include timothy grass, Kentucky bluegrass, Johnson grass, Bermuda grass, redtop grass, orchard grass, and sweet vernal grass.

Trees that produce allergenic pollen include oak, ash, elm, hickory, pecan, box elder, and mountain cedar. Of course, where you live determines what you're exposed to. For instance, birch trees are most prevalent in the northern United States, elms in the eastern part of the country, cedars in the West and in south Texas, and evergreens in New England. Oaks are ubiquitous, with some form of oak growing in every state except Hawaii and Alaska.

revealing **research**

Watch Out for Global Warming

Along with rising oceans, growing deserts, and erratic weather, add increasing allergies to the repercussions we can expect as our planet warms. A study published in the March 2002 issue of the journal *Annals of Allergy, Asthma and Immunology* found that ragweed grown in an atmosphere with double the current carbon dioxide levels (the expected result of global warming) would produce 61 percent more pollen than normal. The report isn't just theory; the researchers actually grew ragweed in a North Carolina pine forest into which they had pumped excess carbon dioxide. The pine trees also produced triple the normal number of pine cones and seeds, suggesting that the more carbon dioxide in the atmosphere, the more plants. This could not only result in more pine allergens, the researchers noted, but could also play havoc with current relationships among plants, inducing the growth of more weeds and thus even more potent allergens.

One clue to the cause of your allergy is when it occurs. Different plants pollinate during different times of the year in different parts of the country. For instance, spring comes early in the South, so seasonal rhinitis might start there in February and March, while people in Maine enjoy a sneeze-free existence through May. You can check a regularly updated pollen map of the United States by going to www.accuweather.com and looking in their health section. Or contact the National Allergy Bureau of the American Academy of Allergy, Asthma, and Immunology at www.aaaai.org/nab for information on pollen preponderance in your area and a clue as to what's blooming.

Newspaper and television weather maps also often provide pollen counts for your immediate area. A pollen count is simply a measure of how much pollen is in the air. It represents the concentration of all the pollen (or one particular type, like ragweed) in the air in a certain area at a specific time, expressed in grains of pollen per square meter of air collected over 24 hours. Pollen counts tend to be highest early in the morning on warm, dry, breezy days and lowest during chilly, wet periods—although thunderstorms can actually spread pollen farther. Keep in mind, however, that the pollen count reflects the *previous* 24 hours, not the coming day. Also note that while the amount of pollen makes a difference in the severity of your symptoms, the type is just as important. For instance, it takes just a little pollen from grasses (such as bluegrass or Bermuda grass) or trees (such as oak and elm) to trigger allergies, while it generally takes much larger quantities of pollens such as eucalyptus, which are heavier and don't disperse as easily.

But don't despair; later in this book we'll tell you how you can still enjoy the great outdoors despite your allergies.

Formidable Fungi: Molds

Mold has received a lot of bad press in recent years, with lawsuits relating to mold growth in homes—especially multi-million-dollar celebrity homes—grabbing headlines. We'll talk more about so-called sick building syndrome, believed to be caused in part by mold, later. For now, we're going to focus on the role common mold spores play in your allergies.

When Allergies Bloom

Here are rough timetables for when the most common plant allergens are in bloom in nine different climate regions of the United States. Note that flowers, with their oversize pollen grains, rarely cause allergies.

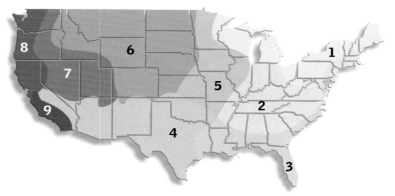

Area		Ragweed	Trees	Grasses
1		July-September	February-June	May-November
2		August-September	March-June	June-November
3		August-October	April-June	May-September
4		July-October	March-July	May-November
5		August-October	March-June	May-October
6		June-November	January-July	April-November
7		June-September	January-April	April-October
8		June-November	March-June	May-October
9		August-September	March-June	May-August

There are thousands of types of molds and yeasts in the fungus family. Molds are made of many cells that grow as branching threads called hyphae; yeasts are single cells that divide to form clusters. Although both can probably cause allergic reactions, only a small number of molds are recognized offenders.

If you're allergic to mold, your symptoms may get worse from spring to late fall. Just as with plant pollens, there is a mold "season," which peaks from July to late

allergy **sufferers ask**
What about That Yellow Stuff on My Car?

Most likely, it's pine tree pollen. In the spring, it blankets some areas of the country with a thick layer of yellow dust, coating cars, sidewalks, and buildings and painting puddles yellow when it rains. But it's probably not the cause of your misery. The chemical composition of pine pollen appears to make it less allergenic than other types. Also, because it's heavy, it tends to fall straight down and doesn't scatter, so it rarely reaches human noses.

summer, but unfortunately, the first freeze doesn't end the problem with molds as it does with pollen. Molds are tenacious little fungi that are able to grow at subfreezing temperatures. Even snow, while lowering the outdoor mold count dramatically by covering mold, doesn't kill mold spores. Come spring, the molds revive from their dormancy, thriving on the vegetation that's been killed by the winter cold. Small wonder that they're believed to be the oldest form of life on the planet!

In warm parts of the country, however, mold allergies can be perennial, or year-round, as can allergies caused by indoor molds. And mold is everywhere, with thousands of mold species throughout the world, even in icy Antarctica. In fact, when it comes to number, molds outnumber pollens, possibly because it's easier for them to grow. They don't need much: just moisture, oxygen, and a few other readily available environmental chemicals. And they can grow on anything, from rotting logs and fallen leaves to compost piles, grasses, and weeds and on grains such as wheat, oats, barley, and corn, not to mention your shower curtain. Anywhere there's the slightest bit of dampness in your house—the basement, bathroom, refrigerator drip tray, or even houseplants—there's likely to be mold.

It's not the mold itself that causes the allergic reaction, but its spores, which could be described as the mold's form of pollen. Each spore that germinates results in new mold growth, which can in turn produce millions of spores. These spores are so small that they easily evade the protective mechanisms of the nose and upper respiratory tract to reach the lungs. In some people, eating mold-containing foods, such as cheese, mushrooms, and dried fruit, can also bring on allergic symptoms.

Only a few types of mold get the allergen label. In general, Alternaria and Cladosporium (Hormodendrum) are the allergenic molds most commonly

A Mold Allergy on Steroids: Aspergillus

Although allergic rhinitis caused by mold is relatively benign, there is a certain kind of mold that can cause a more severe respiratory reaction. Called Aspergillus, this form of mold, found throughout the environment, may lodge in your airways or in a distant part of your lung and grow until it forms a compact sphere known as a fungus ball. Aspergillus mold can also lead to asthma or to a lung disease resembling severe inflammatory asthma, called allergic bronchopulmonary aspergillosis. The latter condition, which occurs rarely in only a minority of people with asthma, is characterized by wheezing, low-grade fever, and coughing up of brown-flecked masses or mucus plugs. Corticosteroid drugs are often used to treat the reaction; immunotherapy (allergy shots) doesn't do much good.

found indoors and outdoors throughout the United States. Aspergillus, Penicillium, Helminthosporium, Epicoccum, Fusarium, Mucor, Rhizopus, and Aureobasidium (Pullularia) are also common allergy triggers. There is no relationship, however, between a respiratory allergy to the mold Penicillium and an allergy to the drug penicillin, which is made from mold.

Not sure if molds are to blame? Think about your symptoms. Do they tend to occur most of the year, worsening in the summer, when you're near fields or just after gardening? It could be a mold allergy.

Although mold spores are counted just like pollen, the information isn't quite as helpful. One reason is that the number and types of spores actually present in the mold count may change considerably within 24 hours, depending on the weather. Many of the common allergenic molds are of the dry spore type, meaning they release their spores during dry, windy weather. Other fungi need high humidity, fog, or dew to release their spores. Although rain washes many larger spores out of the air, it also causes some smaller spores to be shot into the air. So don't count on a mold spore count to tell you when it's safe to come out of the sauna.

Dust Mites and Cockroaches

If you ever got a good look at what lives on the ostensibly clean surfaces of your home, it might make you sick. Billions of microscopic, eight-legged creatures called dust mites call your bed, carpeting, drapes, and furniture "home." Their favorite food? Flakes of your dead skin. Want to hear another gross fact? Those bits of dust you see floating in shafts of sunlight include dead dust mites and their droppings.

Dust mites just love dark, warm, humid spaces, such as upholstered furniture, mattresses, comforters, pillows, rugs, drapes, and stuffed animals. In fact, you can figure that millions are making themselves comfortable in your pillows. That's why you may find that your allergies worsen when you're in bed or on the couch.

You're actually allergic not to dust mites but to their excrement. The same goes for cockroaches, another major cause of allergic rhinitis. While dust mites are ubiquitous, cockroaches are more selective and are most commonly found in crowded cities and in the southern United States. Minuscule mite and cockroach droppings, which you can't see, seem to have this uncanny ability to drive your immune system batty. Never fear! We'll tell you more about how to stay one step ahead of the bugs and dust bunnies in chapter 8.

Animal Dander

The jury is still out on pets and allergies. A growing body of research suggests that having a cat or dog in the house when you're very young may actually prevent the development of asthma or allergies, even if you have a genetic tendency toward them. For instance, Claudia Rock, a researcher at the University of Wisconsin-Madison, studied nearly 300 children who were at risk for developing allergies because of their family histories. A year after their birth, her study found that babies were not any more sensitive to allergens if they had a cat or other animal in their home than if they didn't, and if they had a dog, their sensitivity significantly *decreased.* Exposure to dogs, the researchers found, increased levels of cytokines, chemicals that put the brakes on the body's reactions to allergens.

Household pets are still among the most common source of allergic reactions, however, and some allergists won't even begin treatment until a patient agrees to give up the family dog or cat. Plus, it can take as long as two years after you get a pet for the allergy to develop.

Don't blame your pet's fur or hair, and don't bother getting a hairless cat or a Chihuahua, thinking that will solve the problem. It's not the fur that makes you sneeze but rather proteins that are secreted by oil glands in the animals' skin and shed in dander, as well as proteins in their saliva, which sticks to the fur when the animal licks itself. Another source of allergy-causing proteins is animal urine. When the substance carrying the proteins dries, they are free to float into the air.

Research suggests that having a cat or dog in the house when you're very young *may actually prevent the development* of asthma or allergies.

Cat dander is particularly ubiquitous. First, there's the basic lifestyle of cats: They lick themselves more, may be held more, spend more time in the house close to humans, and do their bathroom duties in litter boxes in the house. Their dander also seems to hang in the air longer than dog dander—and it spreads faster than melted butter. Let your girlfriend bring her cat over for the weekend, and within 30 minutes of the feline's entrance into

What Is Dust?

Take one part mold, a few dust mites and their fecal matter, plus some animal hair and dander, then throw in minuscule bits of upholstery, lint, and other fibers and mix well with bits of human skin, plants, food remnants, and insect droppings. Voilá! You've got dust. Dust is who you are, where you live, what you do. You can go on vacation, leaving an immaculate house with every surface shining, and when you return, you'll still have house dust. It took scientists years to figure out the recipe and to realize that people aren't allergic to dust bunnies per se, but to specific components in the fluff.

your home, the air will be filled with allergy-causing proteins.

Some studies also find that intact male cats produce more allergy-causing proteins than female cats—yet another reason to have your kitten neutered. Another study found that dark-haired cats seem to cause more severe symptoms in their allergic owners than light-haired cats, so you may want to opt for a light-colored tabby rather than a black cat if you're determined to be a cat owner.

Pet allergies aren't restricted to cats and dogs. Even small pets, such as guinea pigs, gerbils, and birds, can cause allergic reactions, as can mice and rats. And just getting rid of your pet won't magically clear up your nose. Animal dander can remain on furniture, bedding, drapes, and other surfaces for months after the pet is gone. You're also at risk even if you've never owned a pet, since animal proteins are stickier than SuperGlue. You can be exposed to pet proteins from the clothes of pet-loving colleagues at work or even the gal at the next table in the coffee shop. When researchers from Johns Hopkins University in Baltimore measured air-borne concentrations of cat allergens in homes with and without feline occupants, they found low levels of cat allergens in the homes without cats, "as well as in every other building where it has been sought, including newly built homes, shopping malls, doctors' offices, and even hospitals."

Despite the agony of allergies, many pet owners would rather live with the symptoms than give up their beloved animals. About one-third of the estimated 6 million people who are allergic to cats have cats in their homes. For those diehard pet owners, the only option may be immunotherapy shots (described in chapter 7), drugs, and lots and lots of tissues.

the eyes have it

The red, itchy eyes of allergies may be related to more than just your nose; you may have an eye allergy as well. Doctors estimate that such allergies affect about 82 percent of Americans, only half of whom seek help for their symptoms. Think you're immune because you don't have nasal allergies? Think again. A survey by the American College of Allergy, Asthma, and Immunology in 2002 found that of the 82 percent of people who reported itchy, watery eyes, just 37 percent said they also had nasal allergies. Sufferers described their symptoms as "feeling like they had sand in their eyes" and said that symptoms interfered with their daily activities. Sometimes an allergic attack can be so intense that the actual surface of the eye swells, a condition called chemosis.

Eye allergies, or allergic conjunctivitis, result from the same immune system malfunction that causes nasal allergies, this time affecting the mast cells in the eye (there are plenty to go around, with more than 50 million in each eye). The triggers are similar to those that cause nasal allergies—pet dander, mold, pollen, and dust mites—and the condition can be either seasonal or perennial. There are also three other forms of allergic conjunctivitis that may affect your eyes.

■ **Vernal conjunctivitis.** This condition tends to occur in the spring, most often in boys under 10. Left untreated, it can result in scarring that could lead to vision loss. Symptoms include intense itching, sensitivity to sunlight, blurred vision, and stringy or ropy mucus discharge.

■ **Atopic keratoconjunctivitis (AK).** This form is very closely associated with the skin condition atopic dermatitis (you'll read more about skin-related allergies in chapter 14). Ninety-five percent of people with AK have atopic dermatitis, and almost 90 percent have asthma. It occurs most often in adolescence or early childhood. Symptoms include burning and tearing, along with corneal ulcers or cataracts; red, oozing lesions around the eye; mucus discharge; and sensitivity to light.

■ **Giant papillary conjunctivitis.** This form results from a combination of allergies and overuse of contact lenses, causing intense itching, tearing, burning, and redness.

Treatment for run-of-the-mill allergic conjunctivitis ranges from

allergy **sufferers ask**

What Is a Sneeze?

It's as much a part of allergies as a stuffy nose, but what, exactly, *is* a sneeze? Well, it's an involuntary violent expulsion of air through your nose and mouth involving many upper-body muscles. The sneeze sequence is probably hardwired in your brain and spinal cord, which is one reason it's so difficult to suppress a sneeze once the irritation message is sent to the brain.

The sneeze occurs when the nervous system in your nose (which you probably didn't even know you had) is stimulated, causing a sudden contraction of dozens of muscles in your face, chest, and abdomen. This contraction forces air out of your nose extremely fast, with the goal of getting rid of the irritation. How fast? One estimate says a sneeze emerges about as fast as the best professional baseball pitcher can throw a fastball, i.e., about 100 mph. But sneezing comes in handy if you have a stuffed nose. The acceleration of air through the nose causes a drop in pressure, and this tends to draw excess mucus and other fluids from the sinuses, having the same effect as when you blow your nose.

And yes, sometimes looking at a light can bring that just-on-the-edge sneeze to the forefront of the achoo-a-meter. Another bit of sneezing trivia: None other than Thomas Edison studied the sneeze, and in 1897, he created one of the first "action" movies of the time by filming a series of still shots of a sneeze in sequence, then replaying them rapidly one after another.

over-the-counter eyedrops, such as tear substitutes and decongestants/antihista-mines meant especially for the eye, to prescription eyedrops. The more serious forms of conjunctivitis require more aggressive approaches using a variety of prescription drugs. We'll talk more about the specific treatments available for allergic conjunctivitis in chapter 7.

allergies through a lifetime

It's long been a common misconception that people outgrow their allergies, or that if you didn't have allergies as a child, you won't get them as an adult. In fact, during the first year or two of life, children rarely develop allergic rhinitis. They're more prone to food allergies, particularly to milk and peanuts. That's probably because very young children aren't exposed much to the outdoors. As they grow and have more exposure to both outside allergens (pollens and grasses) and indoor allergens (pet dander, dust mites, and cockroach droppings), the allergies begin. Conversely, as children grow older and their immune systems become better able to regulate the production of IgE, they may no longer react to certain food allergies.

Puberty provides another impetus for the development of allergies, with some adolescents pegging the start of their allergies to their spurt of reproductive hormones.

One positive side effect of aging is that many people find that their allergies disappear as they grow older. The reason, researchers suspect, is that people tend to produce less IgE as they age.

putting it into perspective

Whether your symptoms are triggered by cat dander or pollen, mold or dust mites, the Breathe Easy Plan will help you find a way to live in this world without hiding out because of your allergies. We'll get into the plan in part 3. If your only problem is allergic rhinitis, you may want to skip to that part now, but if you have asthma or food allergies, keep reading. We bet the next two chapters are packed with information about these two conditions that you never knew.

chapter **four**

all about
asthma

"Having an asthma attack requires a laborious intake and outtake of breath, which induces a maddening wheeze and whistle as each breath is drawn and exhaled. My lungs feel sticky, and it's like the air is fighting its way to open the passages. As it opens those passages, there's often a release of mucus, which causes a constant need to cough or clear my throat. Sometimes it feels like the air is sandpaper and is actually scraping against my lungs. Whether it's real or psychological, the attack is followed by an immediate feeling that I'm not getting enough oxygen and a bit of accompanying panic. At that point, the only thought in my head is getting to my inhaler, which immediately eases the breathing process."

—Gwen Moran, *37, New Jersey–based writer and consultant*

As Moran and other asthma sufferers describe, having an asthma attack feels as if you're suffocating. That's why ancient Greek and Roman physicians used the word *asthma*, meaning "gasping," to describe shortness of breath. Ironically, the problem isn't only that you can't get enough air into your lungs; it's also that your lungs become so inflamed and congested that you can't get the air that's in them *out*. In fact, if you threw the lungs of someone in the midst of an asthma attack into a swimming pool, they'd float, thanks to all the trapped air.

Asthma is an ancient disease, dating back to the twelfth century, when Moses Maimonides, a renowned rabbi, philosopher, and physician who practiced in the royal courts of Egypt and Syria, wrote a treatise on it. Among his recommendations: moderation in food, drink, sleep, and sexual activity; avoiding polluted city environments; and, as a specific remedy, chicken soup. Not bad advice, given that inhalers and anti-inflammatory medications didn't exist back then!

About 800 years later, the treatments are more sophisticated, but the disease remains a conundrum. Today, identifying the cause (or causes) of asthma is as hard as blowing up a balloon during an attack. And because the causes are hard to pinpoint, doctors often misdiagnose the condition. They may say the problem is chronic bronchitis, pneumonia, or hyperactive lungs. This misreading delays the proper treatment.

The confusion stems from the disease itself. Unlike singular diseases such as chickenpox, asthma has many forms, all caused by different organisms but all triggered by a similar effect on the lungs.

Stated simply, asthma is a disease in which the airways of the lungs become hypersensitive to one or many irritants. When exposed to such irritants, the airways constrict, the lining of the bronchial tubes swells, and mucus production increases, making it hard for air to get into and out of the lungs. Repeated asthma attacks cause permanent scarring and compromise lung function over time.

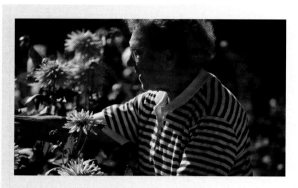

Over 65? Read This

You may have asthma and not know it. A study of 4,581 people age 65 and older, published in 1999 in the journal *Chest*, found that not only was asthma underdiagnosed in this group, it was also undertreated in the majority of those with the disease. This and other studies also found that asthma contributes to a decreased quality of life in the elderly, with those who have severe asthma reporting more negative feelings about life in general, describing their health as being poor, and having a greater degree of impairment during daily activities. At the same time, researchers in one study found high levels of potential asthma triggers in the homes of the elderly people tested, from carpeting, older furnishings, high indoor relative humidity, and nonencased mattresses. Ironically, the researchers noted, the poor quality of life many of the people reported meant that they were less likely to do the kind of housekeeping, such as dusting and vacuuming, that could reduce allergen levels in their homes and thus ease severe asthma.

The message for you? If you experience trouble breathing, chronic cough, wheezing, or any other asthma symptoms, insist that your doctor evaluate you for asthma and treat you aggressively. Age is not a reason to ignore asthma.

Our understanding of asthma has continued to evolve, even in just the past 10 years. Historically, doctors thought asthma was a disease of the smooth muscles that wrap around the airways in a lung. A trigger would cause the muscles to go into spasms, narrowing the airways and thus limiting the flow of air. Such triggers included allergens, air pollution, exercise, cigarette smoke, and cold air. Since these episodes waxed and waned over time—and disappeared after treatment—asthma was viewed as an intermittent illness that required minimal treatment between episodes.

Today, that view has been turned on its head. Doctors now know that asthma is a chronic condition and that even without symptoms, the disease is still active.

Some other new understandings about the disease include:

■ **Inflammation of the airways is a persistent feature of asthma**—even between attacks—and plays a critical role in changing overall lung function. Translation: Your asthma is changing the way your lungs work every minute of every day, even if you feel just fine and are breathing well. That's why most people with asthma require medication daily, not just during an attack.

■ **Complex reactions within the airways are a big part of an asthma attack.** These reactions are based in the immune system, meaning they involve many of the cells that play a role in allergies: eosinophils, T lymphocytes, macrophages, neutrophils, and basophils as well as mast cells and epithelial cells, which line the airways. It's these reactions that create the mucus and inflammation that further restrict breathing capacity.

Our improved understanding of asthma, however, still leaves us light years away from truly knowing what causes it. One of our greatest questions: Just what *is* the relationship between inflammation and asthma?

For instance, we know that asthma is always associated with inflammation of the lungs and that the intensity of the inflammation determines the severity of the symptoms. We also know that there can be a spiraling effect in asthma: Inflammation makes the hypersensitivity worse, which triggers more asthma attacks, which brings on more inflammation. No one is quite sure what triggers this inflammatory response. We do know, however, that over time and without proper treatment, the inflammation can eventually change the physical appearance and function of your lungs, leading to the replacement of normal tissue with nonfunctioning scar tissue that no amount of treatment can reverse.

Currently, asthma is divided into four main types, each of which behaves somewhat differently, is triggered differently, and may respond to different treatments or interventions.

■ **Allergic asthma (sometimes called extrinsic asthma).** This is the most common form; if you have allergies, you probably have allergic asthma. Attacks are triggered by allergens such as seasonal pollens or perennial inhalant allergens such as dust mites and animal dander. Allergic asthma often begins in childhood and stays with you for life.

■ **Nonallergic asthma (sometimes referred to as intrinsic asthma).** This form of asthma results from something within your body, such as a sinus infection or gastroesophageal reflux (heartburn). It generally develops later in life, and very little is known about its causes. One thing that is known: It's often more difficult to treat than allergic asthma.

■ **Mixed asthma.** You can have asthma that's triggered by both allergies and nonallergic factors. For instance, your allergy to grass and ragweed triggers your asthma, but you have symptoms even during the winter, when there is no pollen.

■ **Acute severe asthma or potentially fatal asthma.** If you have experienced this form of asthma, you know it. This life-threatening condition used to be called status asthmaticus. It's a type in which attacks come on suddenly and very intensely but don't respond to the usual treatment. With this form, you often have so much trouble breathing that you become exhausted and collapse. You're also in significant danger of death; people with acute severe asthma can go downhill very fast and die within the first 24 hours of an attack. One regional survey of fatal or near-fatal asthma attacks found that half occurred suddenly and unexpectedly, without any obvious predisposing factors. In the other half of attacks, psychosocial factors (such as stress), running in cold weather, overreliance on inhaled bronchodilators, and delays in seeking care were contributing causes.

inside an asthma attack

"Imagine yourself after you've run a race, and you've put everything you have into getting to the end. When you stop to catch your breath, you can't. It's sort of like that—no matter how hard or deep you breathe in, you just can't get enough oxygen."

—***Diana Burrell***, *38, Chelmsford, Mass.*

"I've never had a full-blown asthma attack (thank God), but when my asthma is in full force, like when I have a cold, it feels like an elephant is sitting on my chest, and it takes all of my effort to move it so I can breathe in and out. Also, I have so much gunk in my lungs that no amount of coughing can move it so I can breathe clearly."

—***Leah Ingram***, *37, New Hope, Pa.*

"The things I recall about my worst attacks:
• The horrible whistling from deep down in my chest, which only reminds me of how bad an attack I'm experiencing

• How conscious I am of each breath in and out; it's so much work that even bending over to pick up something is incredibly difficult

• Not only the tightness in my chest, but a soreness, too, that comes from using my whole body to try to take in more air

• The feeling of helplessness as I use my nebulizer to get more medication in, but I realize it's not working, and I need either my doctor or the ER."

—*Debbie Feit*, 36, Farmington, Mich.

An asthma "attack" starts with a trigger, just like an allergy attack. It can be an allergen (recall that the majority of people with asthma also have allergies) or something as seemingly innocuous as breathing in the first cold air of winter. The trigger irritates your airways. If you don't have asthma, you can just cough and be done with it. If you do have it, this irritation results in the release of chemicals such as histamines and leukotrienes from the mast cells found in the lining of your airways.

Warning Signs of an Asthma Attack

Yours may differ, but signs generally include at least one of the following:

• Decline in blowing power
• Chronic cough, especially at night
• Difficult or rapid breathing
• A feeling of chest tightness or discomfort
• Mucus in your chest that you can't cough out
• Becoming out of breath more easily than usual
• Wheezing
• Fatigue
• Itchy, watery, or glassy eyes
• An itchy, scratchy, or sore throat
• A tendency to rub or stroke your throat
• Sneezing
• Feeling that your head is stopped up
• Headache
• Fever
• Restlessness
• Runny nose
• A change in the color of your face
• Dark circles under your eyes

This triggers tightening of the muscles around your bronchial tubes, the small branches in the lung, which accounts for the tightness and pressure asthma sufferers feel. The underlying inflammatory process inherent in asthma may also lead to bronchial spasms, in which the muscles around your bronchial tubes twitch, preventing air from entering or leaving the lungs and helping to explain the wheezing (as you struggle to get air in or out through clogged airways) and the feeling of choking or drowning many people with asthma describe.

Thanks to the inflammation that's been triggered, mucus and fluids quickly build up in your lungs. They overwhelm the cilia, the tiny hairlike projections on certain cells that keep the lungs clear by pushing the fluids on. This forms the "gunk" that people describe as part of an asthma attack.

The result so far: You try to cough to clear out the gunk, but at the same time, you gasp for air. All of this is just phase I of an asthma attack. It doesn't end there.

(continued on page 56)

What We Think about Asthma

We asked nearly 300 people with asthma how they perceive and manage their condition. Here are some of their responses.

■ How often do you have an asthma attack?

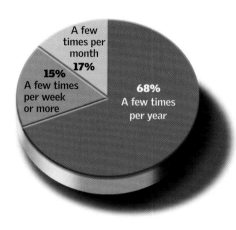

A few times per month 17%

15% A few times per week or more

68% A few times per year

■ In which seasons do you suffer from asthma?

Spring	84%
Fall	76%
Winter	73%
Summer	64%

■ When or where are you more susceptible to an attack?

Outdoors	64%
Nighttime	53%
Indoors	45%
At home	43%
While exercising	42%
Daytime	38%
At work	20%
None of the above	5%

■ Which of the following cause you to have an asthma attack?

Smoke	59%
Dust	56%
Mold/mildew	52%
Pollen	51%
Cold air	47%
Change of seasons	45%
Common cold/influenza	44%
Chemicals, paints, etc.	41%
Hairspray, perfumes, etc.	40%
Pets/animals	35%
Stress, tension, anxiety	31%
Exercise/sports activity	29%
Humidity	23%
Food	4%
Other	2%
None of the above	3%

■ Do you see a doctor who specializes in the treatment of asthma on a regular basis?

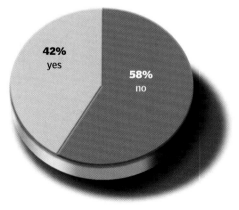

42% yes

58% no

■ Which of the following best describes the type of asthma attacks you experience most often?

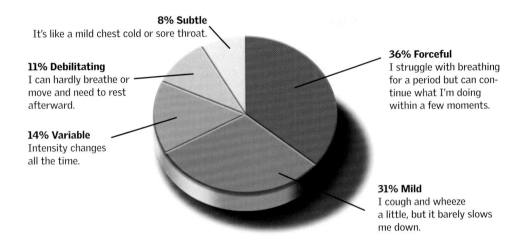

8% Subtle
It's like a mild chest cold or sore throat.

11% Debilitating
I can hardly breathe or move and need to rest afterward.

14% Variable
Intensity changes all the time.

36% Forceful
I struggle with breathing for a period but can continue what I'm doing within a few moments.

31% Mild
I cough and wheeze a little, but it barely slows me down.

■ Which of the following do you or someone in your household use to prevent, treat, or alleviate asthma?

Treatment	Always/ Sometimes	Most Preferred
Medication for attacks, such as bronchial inhalants and other fast-acting drugs	96%	55%
Preventive medication	87%	32%
Restricted activities	72%	0%
Frequent hand and face cleaning	66%	2%
Frequent cleaning of sinks, surfaces, and floors	63%	1%
Allergen-fighting home products (air filters, mite-resistant mattress covers, etc.)	59%	2%
Breathing exercises	56%	0%
Air cleaner	52%	2%
Vacuum with HEPA filter	47%	0%
Filter for drinking water	45%	0%
Peak Flow Meter	45%	0%
Air-filter mask when cleaning, working, or gardening	40%	0%
Meditation/relaxation techniques	38%	0%
Hot herbal tea	34%	2%
Restricted diet	23%	0%
Biofeedback	19%	0%
Herbs/essential oils	10%	1%
Yoga	6%	0%
Acupuncture	3%	0%
Other	24%	0%

Source: Reader's Digest Survey, March 2003

As this occurs, your immune system senses that something's wrong and rushes in to fix things. Instead, it only makes a bad situation worse. Various immune system cells release chemicals that activate the immune system's neutrophils and eosinophils. They then release chemicals that cause inflammation. The result: the chronic inflammation characteristic of asthma.

These chemicals can also hamper how well the smooth muscles in your lungs respond to signals from the nervous system to loosen their grip on the airways. What's more, they can prevent blood from picking up oxygen (starving your entire body of this vital element) and increase mucus secretion (gunking up the works even more).

Over time, these effects can result in permanent changes in your lungs, called airway remodeling. This is due to leakage from tiny blood vessels, overgrowth of smooth muscle cells, and thickening of the airway walls as scar tissue forms and other changes occur. The result: irreversible alterations in your airways and permanent loss of lung function.

Constricted Airways

An irritant lands in one of the bronchioles. For a person with healthy lungs, a cough moves it on, or cilia sweep it away. But for a person with asthma, the irritant causes the release of histamines and other chemical responses that start the domino chain of an asthma attack.

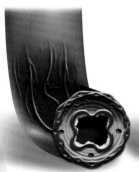

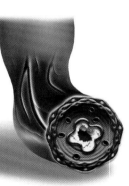

NORMAL AIRWAY
Muscles are relaxed, blood vessels are smooth, and a thin coat of mucus helps keep things flowing through.

DURING AN ASTHMA ATTACK
Muscles constrict, muscus membranes swell, and extra muscus builds up in an overwrought and cascading response to the trigger. The result is shortness of breath, coughing, wheezing, and other symptoms of asthma.

when asthma turns fatal

As the incidence of asthma has risen, so has the death rate from the disease. There are more than 5,000 deaths annually due to asthma, and asthma-related deaths among children 5 to 14 years of age more than doubled from 1979 to 1995. Complicating attempts to battle back is the absence of a way to predict which people with asthma face an increased risk of death. For instance, in one report on 51 asthma deaths in children under age 20, researchers found a third had "trivial or mild" asthma, while a third had no previous hospitalizations. Sixty-three percent collapsed suddenly minutes after developing shortness of breath, and 78 percent died before reaching the hospital. For half of those who died, the final attack lasted less than 2 hours.

There are some clues, however, as to whether asthma may suddenly become severe and life-threatening. Researchers have found that many who died from the disease had histories of severe asthma, with some previously requiring breathing tubes. It's also possible that people who have life-threatening episodes aren't able to normally sense when their oxygen levels are dropping, thus delaying medical treatment. Or, too often, they may think they're doing fine and wean themselves off their daily medications. This is very dangerous, and it can't be emphasized enough that asthma does *not* go away.

Death from asthma is usually related to either respiratory arrest, in which breathing suddenly stops, or pneumothorax, in which air leakage causes the lungs to collapse.

common causes of asthma and asthma attacks

Before we get into the details, you need to understand the difference between something that causes the disease called asthma and something that triggers an asthma attack. Most research has been conducted on what triggers attacks or makes symptoms worse in someone who already has asthma. The scienific investigation into the underlying cause of the disease itself is just catching up, so here we'll describe mainly the irritants that trigger an asthma attack or worsen symptoms. Keep in mind, though, that even when you're not having symptoms, the disease is still silently menacing your lungs.

The Air We Breathe

You don't need a book to tell you that most Americans breathe some pretty dirty air. But did you know that breathing polluted city air is almost as damaging to your health as living with someone who smokes cigarettes?

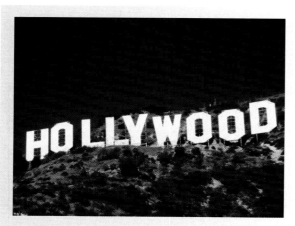

The 8 Most Polluted Areas in the United States

The American Lung Association ranks the following geographic areas as having the most polluted air in the country.

1. Los Angeles/Riverside/Orange County, Calif.
2. Bakersfield/Fresno/Visalia/Tulare/ Porterville, Calif.
3. Houston/Galveston/Brazoria, Tex.
4. Atlanta, Ga.
5. Merced, Calif.
6. Knoxville, Tenn.
7. Charlotte, N.C., and Rockville, S.C.
8. Sacramento, Calif.

The cleanest big cities include Bellingham, Wash., Colorado Springs, Colo., and Lincoln, Neb. To find out exactly how dirty (or clean) your city's air is, go to the American Lung Association website at http://lungaction.org/reports/stateoftheair2003.html and click on your state.

Admittedly, air quality in the United States has improved since the passage of the Clean Air Act in 1970, but some cities, such as Los Angeles, now find they're losing ground in the battle against air pollution for the first time in more than a decade. In May 2003, the American Lung Association reported that because the government doesn't fully enforce clean air laws, more than half of all Americans breathe polluted air that damages their health. According to the association, more than 7.4 million adults with asthma and nearly 2 million children suffering from asthma attacks live in counties that received an F grade in ozone air pollution. This represents 70 percent of the 10.6 million American adults with asthma and 69 percent of the 2.8 million children who have had an asthma attack and live in counties with an ozone monitor. Fully enforcing the standards of the Clean Air Act, the Lung Association notes, would prevent 15,000 premature deaths, 350,000 cases of asthma, and 1 million cases of decreased lung function in children.

Specific outdoor air-related asthma triggers include:

■ **Ozone.** Ozone is a respiratory irritant that forms when sunlight acts on automobile exhaust fumes and industrial pollution. High levels of ozone, which typically occur on hot summer days, are to people with asthma what a burning cigarette is to a drought-stricken forest. That's why many cities issue ozone alerts when levels are high, warning people with respiratory conditions such as asthma to stay inside in air conditioning. In fact, scientists suspect that high ozone levels may be one reason for our current asthma epidemic: A 2002 study found that children who played a lot of outdoor team sports in areas of high ozone concentration were up to three times more likely to develop asthma than those who didn't participate in such sports. The study offered the first evidence suggesting that ground-level ozone is a "causative factor" in the development of childhood asthma rather than one that just aggravates it.

■ **Particulate matter.** First, there are the fine solids in the air, such as dirt, soil dust, pollens, molds, ashes, and soot. Then there are the aerosols that form in the atmosphere from the by-products of combustion: volatile organic compounds (VOCs), sulfur dioxide, and nitrogen oxides. Particulate pollution comes from diverse sources such as factory and utility smokestacks, vehicle exhaust, wood burning, mining, construction, and agriculture.

When it comes to asthma and other respiratory illnesses, the main concern centers on fine particles, those less than 2.5 microns in diameter. (For comparison, a human hair is about 75 microns in diameter.) You can easily inhale them into your lungs, where they can be absorbed into the bloodstream or remain embedded in your body's cells for long periods of time. One study found a 17 percent increase in the risk of death from asthma and other respiratory conditions in areas with higher concentrations of small particles.

■ **Indoor air pollution.** Hard as it may be to believe, the air we breathe inside our homes, offices, and other buildings has more pollutants than the air we breathe outside. Sources of these air pollutants include combustion sources such as gas stoves, fireplaces, and cigarettes, plus treated woods, paints, furnishings, carpets, and fabrics. And don't forget consumer products, such as sprays, pesticides, window cleaners, and even laundry soap. That's in addition to known indoor allergens such as animal dander, cockroaches, dust mites, molds, and fungi.

In fact, a 2002 study published in the journal *Environmental Health Perspectives* found that more than a half-million children under age 6 with asthma would not have the disease if such common indoor risk factors as pet dander, molds, cigarette smoke, and gas stoves were removed from their homes.

revealing **research**

Causes of Asthma Are Mixed

Looking for the cause of asthma is like searching for the proverbial needle in a haystack. The possibilities are endless, and each month brings another theory. For instance, a Swedish study suggests that women exposed to high levels of pollen in the last trimester of pregnancy are more likely to have children with asthma, possibly because the antibodies the mother produces in response to the pollen may cross to the fetus and make allergies and asthma more likely. Another study examining children's two upper baby teeth—which provide a good picture of nutrition in the womb—suggests that babies who don't receive enough of the minerals iron and selenium while in the womb may have a higher risk of wheezing in early childhood and possibly of developing asthma later on.

With our growing understanding of the genetic underpinnings of disease, researchers are also isolating numerous genes associated with asthma, with nearly 300 linkages so far.

Irritants

Irritants are exactly that: external conditions or substances like smoke that are irritating to almost everyone. For a person without asthma, an irritant might evoke a cough; for a person with hypersensitive lungs, it could trigger the muscle spasms and inflammation that launch an asthma attack. Common irritants include cigarette smoke, cold air, perfume, and paint fumes.

Then there's the chlorine in swimming pools. Researchers found that the high concentrations of chlorine in the air above swimming pools can irritate the lining of the lungs, making it easier for pollen, dander, and other allergens or irritants to trigger an asthma attack. Ironically, people with asthma are often urged to exercise in indoor swimming pools, since the warm, humid air is believed to be beneficial for the lungs. If you're a swimmer and you have asthma, talk to your doctor about the relative risks and benefits.

The Weather

Even the weather can exacerbate your asthma. For years, emergency room physicians throughout the world knew that thunderstorms brought in a rush of

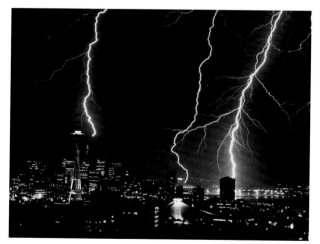

patients with asthma attacks. In 2003, their anecdotal observations were scientifically validated after researchers at the University of Ottawa Health Research Institute in Canada examined four years of records from the Children's Hospital of Eastern Ontario that correlated asthma attacks with information on weather patterns, airborne allergens, and pollution collected at a nearby airport. They found that asthma-related hospital visits jumped 15 percent during thunderstorms, from an average of 8.6 visits on clear days to 10 on stormy days. The reason? Researchers suspect the rise is related to an increase in airborne fungal spores, which nearly double during thunderstorms. In fact, when levels of these spores were high—storm or not—asthma-related hospital visits increased. Another reason may be the creation during thunderstorms of ozone, which, as mentioned earlier, is a well-known asthma trigger. Some studies also suggest that changes in barometric pressure affect asthma.

Research suggests that the *rise in asthma attacks during thunderstorms* could be related to the creation of ozone, an increase in airborne fungal spores, or changes in barometric pressure.

Cold, dry air is another weather-related asthma trigger, particularly for those with exercise-induced asthma, while wind increases asthma flares because it sends more pollen and mold spores airborne, where they can be breathed in by an allergic person and trigger an asthma attack.

Forget a move to Florida, though; the humidity there can be just as bad as the bracing winter air of Vermont. No one knows why, although one reason may be the increased mold and fungal spores that thrive in warm, humid environments.

Emotional Anxiety and Stress

In the mid-twentieth century, some physicians thought asthma and other chronic diseases were psychosomatic—caused by emotional conflicts. Today, we know that's not true. For instance, lung transplants using lungs from donors with asthma result in the recipients developing asthma. Obviously, the disease occurs at the cellular level.

Still, there's no question that stress and emotional anxiety can trigger asthma symptoms; some studies even suggest they may contribute to the initial development of the disease. For instance, an eight-year study of 150 children with a genetic risk for asthma found that those whose parents had difficulty managing the struggles of parenting them during their first year were more likely to develop asthma than those who had a smooth first year. Researchers suggest that a parent who has problems coping may expose the infant to greater emotional stress, which may alter both the immune and inflammatory responses. Another theory is that parents who cope well with parenthood may recognize thier child's medical problems earlier, reducing the duration of any airway inflammation.

Then there are the effects of stress on people who already have asthma. When researchers from the Centers for Disease Control and Prevention in Atlanta surveyed New York City residents a month after the terrorist attacks of September 11, 2001, they found that of the 134 people who had been diagnosed with asthma, 27 percent said their symptoms got worse after the attacks. Even after accounting for the debris that blanketed southern Manhattan after the attacks, those who had had two or more life stressors (such as a divorce, move, illness, or job change) *before* 9/11 were more likely to report their asthma symptoms had worsened than those who hadn't experienced such stressors. Another study, of college students with mild allergic asthma, found they had a greater reaction to allergens just before exams, when stress levels were higher.

The connection between stress and asthma varies. One explanation has to do with the complex effects of stress on the immune system, which dampen its ability to control inflammation (a key problem in asthma). It may also have to do with the fact that people who are under a lot of stress are less likely to take the kind of preventive steps that can reduce asthma symptoms. And then there's the kind of shallow, tight breathing you tend to do when you're stressed. If you hyperventilate, you may think you're having an asthma attack when you're actually just breathing too fast.

Other Illnesses

Often, asthma exists in conjunction with other illnesses, most commonly gastroesophageal reflux disease (GERD), acute or chronic sinusitis, and other infections, such as the common cold. Here's what you need to know.

Gastroesophageal reflux disease

Studies have shown that as many as 70 percent of people with asthma have GERD, a chronic form of heartburn, compared with 20 to 30 percent of the general population. GERD occurs when the esophageal sphincter, which normally keeps food and acid in your stomach where they belong, repeatedly fails to close tightly enough, allowing stomach acid to flow back, or reflux, into the esophagus and create that burning feeling.

Heartburn is just one symptom of GERD, however; others include cough, chronic sore throat, bad breath, and laryngitis. The condition can also be symptomless, when it's known as silent reflux. But if you have asthma and GERD, and GERD is undiagnosed or untreated, it may lead to serious repercussions for your asthma. The connection between the two is still being debated, but doctors suspect that changes in chest pressure that occur during asthma help relax the esophageal sphincter. The effects work the other way, too: Acid in the esophagus can irritate the lungs, either by being breathed, or aspirated, into them or by stimulating the bronchial nerves to go into spasms. To make the correlation even more complicated, some studies also show that theophylline, a medication sometimes used to treat asthma, may worsen GERD symptoms.

We'll talk more in later chapters about environmental and dietary changes you can make to alleviate GERD as an asthma trigger. For now, though, if you often have heartburn (particularly when you lie down), have increased asthma symptoms after meals, and have respiratory symptoms such as frequent coughing and hoarseness, ask your doctor to evaluate and treat you for GERD. One review of 12 studies found that treating reflux improved asthma symptoms in 69 percent of the 326 patients enrolled in the studies. Another study found that children who have both GERD and asthma could cut their use of asthma medication in half if they were effectively treated for reflux.

Sinusitis and allergic rhinitis

Nose constantly running? Feel like someone shoveled concrete behind your eyes? You probably have either sinusitis (inflammation of the sinuses) and/or allergic rhinitis, which we described in detail in chapter 3. Both are the nemesis of anyone with asthma, guaranteed to aggravate symptoms. During a sinus infection, mucus draining into the nose, throat, and lungs can cause asthma symptoms, while the inflammatory response triggered by an allergen (and causing allergy symptoms) spills over to the lungs, making asthma symptoms worse. However, you can have asthma without having allergies. That's why an asthma diagnosis shouldn't make you give up your cat; Tabby needs to go only if you're allergic to her dander.

Infections

Infection with the rhinovirus, which causes the common cold as well as other respiratory illnesses, can cause wheezing, often sending an asthma sufferer into a full-fledged attack. Other infectious agents linked to asthma symptoms include respiratory syncytial virus (RSV), *Chlamydia pneumoniae*, and *Mycoplasma pneumoniae*. In fact, asthma patients infected with mycoplasma have six times more mast cells in their lung tissue than uninfected asthma patients, meaning they have a much greater risk of inflammation. Some researchers suspect that many asthma attacks attributed to colds could instead be the fault of this bacterial infection. In some cases, a course of antibiotics may make a huge difference in your ability to control your asthma symptoms.

Your Job

In the early 1700s, Italian physician Bernardino Ramazzini studied bakers exposed to wheat and rye flour, mill workers exposed to grain dust, and farmers sensitive to animal dander and described a link between their asthma and their occupations. All had what today would be called work-related asthma.

Work-related asthma accounts for about 10 percent of all cases of adult asthma and includes both work-related aggravation of existing asthma and new cases of asthma triggered by something at work. There are two types.

revealing **research**

Migraine? Get Your Lungs Checked

If you're susceptible to migraines and tend to cough a lot, ask your doctor to evaluate you for asthma. A study published in the *British Journal of General Practice* in 2002 found that people with migraines are 59 percent more likely to have asthma. The researchers compared the prevalence of asthma in nearly 65,000 migraine patients with that in the same number of people without migraines. Although they don't know if the link is coincidental or related to some physiological effect, they suspect that both conditions may be linked to problems with the smooth muscle that lines both blood vessels (which play a role in migraines) and airways. Other research suggests that asthma is more common in children of mothers who have migraines than in those whose mothers are migraine-free.

Interestingly, doctors also report that propranolol (Inderal)—a beta-blocker commonly used to treat migraines—makes asthma symptoms worse, while people taking a drug called montelukast (Singulair) to control their asthma reported fewer headaches.

■ **Reactive airway dysfunction syndrome (also known as irritant-induced asthma).** This form usually develops after a single intense exposure to an irritant chemical, such as ammonia, chlorine gas, or hydrochloric acid, often during a chemical spill. The symptoms may be a one-time occurrence, or they may reoccur if you're exposed to lower levels of the irritant.

■ **Allergic occupational asthma (also known as latency-associated asthma).** People with this form of work-related asthma become sensitive to a specific chemical agent in the workplace over time. It could take a few weeks for the condition to develop, or as long as 30 years.

Medications

Each time you go to the doctor, you're asked about any allergies to medications. You probably don't even think about aspirin, but if you have severe

Is Your Job Stealing Your Breath?

The following occupations and agents are associated with allergic occupational asthma, according to *American Family Physician*, the journal of the American Academy of Family Physicians.

Occupation	Allergic to...
Bakers, farmers, flour mill workers, and grain elevator workers	flour and grain dust
Silk-processing workers, research laboratory workers, and insect-raising facility workers	insects
Prawn, snow-crab, and fish processors	seafood and other marine organisms
Laboratory workers and animal handlers	animal dander
Detergent producers, food industry workers, and blood-processing lab workers	various enzymes
Carpet manufacturing workers, pharmaceutical industry workers, latex glove manufacturing workers, and health care workers	latex and gums
Plastic, rubber, or foam manufacturing workers; spray painters; foam insulation installers	diisocyanates such as toluene, diphenylmethane, and hexamethylene
Solderers and electronics industry workers	abietic acid
Woodworkers, foresters, and artisans	plicatic acid in Western red cedar wood dust
Refinery workers	metals such as chromium, platinum, and nickel
Textile workers	dyes
Plastic and epoxy resin workers	anhydrides, such as trimellitic and phthalic anhydride
Adhesive handlers	acrylates
Health care workers	glutaraldehyde and formaldehyde
Pharmaceutical industry workers	certain pharmaceuticals

asthma and/or nasal polyps, you may have a form of asthma known as aspirin-sensitive asthma, in which that most common of all drugs actually makes your asthma symptoms worse.

Overall, 5 to 20 percent of adults with asthma have attacks triggered by sensitivities to aspirin and other drugs like it, known as nonsteroidal anti-inflammatory drugs, or NSAIDs. These include ibuprofen (Motrin and Advil) and naproxen (Aleve and Naprosyn). The older you are, the more likely you are to experience this reaction, and it can be quite serious. Studies found that anywhere from 3 percent of patients with asthma seen in a private allergy practice to 39 percent of adults with asthma admitted to an asthma-referral hospital experienced severe and even fatal asthma attacks after taking aspirin or other NSAIDs. Some doctors say these attacks are the worst they see.

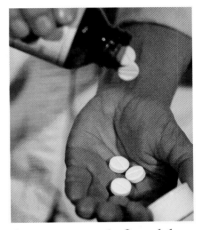

As many as one in five adults with asthma have attacks triggered by **sensitivities to aspirin** and other drugs like it.

Aspirin and the like are believed to affect sensitive individuals because of their effects on an enzyme called COX-1, known to play a role in the production of chemicals that help your lungs work properly. By preventing the COX-1 enzyme from doing its job, NSAIDs also prevent production of these critical chemicals.

There is some good news, though: Several studies have found that the newer, prescription-only pain relievers known as selective COX-2 inhibitors have no effect on aspirin-sensitive asthma sufferers, suggesting that they may be able to use these drugs for pain relief. For now, COX-2 inhibitors are approved only for arthritis. Two popular versions of the drugs are celecoxib (Celebrex) and rofecoxib (Vioxx).

Other medicines known to worsen asthma symptoms include beta-blockers often used to treat high blood pressure, such as propranolol (Inderal), and those prescribed for glaucoma, such as timolol maleate (Timoptic).

Chemicals

This category encompasses chemicals that you're not allergic to but are sensitive to. They include sulfites, which are often used to preserve foods and beverages, including tuna, salad-bar food, processed potatoes, shrimp, dried apples and raisins, lemon juice, grape juice, beer, and wine. Today, most foods containing sulfites carry warning labels, but if you're not sure a food is safe, avoid it.

Another chemical you may want to watch out for is tartrazine, a dye found in numerous foods and medicines, including cough syrups and liquid cold and flu remedies. Check ingredient lists for tartrazine.

asthma and women

Although the overall incidence of asthma is increasing, women are being hit in disproportionate numbers. Between 1982 and 1996, the prevalence of asthma in women rose by 97 percent, compared with a 29 percent increase in men. Some of that increase may be due to improved diagnosis, but some is probably related to gender differences.

Although boys are twice as likely to develop asthma as girls, that discrepancy vanishes once puberty hits. The lifelong prevalence of asthma is 9.5 percent for women and 8.7 percent for men. The gender differences continue in other asthma-related areas, with women being 44 percent more likely to have an asthma attack than men and accounting for 65 percent of asthma-related deaths each year. African-American women have it even worse: They're 2.5 times more likely to die from asthma than Caucasian women.

As with so much in medicine, experts aren't quite sure why this gender discrepancy exists, but they do have some good ideas. Hormones, of course, are thought to play a role, and up to 40 percent of women with asthma find that their symptoms worsen just before and during menstruation. The aggravation is probably due to the effects of progesterone, levels of which rise sharply and then drop abruptly toward the end of the menstrual cycle, just before menstruation begins. Scientists don't understand exactly how progesterone affects asthma, but the hormone does play a role in inflammation. There's also some evidence to suggest that oral contraceptives—which contain estrogen, progesterone, or both—can make asthma worse.

A woman's weight also contributes to her risk of asthma, with a 1999 study published in *Archives of Internal Medicine* finding that women who gained weight after age 18 were at increased risk of developing asthma. The study, part of the long-term, ongoing Nurses' Health Study tracking the health of nearly 86,000 women, found that the higher a woman's body mass index (BMI), the greater her risk of asthma. The risk was almost three times greater for women whose BMI was 30 or more than for those whose BMI was less than 20. (A healthy BMI is between 19 and 25.)

Asthma may also get worse or improve during pregnancy. In

The American Lung Association: From TB to Asthma

The National Tuberculosis Association, founded in 1904, was the first American charity to focus on a single disease. With the decline of TB in the mid-twentieth century, the organization changed its mission to include asthma, becoming the American Lung Association in 1973. Today, the association fights lung disease in all its forms, with special emphasis on asthma, tobacco control, and environmental health. It provides grants for scientific research, serves an advocacy role, and disseminates information to the public about respiratory illnesses. Check it out on the Web at www.lungusa.org.

Why Does my Asthma Get Worse at Night?

Do you often wake up in the middle of the night gasping and wheezing? Do most of your asthma attacks occur at night? You may have sleep, or nocturnal, asthma, which affects about 70 to 80 percent of people with asthma. Symptoms generally include shortness of breath or coughing and wheezing at night, and may help explain why 80 percent of severe asthma attacks occur between midnight and 8:00 A.M.

Unless you have GERD (described on page 62), your symptoms probably aren't related to lying down but rather to the time of day. Asthma, like many diseases, follows the clock or, as they say in medicalese, has its own chronobiology. The study of chronobiology focuses on biological processes that have time-related rhythms.

Basically, it turns out that your lungs work better at certain times of the day, whether you have asthma or not. They're at peak efficiency around 4:00 P.M. and begin falling down on the job (so to speak) around 4:00 A.M. If you have normal lungs, you don't notice these changes in efficiency, but if you have asthma, your lung function can change as much as 50 percent throughout the day.

Researchers don't agree on whether nocturnal asthma represents a worsening of asthma or whether it's actually a separate form, like exercise-induced asthma. They do know the symptoms are related not to lying down but to the time of day or night when you sleep, so even if you work nights and sleep days, you can still experience sleep asthma. They've also found that the chronobiology of asthma, and hence the propensity for nocturnal symptoms, gets worse with age. As to the cause—well, there are several theories, but no one answer. Changes in hormones related to sleep and circadian rhythms, which may affect the relaxation of smooth muscles (like the lungs), and inflammation may play a role.

If you have nocturnal asthma more than once a week, it's a sign your asthma isn't being treated properly. Drugs used to treat nocturnal asthma include theophylline and salmeterol (Serevent). You'll learn more about these drugs in chapter 7.

general, one-third of pregnant women with asthma tend to improve, one-third get worse, and one-third stay the same, with all returning to their pre-pregnancy asthma status once they deliver. No one really knows why these changes occur, but factors such as increased stress, infections, increased production of inflammatory chemicals known as prostaglandins, and increased resistance to the steroids often used to treat asthma are all reasons why an expectant mother's asthma may get worse. Of course, that doesn't explain why asthma improves in some pregnant women.

Women with asthma can have safe and normal pregnancies as long as they keep their asthma under control. This is crucial because asthma attacks cause a decrease in blood oxygen levels, which can affect the amount of oxygen the baby receives. There's also some data that suggests that poorly controlled asthma may affect the size of the baby. For that reason, doctors may decide to use medications in pregnant women. Generally, they prefer inhaled medications because less of the drug reaches the baby. Also, medications that have been used for many years by the mother are less likely to have risks for the baby. The same medications are

Can I Outgrow Asthma?

The idea that you can outgrow asthma stems from the fact that many infants and young children wheeze when they have viral respiratory infections, garnering a diagnosis of asthma. As they grow older, they stop wheezing when those infections hit, suggesting that they've "outgrown" their asthma. Chances are, they never had asthma in the first place. The bottom line: It's rare to outgrow asthma.

also generally safe to use while breast-feeding. We'll talk more about medication use during pregnancy in chapter 7.

living with asthma

Study after study confirms that with the proper treatment—both medical and environmental—you can live a normal life with asthma, avoiding the lung-scarring and life-threatening repercussions of this chronic disease. Unfortunately, too few people with asthma receive proper treatment or comply with treatment advice. A 1998 national survey of 2,509 asthma sufferers and 512 doctors found that the nation fell far short of national government guidelines for asthma care. For instance:

■ **National goal: No missed school or work because of asthma.** Yet 49 percent of children and 25 percent of adults with asthma missed school or work due to their disease in the previous year.

■ **National goal: Asthma symptoms should not disrupt sleep.** Yet almost one in three asthma patients (30 percent) was awakened with breathing problems at least once a week.

■ **National goal: Maintain normal activity levels.** Yet 48 percent of those surveyed said asthma limited their ability to take part in sports and recreation, 36 percent said it limited their normal physical exertion, and 25 percent said it interfered with their social activities.

Here's where the Breathe Easy Plan comes in. We'll not only show you how to get the right diagnosis but also educate you about treatment options so you can work with your doctor to ensure you're getting the right treatment; tell you how to use medications properly; and help you evaluate your life to change those things that may be making your asthma worse. Well…maybe we can't help you change the weather.

chapter five

all about
food
allergies

Remember the good ol' days, when a peanut butter and jelly sandwich was lunch, not a potentially life-threatening experience? Today, some schools are so afraid that a child's peanut butter sandwich will trigger a lethal allergic reaction that they've banned the sticky stuff altogether.

They have good reason to be fearful. An increasing number of children in the United States are allergic to peanuts—about 3.3 percent in 1996 compared with 1.1 percent in 1989—while an estimated 3 million Americans overall are allergic to them, making peanuts the most common food allergen in this country. But it's far from the only one: Overall, an estimated 5 to 8 percent of kids and about 1 to 2 percent of adults have some kind of food allergy, with the "trigger" foods varying widely.

Food allergies, whether to peanuts, shellfish, dairy products, or egg whites, are serious, much more so than everyday allergic rhinitis. They are the leading cause of anaphylaxis, the life-threatening reaction that causes difficulty breathing, swelling in the mouth and throat, a sudden drop in blood pressure, and, in some cases, loss of consciousness. Each year, food allergies account for an estimated 30,000 emergency room visits, 2,000 hospitalizations, and as many as 200 deaths from anaphylaxis.

What You Need to Know about Food Allergies

- It's rare to react to more than three foods.
- Except in gastrointestinal allergies, most food allergy symptoms develop within an hour of ingesting the allergen.
- All food allergies generally cause similar symptoms, affecting the skin, gastrointestinal system, and/or respiratory system.
- Subjective or behavioral symptoms (such as hyperactivity) as a sole manifestation of food allergy are rare.
- Allergic reactions to dyes and additives are also rare.

That's why people with severe food allergies carry a strong antidote with them at all times. The drug, racemic epinephrine, is a synthetic version of the naturally occurring hormone epinephrine, which counteracts anaphylaxis. It comes in the form of a pen (EpiPen) or a dual pen and needle-and-syringe kit (Twinject).

There's also increasing evidence that food allergies may be a risk factor for severe asthma in children, with one study finding that 56 percent of children with serious asthma also had food allergies, compared with just 10.5 percent of those with mild asthma. The results suggest that life-threatening asthma attacks may be triggered by food allergies in susceptible patients with asthma, say researchers.

As for the rising rate of food allergies, it's probably explained by the fact that we're exposed to potentially allergenic foods both more often and earlier in life. For instance, researchers suspect that one reason for the increase in peanut allergies in Great Britain is the use of peanut oil in baby lotions. In the United States, it's our love of peanuts and peanut butter. As soy products become more prevalent, experts expect we'll see the rate of soy allergies jump.

The kicker? Unlike allergic rhinitis or asthma, there is no effective treatment for food allergies. All you can do is avoid the food in question, and that takes a Herculean effort in today's world. Food allergens can be so pervasive, in fact, that some people have had serious reactions just from walking through a fish market or kissing someone who had recently eaten seafood. For some, even inhaling the fumes from frying or steaming foods to which they're allergic can trigger a reaction.

food allergies defined

If you have a food allergy, blame your parents: It's an inherited predisposition. In other words, if your family has a history of allergies, you are much more likely to develop a food allergy than, say, the daughter of parents who wouldn't know an allergy from an alligator.

The development of a food allergy begins with one simple step: exposure to the food. If you never touch or eat a peanut, you'll never develop a peanut allergy. Even that first peanut butter cracker may be innocuous, but as you digest it, it triggers your immune system to produce IgE antibodies that will be activated the next time you eat the food.

Actually, it's not the food per se that triggers the reaction but rather proteins within the food that cooking, stomach acids, or digestive enzymes don't break down. These proteins are absorbed through the gastrointestinal lining into your bloodstream, where they travel through your body.

From there, you know the drill: The proteins interact with the IgE molecules on the surface of mast cells, triggering the cells to release inflammatory chemicals such as histamine. *Where* those chemicals are released determines your reaction. For instance, the mast cells on your skin are most likely to be

Watch What You Eat: Common Food Allergens

Theoretically, any food containing protein can contribute to a food allergy. In reality, just seven foods account for more than 90 percent of the food allergies in the United States.

1 **Peanuts.** These are the leading cause of severe allergic reactions to food, including food-related anaphylaxis.

2 **Seafood.** If you have a seafood allergy, chances are you react to shellfish, generally shrimp, crayfish, lobster, or crab. Some people, however, are also allergic to both fresh- and saltwater fish. Once you have a seafood allergy, you'll probably have it for life.

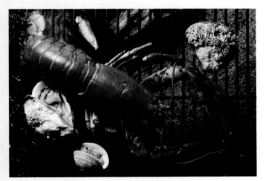

3 **Tree nuts.** Almonds, Brazil nuts, cashews, hazelnuts, and walnuts are in this category.

4 **Eggs.** The whites in particular cause reactions. Between 1.6 and 2.6 percent of children are allergic to eggs, but those with atopic dermatitis—dry, scaly, itchy skin—are more likely to be allergic to eggs.

5 **Cow's milk.** The main culprits are the proteins in milk, such as lactoglobulin, lactalbumin, casein, and whey. Milk allergies almost always begin in the first year of life, soon after cow's milk or cow's-milk-based formula is introduced to a child's diet. Milk allergies affect about 2.5 percent of infants, with about 1 percent of all children developing IgE-mediated milk allergies and approximately 1.5 percent developing non-IgE-mediated reactions.

6 **Soy.** The prevalence of soy-based formulas and baby foods today is leading to an increase in soy allergies among babies, with gastrointestinal symptoms most common.

7 **Wheat.** Don't confuse a wheat allergy with gluten sensitivity. Gluten is the component of wheat, barley, rye, and other grains that provides the "glue" holding the grain together. It's associated with a disease called gluten-sensitive enteropathy, or celiac disease, caused by an abnormal response to gluten. A wheat allergy, on the other hand, means you're allergic to certain proteins in wheat. If you eliminate wheat from your diet and your symptoms disappear, you have a wheat allergy; if the problem persists even after you substitute other grains, chances are your symptoms are related to gluten. Of course, an allergy test is generally the best way to tell what's plaguing you.

affected by food allergies, leading to hives or atopic dermatitis (eczema), a skin condition characterized by itchy, scaly, red skin. If mast cells in your ears, nose, and throat are activated, your mouth may itch, and you may have trouble breathing or swallowing. If they're activated in your gastrointestinal tract, you may have abdominal pain, diarrhea, or vomiting. If it happens in your lungs, you could have an asthma attack.

The reaction can take as little as a few seconds (the tingling you feel in your mouth as you eat the food) or as long as an hour (a full-blown allergy attack, possibly culminating in anaphylaxis).

This sequence is known as IgE-mediated food allergy, for the obvious reason that IgE antibodies are integral to the reaction. You can also have a *non*-IgE-mediated food reaction. This occurs when a food triggers the production of T cells, which in turn call in other substances that activate your immune response, including inflammation. Most non-IgE-mediated food reactions result in gastrointestinal symptoms, such as gas, and are not life-threatening.

A third possibility is a combination of IgE-mediated allergy and non-IgE-mediated food sensitivity. For instance, you could have a bona fide allergy to milk and at the same time be lactose intolerant, meaning that you lack the enzyme that enables you to digest the milk sugar lactose.

If you are allergic to one food, you're more likely to be allergic to others. For instance, if you have a history of allergic reactions to shrimp, you're likely to be allergic to crab, lobster, and crayfish as well. Doctors call this cross-reactivity.

Additionally, if you're allergic to ragweed, you may find that during ragweed season, you're also allergic to melons, particularly cantaloupe, honeydew, and watermelon. People who have a birch-pollen allergy may also react to hazelnuts, apples, carrots, and celery. Allergic to latex? Watch out for bananas.

Another form of food allergy is called exercise-induced food allergy. To trigger a reaction with this form, you not only need to eat a certain food but also to exercise soon afterward. As you work out and your body temperature rises, you begin to itch, get light-headed, and soon have allergy symptoms such as hives or even anaphylaxis. The cure is simple: Don't eat for a couple of hours before exercising.

food allergy or food intolerance?

Every time you drink a glass of milk or eat an ice cream cone, you feel bloated, with gas, stomach pain, and diarrhea. Are you allergic to milk? Probably not. Usually only young children are allergic to milk and other dairy products; you're probably lactose intolerant. If you lack the enzyme lactase, your body can't digest lactose, a sugar found in dairy products. Lactose intolerance affects 1 out of 10 people, though it is much more prevalent among African-Americans.

Don't feel too bad about your missed self-diagnosis, though. Although only between 1 and 2 percent of American adults have food allergies, as many as 30 percent *think* they do. Similarly, although between 5 and 8 percent of American children have food allergies, nearly one-third of parents blame foods for a multitude of symptoms in their children. This means there are millions of people depriving themselves of nutritious, delicious foods for absolutely no reason.

Instead of an allergy, what they probably have is a food intolerance—an abnormal response to a food that is not an allergic reaction. It differs from an allergy in that it doesn't involve the immune system but rather an inability to digest the food.

It's understandable that people might think they have food allergies, since the symptoms mimic those of reactions to infectious agents and other substances, as well as digestive problems. For instance:

■ **Microorganisms.** Foods contaminated with microorganisms, such as bacteria, and their products, such as toxins, can trigger symptoms that mimic an allergic food reaction. In reality, the problem is food poisoning.

■ **Histamines.** Some natural substances, such as histamines, can occur in foods and stimulate a reaction similar to an allergic reaction. For example, histamine can reach high levels in cheese, some wines, and certain kinds of fish, particularly tuna and mackerel. In fish, histamine is believed to stem from bacterial contamination, particularly in fish that hasn't been refrigerated properly. If you eat a food with a high level of histamine, you may experience histamine toxicity, a reaction that strongly resembles an allergic reaction to food.

■ **Food additives.** Compounds most frequently tied to adverse reactions that can be confused with food allergy are yellow dye #5, monosodium glutamate, and sulfites. Yellow dye #5 can cause hives, although it's rare. Monosodium glutamate (MSG) is a flavor enhancer that, when consumed in large amounts, can cause flushing, sensations of warmth, headache, facial pressure, or chest pain. Sulfites, described in chapter 4, can trigger asthma attacks in susceptible people. They give off a gas called sulfur dioxide, which irritates the lungs.

Preventing Food Allergies

The majority of studies suggest that exclusively breastfeeding babies for their first four to six months helps reduce the risk of allergies, particularly to milk or soy. If you're breastfeeding, though, the American Academy of Pediatrics recommends that you eliminate cow's milk, eggs, fish, peanuts, and tree nuts from your diet, if possible, to reduce the possibility that your infant will develop food allergies. Even once he's eating solid foods, hold off on introducing him to these common allergenic foods until he's at least three.

■ **Gluten.** Some people are gluten intolerant, a condition associated with a disease called gluten-sensitive enteropathy, or celiac disease. It's caused by an abnormal immune response to gluten, a component of wheat and some other grains. A blood test that looks for anti-gliadin antibodies can diagnose this problem.

■ **Psychological factors.** Certain foods may be associated with unpleasant memories. Say, for instance, that when you were a child, your family had weekly dinners at the local Chinese restaurant, ordering the same dishes each week: spareribs, egg fu yung, and wonton soup. Those dinners were miserable affairs of yelling and screaming. Today, when you try to eat those foods, you have what seems to you to be an allergic reaction. Since the foods remind you of those awful dinners, they may trigger a physical reaction to the psychological distress.

■ **Diseases.** Some diseases that share symptoms with food allergies (such as vomiting, diarrhea, cramping, or abdominal pain that gets worse when you eat) include ulcers, colitis, and cancers of the gastrointestinal tract.

the challenges of avoiding foods

So, you're thinking, what's the big deal? If you're allergic to peanuts, just avoid peanuts and foods that contain them. Allergic to shellfish? Skip the shrimp on the buffet.

Well, it's not that easy, particularly given our increasing dependence on prepackaged and processed foods. Just consider that up to 50 percent of people who are allergic to peanuts experience an accidental peanut ingestion every four years, even if they're being exceedingly careful. Or that a single-serving juice drink boxed on a packaging line that may be also used for milk products may have enough milk protein contamination to trigger an allergic reaction. The same is true of tofu desserts packaged in ice cream plants. Hugh A. Sampson, M.D., who is director of the Jaffe Food Allergy Institute at Mount Sinai School of Medicine in New York and is considered the medical guru when it comes to food allergies, notes that a banana slice lying against a slice of kiwi may contain enough kiwi protein to provoke an allergic response.

Plus, just figuring out what's *in* certain foods is a challenge akin to translating Swahili. For instance, did you know that arachis oil is peanut oil, or that some commercial brands of egg substitutes contain egg whites? That most commercially processed cooked pastas (including those used in prepared foods such as soup) contain eggs or are processed on equipment shared with pastas that contain eggs? That eggs are often used to create the foam or milk topping on specialty coffee drinks and are used in some bar drinks?

Did you know that flu vaccines are grown on egg embryos and may contain small bits of egg protein? That many medications contain food proteins? And if you're allergic to fish, watch out for Caesar salad dressing and Worcestershire sauce; both contain anchovies.

Then there's milk. Just because the label says a product is nondairy, that doesn't mean it's milk-free. Current labeling guidelines allow the use of the term *nondairy* even for foods that contain milk by-products.

As Dr. Sampson notes, milk and soy proteins are often added to increase protein content or enhance flavor in various foods. Likewise, spices (such as garlic and coriander) and seed derivatives (such as mustard and sesame seeds) are included for flavoring in many prepared foods. Peanut and nut products are added to flavor and thicken sauces (such as spaghetti sauce, gravy, and barbecue sauce) and baked goods. And eggs and milk are frequently added to improve the integrity of other food products (such as egg for meatballs and pasta and milk for bologna and canned tuna).

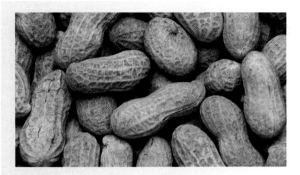

More on Peanut Allergies

There are a lot of myths swirling around about peanut allergies. One is that they are always lifelong. In truth, between 20 and 50 percent of children may outgrow peanut allergies. Another is that merely inhaling the odor of peanuts or sitting next to someone eating a peanut butter sandwich can trigger a reaction. Probably not. One study of 30 children with severe peanut allergies found that none had reactions when a cup of peanut butter was held a foot from their noses for 10 minutes. When a pea-size amount was pressed onto their backs for 1 minute, just one-third had mild reactions.

These results led researchers to predict that at least 90 percent of those with peanut allergies would not react to the types of exposure studied. The study didn't test reactions to whole, roasted peanuts, however, from which dust might become airborne and trigger reactions. That's why many airlines have stopped passing out roasted peanuts during trips; the dust could trigger allergy attacks in passengers.

How about this: In 2003, the FDA approved the use of bandages and dressings containing chitosan, derived from the shells of shrimp, to reduce superficial bleeding. This could prove dangerous to people with shellfish allergies.

And this: Between September 1999 and March 2000, FDA researchers inspected 85 manufacturers of baked goods, ice cream, and candy for allergen labeling and cross-contamination issues. They found that companies unintentionally introduced food allergens into other foods through poor cleaning, back-to-back cooking schedules, or reuse of utensils, and just over half of the manufacturers checked their products to ensure the labels accurately reflected all of the ingredients.

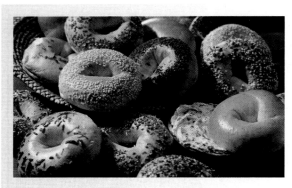

The Other 10 Percent

If 90 percent of food allergies are caused by one of the seven foods listed on page 71, then what makes up the other 10 percent? Seeds, for one. These include sesame seeds, sunflower seeds, cottonseed, and poppy seeds. The problem is much bigger than you'd think. Just consider your local bakery, where 10 varieties of bagels—including poppy seed and sesame seed—sit hole to hole, or the hamburger bun at a fast food restaurant, bristling with sesame seeds. Additionally, sesame and poppy are considered spices by some food manufacturers, so they don't have to be listed as separate ingredients on labels.

The good news? The oils from cottonseed and sunflower seeds are usually highly refined, meaning they're free of proteins, so they probably shouldn't cause a problem for anyone allergic to various seeds.

Even if food labels are accurate, they're pretty darn complicated to read. A 2000 study of attendees at the Food Allergy and Anaphylaxis Network conference found that just 12 percent thought ingredient statements were easy to understand, less than 9 percent thought they were simple enough, and only 2.4 percent thought they gave enough information about allergens.

One mother of two children with severe food allergies notes that she sees food recalls every week for allergen-contaminated products. "Recalls are great," says Beverly Bennett, a freelance writer who lives outside Chicago, "but for the person who has already eaten a tainted food, it's no comfort. You may be rushed to a hospital not even knowing what triggered a reaction."

For instance, her son was taken to the emergency room a few years ago after eating brownies she'd made. "I had no idea the imported expensive chocolate I used was tainted with peanut residue, one of his allergies," she says. In the Bennett house, the rule is to take a bite of processed food, then wait 5 to 10 minutes before eating more, just in case there's a reaction.

diagnosing food allergies

A diagnosis of food allergies requires careful evaluation of your diet and symptoms, as well as medical testing. Even then, since there are no tests for non-IgE-mediated food sensitivities, it may be difficult to get a definitive diagnosis.

Probably the first thing your doctor will do is conduct a detailed medical history about your symptoms: when they occur, how long they last, what treatments worked, whether the reaction is always associated with a particular food, whether anyone else eating the same food got sick, how much you ate before the reaction began, how the food was prepared, and if you ate other foods at the same time as the one that made you ill. You'll also probably be asked to keep a food diary like the one below, in which you track everything you put into your mouth.

These two steps may enable your doctor to reach a diagnosis with no further testing; in this case, he will probably put you on an elimination diet, in which you eliminate the suspect food for a week or two and see if the symptoms disappear. Again, the food diary will come in handy in tracking whether this works. If your symptoms disappear when you eliminate the food, then reappear when you eat it again, it's nearly certain that the food is causing the symptoms.

To confirm the allergy, your doctor may then turn to medical tests that measure the allergic response. These include:

■ **Scratch skin test.** A small amount of liquid extract made from the suspect food is placed on your forearm or back, then your skin is scratched or pricked with a needle. Any swelling or redness, called a wheal, indicates a local allergic reaction, meaning you have IgE on your skin's mast cells specific to the food being tested.

■ **RAST or ELISA blood test.** If you have severe reactions to the suspect food that lead to anaphylaxis, or you get severe skin rashes or hives, your doctor

Keeping a Food Diary

Think you may have food allergies? The best way to tell is to keep a food diary for at least two weeks. It seems tedious, but it's what your doctor will tell you to do, too. Keep track of everything you put in your mouth, including chewing gum, as well as processed and other prepared foods. Be thorough, but within reason. If you have a bad allergic reaction, go back and add greater detail about the ingredients of your most recent meal. This written record should provide the data you need to identify the culprit. You can set up your chart like this one.

Date	Time	Food	Symptoms	Time elapsed between eating the food and start of the symptoms

The Best Cookbooks

Looking for a recipe for chocolate cake that doesn't include eggs or milk? How about tips for shopping, substituting foods, and cooking when you or a family member has food allergies? Check out these cookbooks.
- Food Allergy and Anaphylaxis Network, *Food Allergy News Cookbook,* vol. 1 and 2. Order online at www.foodallergy.org.

  The following are available in bookstores or online from Amazon.com.
- Anne Muñoz-Furlong, ed. *The Food Allergy News Cookbook: A Collection of Recipes from Food Allergy News and Members of the Food Allergy Network*
- Jeanne Marie Martin, *The All Natural Allergy Cookbook*
- Mary Harris, et al., *"My Kid's Allergic to Everything" Dessert Cookbook*
- Marilyn Gioannini, *The Complete Food Allergy Cookbook: The Foods You've Always Loved without the Ingredients You Can't Have*
- Nicolette M. Dumke and William G. Crook, *Allergy Cooking with Ease: The No Wheat, Milk, Eggs, Corn, Soy, Yeast, Sugar, Grain, and Gluten Cookbook*
- Marjorie Hurt Jones, *The Allergy Self-Help Cookbook: Over 325 Natural Food Recipes, Free of All Common Food Allergens*

probably won't use a skin test but rather a blood test such as the RAST or ELISA test, which measures the presence of food-specific IgE in your blood. It takes about a week to get the results.

However, positive skin or RAST/ELISA tests correlate with reactions less than half the time. Conversely, even a negative test can't be trusted, because it may be that you have a non-IgE-mediated allergy, the wrong food was tested, or the test wasn't sensitive enough.

■ **Double-blind food challenge.** Considered the "gold standard" of food allergy testing, this involves placing various suspect and nonsuspect foods in individual opaque capsules. You swallow a capsule, and the doctor waits to see if you have a reaction, then you continue the process until you've taken all the capsules. The study is considered "blinded" because neither you nor the doctor know what food the capsules contain until the test is finished. Again, someone with a history of severe reactions can't be tested this way, and, because the test takes time, it's fairly expensive. Studies show that less than half of all people who suspect they have a food allergy test positive in a double-blind food challenge.

treatment for food allergies

Currently, there is no treatment—in terms of medication, at least—for food allergies. There is hope on the horizon, however, in the form of an experimental drug that locks on to circulating IgE, thus preventing it from locking on to the mast cells. It's like a Star Wars defense system: The IgE is rendered harmless before it can "hit" any targets. In a study published in 2003 in the *New England Journal of Medicine*, researchers reported that the injectable drug kept people who were allergic to peanuts from having serious reactions. You'll learn more about this drug in chapter 7.

There is some evidence that traditional Chinese medicines may have antiallergenic properties, which may be useful for treating peanut allergy. When researchers from Mount Sinai School of Medicine and Johns Hopkins University investigated the effects of a Chinese herbal formula, FAHF-1, on mice that were bred to have severe peanut allergies, they found that the compound completely blocked anaphylactic symptoms and significantly reduced peanut-specific IgE levels after two weeks of treatment, similar to the way allergy shots might work.

Researchers are also on the road to developing a vaccine for peanut allergies, with several groups reporting the production of a vaccine against allergy-causing proteins that proved "very effective" in mice with peanut allergies. Researchers hope to begin testing it in humans within the next few years.

As if that weren't enough, other researchers are trying to genetically alter foods such as peanuts and soybeans to remove the allergy-causing proteins. Someday, the thinking goes, people with food allergies may be able to eat whatever they want—with no reading of complex labels required.

Allergen-Free Eating

It isn't easy, but the following tips, courtesy of the Food Allergy and Anaphylaxis Network (FAAN), the largest research and advocacy group for food allergy sufferers, can help you and your children cope with food allergies.

Learn to substitute. For instance, you can substitute 1 cup of water or fruit juice for each cup of milk in baking and cooking. For each cup of wheat flour, substitute either $7/8$ cup rice flour, $5/8$ cup potato starch flour, 1 cup soy flour plus $1/4$ cup potato starch flour, or 1 cup corn flour. For each egg called for in a recipe, substitute one of the following:

✓ 1 teaspoon baking powder, 1 tablespoon liquid, and 1 tablespoon vinegar
✓ 1 teaspoon yeast dissolved in $1/4$ cup warm water
✓ $1½$ tablespoons water, $1½$ tablespoons oil, and 1 teaspoon baking powder
✓ 1 packet gelatin and 2 tablespoons warm water (do not mix until ready to use)

Check your steak. Many restaurants put butter on steaks after they have been grilled to add extra flavor; since it melts, you won't see it.

Go Kosher. Two Kosher symbols help if you have a milk allergy. A "D," or the word *dairy*, on a label next to "K" or "U" (usually found near the product name) indicates the presence of milk protein, while "DE" indicates the product was produced on equipment shared with dairy products. If the product contains neither meat nor dairy products, it's Pareve (or Parev or Parve). "Pareve" on a label indicates the product is considered milk-free according to religious specifications.

Watch out for nut butters (such as cashew nut butter). Although you might think they'd make good substitutes for peanut butter, many nut butters are produced on equipment used to process peanut butter, so they can be a somewhat risky alternative. Also, most experts recommend that peanut-allergic people avoid tree nuts as well.

Check the nationality. Of your food, that is. African, Chinese, Indonesian, Mexican, Thai, and Vietnamese dishes often contain peanuts or are contaminated with peanuts during preparation.

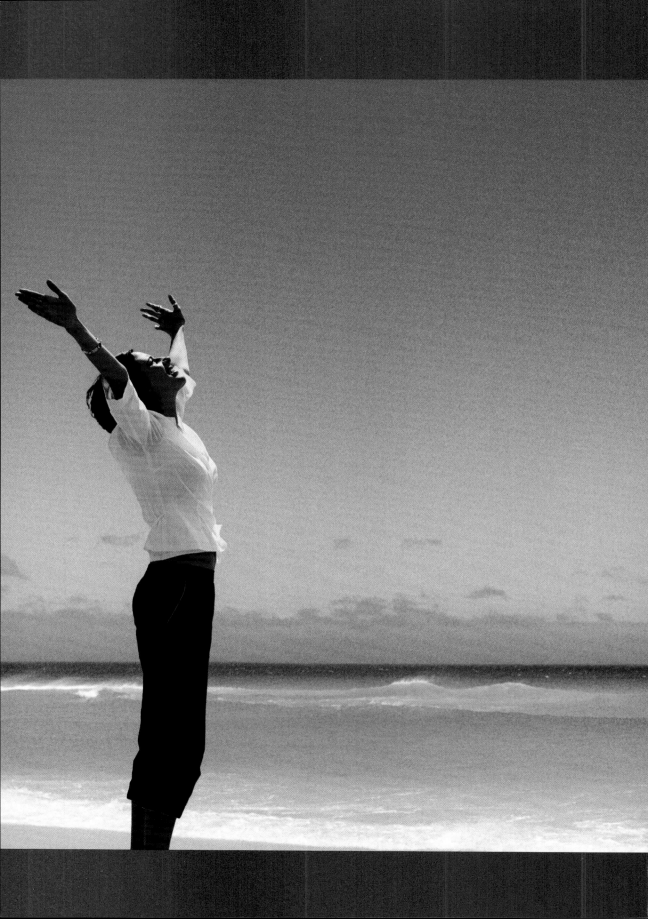

the **solutions**

You CAN control your allergies and asthma. No matter what the severity or cause of your condition, researchers have developed outstanding medications to end the attacks and prevent new ones from occurring. Just as important, there are many, many things in your power to improve your situation.

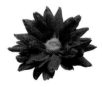

chapter **six**

the right
diagnosis

So you're tired of spending every spring wheezing like some ancient Model T, with your eyes redder than a stop sign and your nose more clogged than Macy's after Thanksgiving. It's time to get a proper diagnosis and get those allergies taken care of.

But wait a minute... you just diagnosed yourself, didn't you? "Hey," you're thinking, "that's pretty good. I don't need a doctor; I can just hustle myself down to the corner Rite Aid and pick up a passel of antihistamines. I'll be just fine."

Hold on there. You've just fallen into one of the biggest traps in the allergy/asthma world: thinking you can self-diagnose and, by extension, self-treat your symptoms.

First, as we discussed earlier, allergies and asthma are pretty good at masquerading as other ailments, and vice versa. For instance, a 2002 survey conducted by the American College of Allergy, Asthma, and Immunology found that 41 percent of those with allergies thought they had colds or viral infections when they first began having allergy symptoms. And in a nationwide survey of 250 allergists, more than 80 percent said they believed self-medicating for allergies was likely to mask more serious health problems. In the same survey,

60 percent of the doctors said that seasonal allergies and allergic asthma are best treated with prescription medications, available only through physicians.

Given that, why is it that another survey, of 501 women with asthma, found that 74 percent didn't see their doctors unless their symptoms got severe? Maybe they didn't think doctors could help: Almost half the women interviewed believed that doctors thought psychological factors were more likely to influence asthma symptoms in women than in men, and more than one-quarter (27 percent) were convinced that clinicians took men's asthma complaints more seriously than they did women's.

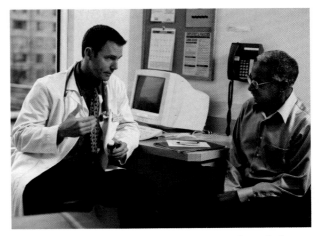

One survey found that 41 percent of those with allergies *thought they had colds or viral infections* when they first began having allergy symptoms.

We can tell you that none of this is true. Times have changed: Doctors *do* care about women's asthma, they *don't* ascribe symptoms to psychological conditions, and treatments are often continuous, not only for when things get bad.

Before you can even talk about treatment, though, you need the right diagnosis. Here's how to get it.

choosing a doctor

Currently, about 65 percent of outpatient chronic care for asthma is provided by general physicians, with allergy and immunology specialists providing about 26 percent and pulmonary specialists about 5 percent. Overall, then, most medical care for moderate or severe asthma is provided by primary care doctors.

Studies have found, however, that expert care (provided by allergy and immunology or pulmonary care specialists) reduced hospitalizations for asthma by an average of 77 percent and emergency room visits by 53 percent. Among the reasons: Specialists are generally more up to date on the latest research, attend more allergy/asthma-specific medical meetings, and are board-certified, which means they've received additional training in asthma and allergic diseases and must take continuing education courses to maintain that certification.

Certainly, start with your primary care physician (most insurance plans mandate that anyway). You'll probably need to switch to an allergy or asthma specialist if any of the following circumstances apply.

- You have trouble getting a diagnosis from your primary care doctor.
- Your symptoms continue despite the treatment prescribed.
- You need specialized allergy testing or allergy shots.
- You have other conditions that make your allergies or asthma symptoms worse, such as polyps, gastroesophageal reflux, or chronic bronchitis or emphysema.

Finding a specialist is easy. Start with recommendations from your primary care physician, friends, and relatives. If that doesn't work, go to the website of either of the two major professional associations—the American College of Allergy, Asthma, and Immunology (www.acaai.org) or the American Academy of Asthma, Allergy, and Immunology (www.aaaai.org). Both allow you to search for a board-certified allergist by zip code.

When choosing a doctor, look for the following:

- A practice that isn't too busy. You don't want to wait months for an appointment, nor do you want to sit for hours in the waiting room.
- A doctor who has a hands-on approach and doesn't turn you over to ancillary staff after your initial visit.
- A doctor you can talk to, who doesn't make you feel rushed, who answers your questions and explains things using language you can understand, and who works with you to craft a treatment plan.
- A doctor who keeps up with the latest research on allergies and asthma by attending meetings, reading journals, and so on.

Cold or Allergy?

So you think you have allergies. Well, are you sure? Although allergies are one of the most prevalent medical conditions in the United States, and although their incidence in the population is rising faster than a thermometer in July, other conditions, such as colds, are great at mimicking them.

Before you make that appointment with your doctor, take a few minutes to answer the following questions.

1. Do your symptoms, including sneezing, congestion, runny nose, watery eyes, fatigue, and headaches, occur simultaneously?　　　　　　　　　　yes ☐　no ☐
2. Is the duration of your symptoms variable—for instance, sometimes a month or more and sometimes just a couple of days or even hours?　　yes ☐　no ☐
3. Is the mucus discharge from your nose clear?　　　　　　　　　　yes ☐　no ☐
4. Do you sneeze frequently, particularly two or three times in a row?　　yes ☐　no ☐
5. Do your symptoms occur more often in spring through fall?　　　　yes ☐　no ☐
6. Are your nasal symptoms unaccompanied by aches and chills?　　　yes ☐　no ☐

SCORING: *3 to 5* yes *answers:* It's quite likely that your symptoms are related to allergies. See your health care provider for further testing. *3 to 5* no *answers:* You probably have a cold or other respiratory ailment. Wait a few days, and if it doesn't clear up on its own, see your health care provider.

- A doctor who takes your symptoms seriously and doesn't dismiss allergic rhinitis or eczema as minor irritations.

Watch out for doctors who dress inappropriately, whose offices seem disorganized or chaotic, who urge you to purchase supplements or allergy products from their office, who order tests as if they were potato chips without giving you a good explanation of why they're necessary, or who keep changing your medications without considering other options (such as environmental changes and allergy shots).

You may want to schedule a get-acquainted visit as you're checking out potential specialists, but you can expect to pay for it. Few doctors can afford to give away their time these days, and insurance usually doesn't pay for such visits.

Once you choose a doctor, check to see whether your insurance covers your visits; if not, talk to the business manager in the doctor's office about fees. Don't be afraid to ask for a discount if you pay cash; many physicians are happy to do this for patients who pay quickly.

allergy & asthma **sufferers ask**

What's Board-Certified Mean?

You can check whether your doctor is board-certified in any of 24 specialties overseen by the American Board of Medical Specialties at www.abms.org/about.asp or by calling 1-866-ASK-ABMS. Allergists should already be board-certified in internal medicine or pediatrics, with additional certification in allergy and immunology conferred by the American Board of Allergy and Immunology.

To gain this certification, they must have completed a two-year fellowship program and passed a rigorous exam. This ensures that they have detailed knowledge of the underlying pathophysiology and the diagnosis, treatment, and prevention of allergic diseases such as allergic rhinitis, allergic asthma, urticaria, anaphylaxis, hypersensitivity pneumonitis, atopic and contact dermatitis, and allergic gastrointestinal disorders, as well as comparable clinical problems in which it doesn't appear allergies are to blame, such as vasomotor rhinitis and nonallergic asthma. They must also have expertise in managing pulmonary complications of certain other diseases, such as chronic obstructive pulmonary disease (COPD). Board-certified allergists must recertify their board standing at least every 10 years by taking an examination.

preparing for the first visit

Your initial evaluation will go much smoother if you take some time to prepare before entering your doctor's office. To help you do this properly, we've prepared a three-part homework assignment. Do all three, and the doctor will not only love you but will also be much more effective at making a fast, correct diagnosis. The assignments:

1. Track your allergy/asthma symptoms, using the symptom tracking log provided.
2. Gather salient health history facts, using the health history form provided.

3. Finally, near the time of your appointment, prepare your answers for the 10 questions your doctor is likely to ask (they're provided on page 89).

Make copies of these forms as needed and do your best to be thorough and honest. Good luck!

■ form one

symptom tracking log

Each time symptoms hit, use this log. Rank each symptom on a scale from 1 to 10, with 1 being barely noticeable and 10 interfering with your ability to function.

Date and circumstances*	Missed school or work	Decreased exercise tolerance	Tight chest/short of breath	Waking up at night	Sneezing	Postnasal drip	Nasal congestion	Itchy nose	Runny eyes	Headache	Wheezing	Cough

*Note whether you were around pets, at work, or working in the garden; sudden changes in the weather; the foods you ate and medications you took; whether you were exercising; and so on.

■ form two
your health history

NAME _____

BIRTHDATE _____   SEX male ☐ female ☐

OCCUPATION _____

MARITAL STATUS single ☐ married ☐ widowed ☐ divorced ☐

CURRENT MEDICATIONS

Prescription: _____

_____

Nonprescription (list all you take regularly, including antacids, pain relievers, and healing supplements):

_____

_____

CURRENT/CHRONIC MEDICAL CONDITIONS _____

_____

PAST MEDICAL PROBLEMS (include year occurred): _____

_____

SURGERIES (include year occurred): _____

_____

ALLERGIES yes ☐ no ☐

To which of the following are you allergic (be specific)?

Insects: _____

Plants: _____

Medications: _____

Foods: _____

Other: _____

TOBACCO USE yes ☐ no ☐ Current use (type/amount): _____

Started (year or age): _____ Quit (year or age): _____

ALCOHOL USE yes ☐ no ☐

Estimated number of drinks (beer, wine, spirits) per day/week: _____

Are you or others you know concerned about your use of alcohol? yes ☐ no ☐

SUPPLEMENT USE

Daily Vitamin: yes ☐ no ☐   Vitamins when needed: yes ☐ no ☐

Are you or others you know concerned about your use of illicit drugs? yes ☐ no ☐

DIET /EXERCISE

My current diet is: very healthy ☐ healthy ☐ variable ☐ unhealthy ☐

Concerns: _____

My current exercise/activity level is: very high ☐ high ☐ moderate ☐ low ☐

Concerns: _____

My current weight is: much too high □   somewhat high □   acceptable □   too low □

Concerns: _____

I have previously used diet or a formal program to gain/lose weight: yes □   no □

I have previously used medication or supplements to gain/lose weight: yes □   no □

FAMILY MEDICAL HISTORY

No knowledge of family medical history □

Race/ethnicity (optional): _____

Relative	Age	Health status	Cause/age at death (if deceased)
Father			
Mother			
Siblings			
Children			
Other			

Please indicate all conditions that apply to members of your family (brother, sister, father, mother, aunt, uncle, grandparent) below and note the relationship or additional concerns.

□ Alcohol/substance abuse: _____

□ Arthritis: _____

□ Asthma/allergies: _____

□ Bleeding/clotting disorder: _____

□ Breast disease (benign): _____

□ Breast disease (cancer): _____

□ Chronic lung disease: _____

□ Diabetes: _____

□ Headaches: _____

□ Heart disease: _____

□ High blood pressure: _____

□ High cholesterol: _____

□ Mental illness: _____

□ Seizures/epilepsy: _____

□ Stroke: _____

□ Thyroid disorder: _____

□ Ulcers: _____

□ Other (specify): _____

_____

_____

mission: diagnosis

Although doctors use several tests for allergies and asthma, they are mainly used to confirm a diagnosis and provide more detailed information. The most important part of any diagnosis is the physical examination and medical history, so it's vitally important that you be completely honest with your doctor during your initial examination, answering every question as completely as possible. For instance, if you suspect you're allergic to cats, hiding the fact that you have a calico kitten at home won't do you any good. Also tell your doctor *why* you think you have a certain allergy; if your mother said that you were allergic to penicillin as a child, and you're now 45, you may not really be allergic to the drug. Be specific; it's not enough to say you think you have allergies; refer to your symptom tracking log so you can provide your doctor with a detailed overview of your condition.

During the physical examination, your doctor will focus on your head—eyes, ears, nose, and throat. Among the signs she looks for are the boggy, pale gray-blue lining of the nose that's characteristic of allergies; any nasal polyps or sinus infection; dark circles under your eyes; redness of your throat; and postnasal drip. Relax, sit still, and open wide.

Diagnosing Allergies

Many doctors can diagnose allergic rhinitis based on just your medical history. That's fine for run-of-the-mill allergies, but if yours are significantly interfering with your life or aren't easily controlled with standard medications, you may need more sophisticated testing to pinpoint the exact cause so your doctor can develop a more targeted treatment plan. This will help you make the necessary lifestyle changes to avoid the allergens and, if you are open to having allergy shots (described in detail in chapter 7), let your doctor know if you're likely to benefit from the treatment and which allergens to include. You're also more likely to require allergy testing if you have allergic asthma, i.e., asthma that's triggered by allergens.

Questions Your Doctor May Ask

1. When did your symptoms begin?
2. What makes them better or worse?
3. When do they typically appear?
4. Have you ever been diagnosed with allergies or asthma?
5. Do you wheeze or cough a lot, particularly at night?
6. Do you ever have difficulty breathing?
7. Are you oversensitive to heat, cold, or temperature changes?
8. Do your symptoms continue when you vacation away from home? Do they get worse?
9. Do you have any relatives with current asthma or allergies?
10. Do you have relatives with a history of allergies?

There are two main types of allergy tests.

1. Skin tests

Gold-standard, immediate-type hypersensitivity (IgE) skin tests are typically used to test for reactions to airborne allergens, foods, insect stings, and penicillin. All skin tests identify the presence of IgE antibodies to a particular allergen. They can also help diagnose drug and chemical hypersensitivities. Although early skin tests used a "scratch" technique, in which the allergen was applied to the skin and the skin was scratched, this technique is no longer often used because it's just not as accurate as the favored prick/puncture test (see below).

Before having any tests, talk to your doctor about which, if any, medications you should stop taking. Generally, you'll need to stop all antihistamines for 24 to 72 hours prior to testing (and sometimes for up to 10 days, depending on the drug), since they may affect the test's accuracy. You may also be asked to stop taking any other drugs with antihistamine properties, including those for schizophrenia, such as chlorpromazine (Thorazine); the anti-nausea medication prochlorperazine (Compazine); and tricyclic antidepressants, such as amitriptyline (Elavil) and doxepin (Sinequan). Your doctor may also consider having you stop taking beta-blockers for the day of your tests. These drugs, such as propranolol (Inderal) and atenolol (Tenormin), block the actions of epinephrine, an emergency medicine used if you have a severe allergy attack. Also, if you're taking long-term or high doses of oral corticosteroids, your doctor may recommend that you stop prior to the tests. Check with your doctor before stopping. Given all of this, it's easy to see why it's so important to take a list of all your medications and dosages to your first appointment.

Before testing for specific allergens, your doctor will perform a

Conditions That Mimic Asthma

One reason it's so important to get the right diagnosis if you think you may have asthma is that several conditions—some of them quite serious—mimic it.

Coronary disease can produce asthma-like constriction of the chest.

Early congestive heart failure can mimic asthma, with shortness of breath and even wheezing (it used to be called cardiac asthma and was treated with aminophylline, an ancient asthma medication).

Recurrent blood clots in your lungs (pulmonary emboli) produce shortness of breath and even some wheezing.

Airway and chest tumors may cause wheezing and coughing.

Immunologic lung diseases, such as pulmonary vasculitis, have asthma-like features.

Vocal cord spasms have symptoms similar to asthma. In one study, when 56 patients diagnosed with asthma were treated with vocal retraining by speech pathologists, more than 90 percent improved.

Hyperventilation, or panic disorder, acute **infectious bronchitis**, and adult mild **cystic fibrosis** are other conditions that mimic asthma.

GERD

"negative control" test with saline solution. You shouldn't have any reaction to this test; if you do, it means you're oversensitive, which makes accurate readings of any other skin tests much more difficult. Additionally, the doctor should conduct a "positive control" test, injecting a bit of histamine, which causes an allergic reaction, under your skin. It should produce a bump; if not, you're underreactive, which also makes evaluating future skin tests difficult. The positive control test is also used for comparison with allergen skin testing to determine how severely you react to the allergen.

■ **Prick/puncture (percutaneous) tests.** These tests are the most convenient, least expensive, and most specific screening method for detecting IgE antibodies, and they tend to be the best for determining the causes of allergic rhinitis. They're usually performed on your upper back or forearm. Using a diluted solution of various airborne allergens common in your geographic area, the doctor or other medical professional places a drop on your skin, then either punctures or pricks the skin with a special tool, allowing the allergen to come in contact with deeper layers of skin.

■ **Intracutaneous tests.** These are generally performed when a prick/puncture test is negative for IgE antibodies but symptoms strongly suggest an allergic mechanism. It involves using extremely fine needles to inject the diluted allergen just below the skin surface on your upper arm or forearm. It's not as bad as it sounds; the needles are so fine that you may feel only a slight burning sensation. These tests are much better for people with low skin-test sensitivity, but they should be performed only *after* a negative prick/puncture test because they carry a slightly higher risk of reaction.

About 15 minutes after performing a skin test, the doctor "reads" the resulting wheal, a small, raised, reddened area like a mosquito bite, and the amount of redness on your arm, measuring the wheal and comparing it with the positive control test performed earlier. A wheal at least 3 millimeters larger than any wheal that appeared after the control test proves the presence of allergen-specific IgE. The larger the prick/puncture skin test reaction, the

Sensitive vs. Specific

If you spent time in the break rooms where allergists congregate at a hospital or clinic, you would hear them talking about a test's sensitivity or specificity. The terms might even enter a conversation with you if you were a patient. Here's what they're talking about.

The more *sensitive* a test is, the more likely it is to identify all people who have the allergy. However, it may also include a fair number of "false positives," which are positive readings for someone who really doesn't have the allergy. The more *specific* the test, the more guaranteed that a positive test is accurate. However, because of its tougher criteria, a highly specific test is likely to miss some who have the disease.

Here's an analogy that might help: If you were to throw out a highly sensitive net to catch tuna, it would catch all the tuna, and perhaps some dolphins and sea turtles as well. A highly specific net would catch only tuna, but you'd also miss plenty of them.

more likely that it's clinically significant. But here's where it gets, uh, sticky: A positive skin test doesn't necessarily mean the allergen tested is the one causing your symptoms; it just means that you have an IgE response to it.

For example, if you have a positive skin test to grass, and you have diabetes, obviously, the test doesn't mean that the grass allergy is the cause of your diabetes. Recall the saying that medicine is as much an art as a science? Well, this is an example of the "art" aspect and why a well-trained doctor is your best bet beyond even the most conclusive tests.

Expect to spend about 2 hours in your doctor's office undergoing skin testing. In some instances, you may require up to 70 prick/puncture tests, followed by up to 40 intracutaneous tests to identify what's causing your allergic rhinitis. Don't be alarmed if you see redness, hardness, or swelling at the site of the test 1 to 2 hours or more after the application of the allergen; this is the delayed allergic reaction we've talked about, which is normal and generally disappears within one to two days.

■ **Patch-type skin test.** Also called delayed-type hypersensitivity skin test, this test is used to see if you have a skin sensitivity, called contact dermatitis, to substances such as rubber, medications, fragrances, hair dyes, metals, and resins. The diluted allergen is put on your upper back, and the site is covered with tape, which is left on for at least 48 hours. Then the patch is removed, and the site is checked for a reaction. The patch is replaced, and the site is checked again at 72 and/or 96 hours (or earlier if a reaction occurs).

2. Blood tests

Radioallergosorbent testing, or RAST, was the first blood test developed for allergen testing. Since then, several others have been approved, including ELISA, modified RAST, Quidel QuickVue One-Step Allergen Screen, and Pharmacia Immunocap. They aren't the preferred testing methods for allergies but are used when skin tests just aren't feasible—for instance, if you have a skin disease that would make it difficult to read the results, or you can't stop taking medications that might interfere with

Question These Tests

There is no scientific evidence that the following tests are effective for diagnosing allergies. If your doctor wants to perform them, ask why and get a second opinion to avoid costly, unnecessary testing.

Cytotoxic test, a blood test to evaluate the effects of allergens on white blood cells

Provocation-neutralization, in which diluted allergens are injected under the skin to elicit a response, then a weaker or stronger dilution is injected to relieve the symptoms

Electrodermal diagnosis, in which an electric current is applied to certain points on your body along with an allergen

Applied kinesiology, in which the practitioner presses down on your arms after you've eaten, held, or had an allergen injected

"Reaginic" pulse test, in which your pulse rate is measured after you've been exposed to a potential allergen

Chemical analysis of body tissues

the test. They're most likely to be performed by primary care physicians who don't have access to a clinical skin-testing laboratory. Few allergists use them because they're just not as accurate as skin tests. Plus, they cost more, it takes longer to get results, and, if the results are inconclusive, they must be repeated.

Diagnosing Asthma

It wasn't until the early 1800s that an asthmatic French doctor, René Laënnec, designed the first crude stethoscope (a rolled-up piece of paper) to listen to a patient's heart

A New Test for Monitoring Asthma

In May 2003, the FDA approved a first-of-its-kind, noninvasive test to measure the concentration of nitric oxide (NO) in exhaled human breath, using a device called the NIOX Nitric Oxide Test System. Nitric oxide levels are higher in the breath of people with asthma because of the inflammation of their airways. Thus, measuring levels of NO is a good way to test whether your anti-inflammatory medications are working.

Although the device is currently used primarily for research, it should make its way into doctors' offices in the not-so-distant future as it becomes simpler to use and the price drops.

and lungs, and not until the 1830s that microscopes allowed doctors to examine patients' lung tissue and secretions. But perhaps the most important diagnostic discovery for respiratory illnesses such as asthma came about in 1850, when British surgeon John Hutchinson developed the spirometer for his research in respiratory physiology. Today, electronic digitized spirometers, along with peak flow meters, are critical tools in any allergy/asthma specialist's arsenal. They're used to monitor the speed and strength of your breathing as well as your lung capacity.

These machines are only tools, however, best used to confirm a diagnosis or track your progress. Most of the work your doctor will do in determining the diagnosis involves talking with you, examining you, and taking a detailed medical history as described earlier. Still, tests do come in handy.

If you have allergic asthma, which is caused entirely or even in part by allergies, you will probably undergo skin testing as described earlier. In addition, there are other tests your doctor will want to conduct, not only to help diagnose your asthma but also to monitor how well you're controlling it once you both agree on a course of treatment.

1. Pulmonary function tests

These tests measure the degree of obstruction in your lungs and involve blowing into a machine that measures your exhaled breath. There are three main types.

■ **Spirometers.** Using a spirometer is fairly easy. You hold the tube in your mouth, inhale as much air as possible, then exhale forcefully for 6 seconds. The spirometry measurements provide clues to the health of your lungs, just as your

Using a Peak Flow Meter

Here's how to use this breath-measuring device at home.

1. Be sure the device reads zero or is at base level.
2. Stand up.
3. Take as deep a breath as possible.
4. Put your mouth around the meter and close your lips around the mouthpiece.
5. Blow out as hard and fast as possible in 1 to 2 seconds.
6. Don't cough, spit, or let your tongue block the mouthpiece.
7. Write down the value you get.
8. Repeat the process two more times and record the highest of the three numbers in your chart.

Today, you can also use an electronic peak flow meter, called the Piko-1. The device stores up to 96 measurements in its memory, which can be downloaded to a computer.

blood pressure and blood cholesterol numbers provide clues to the health of your cardiovascular system. The results are described in terms of:

Forced expiratory volume (in 1 second), or FEV1. This is the amount of air you can force out of your lungs in the first second after you begin exhaling, or your lung velocity. You should be able to get the majority of air out of your lungs in the first second; you want the result to be 85 percent or better. The lower the number, the narrower your airways, particularly the small airways (bronchioles).

Forced vital capacity, or FVC. This is the amount of air you breathe out in 6 seconds after a full inhalation, or your lung capacity. Any remaining air is known as residual volume. As we discussed earlier, people with asthma have a more difficult time exhaling than inhaling. The FVC should be normal in most people with asthma unless the disease is very severe. You want a result of 90 percent or better; any lower means that either you haven't tried hard enough to blow or your lung capacity is reduced, suggesting severe asthma.

■ **Challenge test (bronchoprovocation).** This test is used if spirometry indicates normal or near-normal lung function, but it still seems that asthma is causing your symptoms. First, the doctor gives you a baseline spirometry test, then has you inhale a drug (usually methacholine or histamine), which constricts the airways in some people. Then the spirometry test is repeated. If your airways constrict, the doctor will give you an airway-opening drug. If you're sensitive to methacholine (indicated by a drop of at least 20 percent in your spirometry test) and respond to an airway-opening drug (indicated by an improvement in your spirometry test), you probably have asthma. However, the test isn't always 100 percent accurate. You could have a positive test result and not have asthma; for instance, sometimes people with allergic rhinitis have sensitive airways, resulting in a positive test, but that doesn't mean they have clinical asthma. Conversely, you could have a negative test result and still have asthma. Again, there's that "art vs. science" component of medicine.

■ **Peak flow meter.** This test is to asthma what a thermometer is to fever and a finger prick is to diabetes: It helps you monitor your asthma at home, determining if your medications are working or if you may be headed toward a crash. The peak flow meter is a small, hand-held device that you breathe into. It measures the rate at which you can force air out of your lungs, called your peak expiratory flow rate (PEFR). It isn't very good at measuring small-airway obstruction; it indicates only obstruction in the large airways.

During the test, you breathe in as deeply as you can and then blow into the device as hard and fast as possible. If your asthma symptoms are about to worsen, you'll see your peak flow readings drop. Such drops are a clue that you probably need to increase your medication. Ideally, you don't want your peak flow readings to vary more than 15 percent from the previous reading.

Although your doctor will use the peak flow meter test to assess the severity of your asthma, you should view it as an early warning system, alerting you to the possibility of major problems.

Determining Asthma Severity

A diagnosis of asthma, unlike one for allergies, includes a classification of severity: severe persistent, moderate persistent, mild persistent, or mild intermittent. Here's how your doctor determines your classification, which in turn plays a role in determining your treatment plan.

Severity	Characteristics of symptoms	Occurence of nighttime symptoms	Lung function
Severe persistent	• Continual • Limit physical activity • Frequently worsen	• Frequent	• FEV1 or PEFR less than or equal to 60% of predicted value • PEFR variability greater than 30% (the lower the variability, the more stable your condition)
Moderate persistent	• Daily • Require daily use of inhaled short-acting beta2-agonists • Worsening affects physical activity • Worsen two or more times a week; may last for days	• More than once a week	• FEV1 or PEFR 60–80% of predicted value • PEFR variability greater than 30%
Mild persistent	• Occur more than twice a week but less than once a day	• More than twice a month	• FEV1 or PEFR equal to or greater than 80% of predicted value • PEFR variability 20–30%
Mild intermittent	• Occur two or fewer times a week • No symptoms and normal PEFR between episodes • Episodes are brief (from a few hours to a few days); intensity may vary	• Two or fewer times a month	• FEV1 or PEFR 80% or greater than predicted value • PEFR variability less than 20%

2. Other Tests

In addition to pulmonary function tests, your doctor may perform several other tests, more to rule out other problems than to actually confirm an asthma diagnosis. These include:

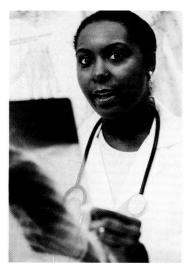

Your doctor may order *CT scans or chest x-rays* to confirm an asthma diagnosis.

■ **Chest x-ray.** An x-ray to view the inside of your lungs helps rule out other possible causes of your symptoms, including bronchitis, pneumonia, and lung cancer.

■ **Sinus x-ray or CT scan.** This test uses x-rays to see if you have nasal polyps (growths in your sinuses) or sinusitis (inflammation or swelling of your sinuses due to infection), both of which may make asthma harder to treat and control.

■ **Sputum evaluation.** It sounds a bit gross, but this test evaluates the mucus you bring up from your lungs, looking for eosinophils, the white blood cells that increase during asthma attacks and are triggered by allergies.

■ **Complete blood count (CBC).** Here, the doctor is looking for elevated levels of white blood cells that could indicate an infection such as bronchitis or pneumonia; high levels of eosinophils also suggest an allergic component to your asthma.

the next steps

By now, you've found a doctor you like, received a diagnosis of allergies or asthma (or both), and find yourself clutching a handful of prescriptions. Welcome to the wonderful world of drugs, which we'll explore in detail in the next chapter.

chapter **seven**

the right
medications

A large part of the Breathe Easy Plan involves lifestyle
changes: changing your environment, your diet, and even the supplements you
take to minimize asthma and allergic reactions. Equally important to the program and to your health is taking the right prescription and over-the-counter
medicines—and taking them the right way for the right reasons.

Unfortunately, far too few people with asthma and allergies understand this
critical tenet. Even those who do take their medicine religiously may not be
aware that they're taking the wrong medication or are taking it at the wrong
times, in the wrong manner, or in the wrong doses. And for what Americans
spend on drugs—overall, about $4.5 *billion* each year for allergy medications
and billions more for asthma drugs—we ought to at least get it right.

Today, there's a host of options available for allergy and asthma treatment,
both over the counter (OTC) and prescription. In this chapter, we'll provide an
overview of each major category. The chapter is divided between medications for
allergic rhinitis and those for asthma. In some instances, a medication may be
used for both.

Before we get too far into the particulars, though, we need to emphasize a
major caveat: *Don't start or stop taking any medication without first talking to your*

doctor. The advice given here is just that—advice. It is not prescriptive, and we aren't telling you what to do. Instead, we hope to arm you with enough knowledge and information to have an educated, informative discussion with your health care provider.

It's also critical that you tell your doctor about *all* medications you're taking, including over-the-counter drugs, vitamin/mineral supplements, and herbs, and about any medical conditions you have other than allergies or asthma. Many drugs recommended for asthma in particular can be dangerous if you have heart disease, diabetes, or liver disease. And if you're meandering through the medication maze on behalf of your child, be sure to ask if the drug is approved for use by children or at least has a good track record with kids. We'll talk more about specific drugs for children later on.

Now... welcome to our virtual medical cabinet!

Medicines for Allergies

If you have allergies today, consider yourself lucky. The past decade has seen a veritable explosion in the numbers and types of allergy medications. In 1997, for instance, 39 percent of Americans used prescription drugs for their allergies, and 47 percent used over the-counter treatments, primarily drugs such as diphenhydramine (Benadryl) that left them drowsy and befuddled.

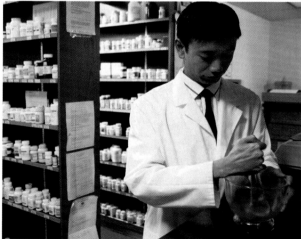

A mere four years later, those figures had pretty much reversed. In 2001, half of those with allergies used prescription medications for relief, compared with 35 percent who used over-the-counter drugs. Put simply, the prescription drugs got much better. Additionally, immunotherapy, or allergy shots, greatly improved in terms of both safety and efficacy.

You can't expect miracles, of course. In a 2001 national survey of allergists and primary care doctors who treat allergies, more than 65 percent said they were only somewhat satisfied with the currently available medications. Also, don't be surprised if you need more than one drug; more than half of allergists and 39 percent of primary care physicians said they prescribe more than one medication to their patients.

If you have allergies today, consider yourself lucky, *because drugs are much improved*. Still, you can't expect miracles.

Their biggest complaint? Oral antihistamines don't act fast enough. As a result, patients end up switching medications or using additional treatments.

Also, different doctors may treat symptoms differently. Despite clear parameters and recommendations from the major allergy societies and national health organizations, there's still no consensus as to the best way to treat allergic rhinitis. Thus, doctors who focus on symptom relief, for instance, may tend to prescribe antihistamines, while those who view inflammation as the principal problem are more likely to favor corticosteroids.

The key is that your doctor works *with* you, taking into consideration your symptoms and health profile, to develop an individualized treatment plan.

antihistamines

- **NONPRESCRIPTION (sedating):** Actifed, Alka-Seltzer Plus, Allerest, Banophen, Benadryl, Diphenhist, BC Multi-Symptom Cold Powder, Chlor-Trimeton, Comtrex, Contac, Dimetapp, Drixoral, Sinarest, Sudafed Plus, Tavist, Triaminic Allergy, Tylenol Allergy Sinus, Vicks NyQuil
- **NONPRESCRIPTION (nonsedating):** Alavert, Claritin
- **PRESCRIPTION (sedating):** Antivert (meclizine), Atarax (hydroxyzine HCL), DAllergy (brompheniramine and pseudoephedrine), Naldecon Children's Syrup (cabinoxamine), Periactin (cyproheptadine), Rynatan/Trinalin (azatadine maleate and pseudoephedrine sulfate), Temaril (phenothiazine), Vistaril (hydroxyzine)
- **PRESCRIPTION (nonsedating):** Allegra (fexofenadine), Clarinex (desloratadine), Zyrtec (cetirizine)

Ah, it's always nice to have a drug whose name tells you what it does. As the name implies, antihistamines counter the effects of histamine, the inflammatory chemical released by your body's mast cells during an allergic reaction. Histamine is to blame for the sneezing, nasal swelling and drainage, and itchy eyes, throat, and nose that are the hallmarks of allergic rhinitis. Today, you're likely to hear antihistamines referred to in two ways: their level of sedation (sedating or nonsedating) and their duration (short- or long-acting).

First-Generation, Sedating Antihistamines

Oral antihistamines, which come as pills, tablets, and syrups, have long been considered a first-line defense against the misery of allergies, with their use dating back to the 1940s. They work well, but with one big problem: Most over-the-counter antihistamines, such as Benadryl, wipe you out. That's because their active ingredients cross the blood/brain barrier, wreaking havoc on your central nervous system. In fact, the active ingredient in Benadryl—diphenhydramine—is also the active ingredient in most over-the-counter sleeping pills. No wonder, then, that people who take Benadryl say they are, on average, 26 percent less effective at work on days they're affected by allergies.

What's more, studies suggest that even those who say medications like Benadryl don't make them drowsy may have impaired reaction time, visual-motor coordination, memory, and learning capacity, as well as poorer performance on arithmetic exercises and driving tests. Just consider a 2000 study that showed the standard 50-milligram dose of Benadryl impaired driving ability (as measured in a driving simulator) as much or more than alcohol, making the subjects legally drunk. Most frightening: Those tested had no sense of impairment after taking the medicine. In other words, they thought they were driving just fine even though they were severely impaired. Also, children who take diphenhydramine score significantly lower on tests of learning ability than those who receive similar amounts of nonsedating antihistamines.

insider information: You can often get relief from allergy symptoms with just half the recommended dose of an over-the-counter, first-generation antihistamine. This reduces the drug's sedating effects.

Thus, many states consider you under the influence of drugs when you're taking an OTC antihistamine. For instance, pilots aren't permitted to fly if they've taken such a drug within 24 hours of a scheduled flight.

These first-generation antihistamines, which include such familiar names as Tavist and Chlor-Trimeton, also don't last terribly long, so you need to take a dose about every 4 hours. Still, they do play a role in the treatment of allergies (Benadryl sales actually increased between 2000 and 2002, despite the fact that newer, less sedating options became available by prescription).

So why their popularity? For one thing, they work relatively fast, providing quick relief. For another, they're inexpensive and, in the case of the OTC

The Hay Fever Treatment Guide

The American Academy of Allergy, Asthma, and Immunology provides primary care physicians with the following step-by-step chart for determining treatment for perennial allergic rhinitis.

With little water discharge (from eyes and nose):	With copious water discharge (from eyes and nose):
• Avoid irritants	• Avoid irritants
• Add a daily topical nasal corticosteroid	• Add a daily topical nasal anticholinergic
If treatment is ineffective after 1 month, consider:	**If treatment is ineffective after 1 month, consider:**
• A short course (3–10 days) of an oral corticosteroid	• Adding a topical nasal corticosteroid
• Adding an oral decongestant	• Referral to an allergy/immunology or ENT allergy specialist for further evaluation and/or co-management
• Referral to an allergy/immunology or ENT allergy specialist for further evaluation and/or co-management	

forms, readily available at any drugstore, supermarket, discount chain, or convenience store.

If you take them, be sure you take them correctly; they're most effective when taken about a half-hour before you expect to encounter the allergen, such as before you visit your sister and her five cats. For chronic allergies, you'll probably do better with timed-release antihistamines that work for up to 12 hours.

Keep taking antihistamines as recommended until you feel better. Sometimes the medication needs to build up in your bloodstream to provide maximum relief. However, if you find that an antihistamine that was working fine suddenly isn't effective, check with your doctor; you may have developed a tolerance and require a different or stronger drug.

Antihistamine Warnings

It's clear that antihistamines have a powerful effect on your brain and body, so those back-of-the-bottle warnings are valid. When taking an antihistamine, heed these words.

- Avoid driving.
- Don't use any motorized equipment.
- Don't drink alcohol.
- Don't take any form of sedative or tranquilizer.
- Watch for side effects such as dryness of the mouth, nose, and eyes.

Second-Generation, Nonsedating Antihistamines

With the advent of the newer, nonsedating antihistamines such as fexofenadine (Allegra) and loratadine (Claritin and Alavert), the picture cleared for allergy sufferers—along with their stuffy heads. The active ingredients in these medications, which also include cetirizine (Zyrtec) and desloratadine (Clarinex), have very little effect on the central nervous system because they are composed of larger molecules that can't get past the blood/brain barrier. Thus, they don't make you tired, irritable, or confused. For instance, a study that tested the effects of Allegra on driving ability found it had no more effect than a placebo. That's why the Joint Task Force on Practice Parameters in Allergy, Asthma, and Immunology recommends these drugs as a first-line therapy for allergic rhinitis.

While these drugs work fairly similarly, some studies suggest that at recommended dosages, Allegra may be slightly more effective at relieving nasal symptoms and may be less sedating than the others. Still, that's probably a subjective finding, given that everyone's allergy symptoms are different. Don't be surprised if you have to try several antihistamines before finding the one that works best for you.

Antihistamine Nasal Spray

In addition to oral antihistamines, there is now an intranasal antihistamine, azelastine (Astelin), approved for both seasonal and perennial allergic rhinitis and available only by prescription. It works quickly and can be used as needed.

Astelin has two main advantages. First is the obvious: It provides targeted therapy, as opposed to oral antihistamines, which must make their way through your digestive system and bloodstream before arriving on the scene. Second, it's the only antihistamine approved for both allergic and nonallergic rhinitis, because it helps with congestion as well as runny nose (which oral antihistamines can't touch).

decongestants

- **NONPRESCRIPTION:** Actifed Allergy Daytime, Allerest, Drixoral Nondrowsy Formula, Edifc/24, Sudafed
- **NONPRESCRIPTION NASAL SPRAYS:** Afrin, Cheracol, Dristan, Neo-Synephrine, Nostril/Nostrilla, Otrivin, Privine, Vicks Sinex Long-Acting
- **PRESCRIPTION:** Dura-Vent (chlorpheniramine and phenylephrine), Entex LA, Guaifed PD, Respaire, and Sinuvent (guaifenesin and phenylephrine), Exgest LA (guafenesin and phenylpropanolamine)

In addition to hitting at the source of your allergy symptoms—histamine—you also want to unclog your nose so you don't feel as if you're packing 10 pounds of cement in there. That's where decongestants come in. They work by restricting the blood supply to the nose and sinuses, thus reducing

insider information: Men with prostate enlargement may have urinary problems while taking decongestants.

swelling, excess secretions, and congestion. They're often combined with antihistamines, as in the oral nonsedating drugs Allegra-D and Claritin-D, and the less sedating acrivastine (Semprex-D) and Zyrtec-D. They also are frequently combined with guaifenesin (an expectorant).

Be aware that if you use OTC decongestant nose drops and sprays for more than a few days, you can get a rebound effect. That is, the more you use, the more you need, until they become ineffective altogether, and your nose and sinuses remain stuffed tighter than a toddler in a snowsuit. Also, use with care if you're taking medication to manage emotional or behavioral problems, such as antidepressants.

saline nasal spray

Don't discount plain old saltwater's ability to relieve stuffiness and congestion. You can buy it over the counter in brands such as Ocean and Salinex or make your own by adding ½ teaspoon of salt and a pinch of baking soda to a

Soothing the Burning, Itching, and Redness of Allergic Conjunctivitis

As you learned in part 1, your eyes are packed with mast cells, which means they're prime targets for allergies. If you have eye allergies, most commonly called allergic conjunctivitis, several forms of eyedrops can provide relief, including these.

Tear substitutes. There are more than 50 different artificial tear preparations available over the counter these days. They temporarily flush out allergens and moisten your eyes. Most contain preservatives, which is fine if you use them less than three times a day. If you use them more often, choose a brand without preservatives, which will be more expensive but safer for your eyes in the long run. Try popping the eyedrops into the refrigerator for extra soothing power.

Decongestants and antihistamines. You can get over-the-counter eyedrop decongestants that

constrict blood vessels in your eyes, thus reducing redness, and antihistamines, which help with itching. A word of warning: Don't use decongestant drops if you have glaucoma, and don't use them for more than two or three days; like nasal decongestants, they can have a rebound effect if overused.

Prescription medications. If over-the-counter preparations don't do it for you, talk to your doctor about prescription eyedrops. There are prescription antihistamine drops, mast cell stabilizers, and nonsteroidal anti-inflammatory drops that help with itching, and corticosteroids for chronic and severe eye allergy symptoms. All carry their own risks of side effects, however. Also, most need to be used twice a day, and some may be recommended for use for only a limited time.

cup of lukewarm water. Then use a bulb syringe like the ones used to clear an infant's nose to spray the solution into your nose a few times. Follow with a good, hard blow.

anticholinergic spray

- **PRESCRIPTION (nasal spray):** Atrovent nasal (ipratropium bromide)
- **PRESCRIPTION (inhaled):** Atrovent 0.03% or 0.06%, nebulized or metered-dose inhaler

Ipratropium bromide (Atrovent) belongs to the tongue-twisting class of drugs known as anticholinergic agents. They block the effects of acetylcholine, a neurotransmitter that stimulates mucus production, which makes them great for combating runny noses. Available only in a prescription spray, Atrovent is officially approved only for treatment of allergic rhinitis (for which runny nose could be called the mascot), but it does work quite well in some cases of asthma and chronic bronchitis because of its ability to dry up mucus secretions. It's particularly effective for older people with asthma who also have emphysema or chronic bronchitis or for those who don't respond completely to the common asthma medications known as beta2-agonists described on page 114.

cromolyn sodium spray

- **NONPRESCRIPTION AND PRESCRIPTION (nasal spray):** Nasalcrom
- **PRESCRIPTION (inhaled):** Intal metered-dose inhaler or nebulized

Rather than treating the symptoms of an allergic attack, this nasal spray stops attacks before they start by preventing the release of chemicals such as histamine from mast cells, thus serving as an anti-inflammatory agent. It has few side effects when used as directed, and it significantly helps some people with allergies. The standard cromolyn nasal spray, Nasalcrom, available without a prescription, is not as effective as steroid nasal sprays

insider information: Cromolyn sodium works best if you start using it two to four weeks before you're exposed to allergens.

(described on page 109), but it will help many people with mild allergies. It's also one of the preferred first-line therapies for pregnant women who have mild allergic rhinitis.

Be patient, though; it may take up to three weeks before you experience the full benefit, and cromolyn sodium doesn't work for everyone. Another drawback is that you have to use it up to four times a day, which can be irksome. Side effects are minimal, though. The possibilities include nasal congestion, coughing, sneezing, wheezing, nausea, nosebleeds, dry throat, and burning or irritation.

Going Over the Counter: What It Means for You

In late 2002, the first of the nonsedating antihistamines—loratadine (Claritin)—became available over the counter (OTC). At first glance, this may seem like a good thing for people with allergies; now they have access to a longer-lasting, nondrowsy medication without having to see a doctor. But it also means that most health insurance plans now refuse to pay for Claritin, even if it's prescribed in stronger, non-OTC forms. In fact, many plans refuse to cover other second-generation antihistamines such as cetirizine (Zyrtec), even though they are only available by prescription.

For consumers, that means a month's supply of Claritin that once cost a co-payment of $10 to $15 is now twice that much in many instances. The drugs that still require prescriptions could cost $80 or more a month. That's driving some people back to the older forms of antihistamines or to combination antihistamine/decongestants, with all their attendant problems. It also means fewer doctor visits, so problems aren't caught as early as they might have been.

If you're thinking of taking a cheaper, sedating antihistamine at night and saving the more expensive, nonsedating medication for daytime, watch out. You're still likely to be woozy in the morning. Studies find that a sedating antihistamine and its by-products linger in the body the next morning, decreasing alertness.

emergency medications

- **PRESCRIPTION (injected):** Adrenalin chloride (epinephrine)
- **PRESCRIPTION (nebulized):** Brethaire (terbutaline), Vaponefrin (epinephrine)

Anyone with severe allergies knows well the benefits of epinephrine, often called adrenaline and administered via injection in the event of a severe allergy attack or anaphylaxis. If you're severely allergic, particularly to insect stings and certain foods, you should carry epinephrine with you at all times as part of your emergency treatment kit.

Also in that kit should be a list of medications you're currently taking and any that your doctor recommends in the event of an anaphylactic reaction, a list of your symptoms during anaphylaxis, a written treatment plan from your doctor, and your doctor's name and contact information. You may also want to consider wearing a MedicAlert bracelet in case you can't communicate during an attack.

If Your Drug Isn't Covered

In today's managed-care environment, you may find that the drug your doctor prescribes isn't covered by your health plan or requires a higher co-payment. That's because most health plans maintain an approved formulary, a list of drugs covered under your prescription benefit. Usually, the formulary includes at least one drug in the class of drugs you've been prescribed; if that's the case, ask your doctor if it's okay to use the covered medication. Otherwise, you may have to put out more money for a higher co-pay or for the entire cost of the medication, which can get quite expensive.

You can always use the appeal process described in your benefits information to try to change the health plan's restrictions. Another option is to have your doctor write a letter to the medical director of the plan requesting that the prescribed drug be added to the formulary or that special consideration be provided for you because of your unique circumstances. Bottom line: Don't give up.

immunotherapy: long-term allergy treatment

Okay, so the idea of getting a shot once or twice a week for six months or more doesn't have much appeal. Well, what if those shots could enable you to enjoy spring days with no fear of allergy attacks? Keep your beloved pet without investing in a pallet-load of tissues? Prevent asthma attacks and trips to the hospital for emergency care? Suddenly, a simple shot doesn't seem so bad, does it?

Immunotherapy, or allergy shots, has been around since 1911. It's the only treatment for allergies that reduces symptoms over the long term rather than just treating them for a few hours.

Immunotherapy works similarly to a vaccine, albeit one that's given many times over a long period. Each successive injection contains a tiny bit more of the substance to which you're allergic. Eventually, your body becomes desensitized to the allergen, decreasing the IgE reaction to it by blocking IgE anti-

How Do I Know If Immunotherapy Is Right for Me?

Allergy shots are generally considered for people with perennial and seasonal allergies to airborne allergens, such as pollens, pet dander, dust mites, and mold, or to insect stings; those whose symptoms are not well controlled with medication; those who want to avoid long-term use of medication; and those who are willing to make the long-term commitment to treatment. The American College of Allergy, Asthma, and Immunology offers the following guidelines for immunotherapy.

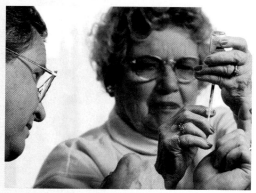

- It should be prescribed only by an allergist, immunologist, or other physician trained in the therapy.
- It should be given only in facilities equipped to treat anaphylaxis.
- You need to be healthy prior to every injection. If you're ill, especially with asthma or respiratory difficulties, you shouldn't receive immunotherapy until your condition improves.
- Tell your doctor about any medications you're taking. Beta-blockers, for instance, block the effect of epinephrine, which may be needed to treat a severe reaction to an allergy shot.
- You should wait at the health care facility for a minimum of 20 minutes after an injection, or longer if you're at high risk for a reaction.

You're probably not a good candidate for immunotherapy if you:

- Have an extreme response to skin tests. This may predict a dangerous allergic reaction to the shots.
- Have uncontrolled or severe asthma or lung disease.
- Are taking certain medications, such as beta-blockers.

And, if you've been having allergy shots for 12 to 18 months and don't have any improvement, you should probably stop.

bodies and minimizing their production and action. Thus, when you encounter the allergen in the future, you have a reduced or very minor response and fewer symptoms. It's somewhat like stepping slowly into a pool of cold water. By the time you immerse your whole body, you've become so used to the cold (or so numb to it), you barely feel it.

And it works. Experts analyzing 24 studies involving more than 900 people with asthma who also had documented allergies found that allergy shots effectively treated allergic asthma in 71 percent, resulting in fewer symptoms, less lung inflammation, and a reduced need for medications. Overall, other studies found that immunotherapy can reduce the sneezing and wheezing of allergic rhinitis by 80 percent and the need for allergy medications by 88 percent.

Other studies suggest that immunotherapy may prevent the development of new allergies and of asthma in children who have allergic rhinitis. Not only that, but another study, presented at the 2000 annual meeting of the American

Academy of Allergy, Asthma, and Immunology, found that allergen immuno-therapy for three years significantly improved patients' overall quality of life even as it reduced costs for doctor's visits.

It sounds great, right? So why doesn't everyone with allergies get allergy shots? For one thing, many people have this aversion to offering up their arms as pincushions. For another, it's pretty intensive therapy. Initially, you may need shots once or twice a week during what's called the buildup phase. This lasts about three to six months, until the target dose of the allergen is reached, after which you need injections every two to four weeks.

It also takes a lot more time than popping a pill. The treatments are usually given in your allergist's office (few primary care physicians give allergy shots), and you'll need to remain there for at least 20 minutes after an injection in case you have a reaction. If the therapy works, you'll probably continue getting shots for three to five years before stopping. The payoff, though, is that your symptoms will remain controlled for several years after you end immunotherapy. If they do return, you may need another course of treatment.

Two types of adverse reactions may occur with immunotherapy.

■ **Local reactions.** You may develop some swelling at the injection site. If you do, try an oral antihistamine and apply ice packs. Also, let your doctor know so the dose can be adjusted next time.

■ **Systemic reactions.** This type of reaction is much less common. It can be mild, marked by sneezing, nasal congestion, or hives. In these mild cases, the symptoms respond rapidly to medications such as antihistamines. Sometimes, however, more serious systemic reactions, such as anaphylaxis, occur. Typically, if you have a reaction, it will occur within 20 minutes of the allergy injection, which is why you need to remain in

An Alternative to Needles: SLIT Immunotherapy

The biggest drawback of immunotherapy is, of course, the needle: By the time you finish immunotherapy, you may have received well over 100 shots. That's why a growing number of physicians in Europe have turned to sublingual-swallow immunotherapy, or SLIT.

Basically, it involves placing drops of the allergen solution under your tongue for a minute or two before swallowing. The treatment remains controversial, however, with opponents insisting there's no way the delicate allergens can survive the rigors of the digestive tract long enough to have any significant effect on the immune system. Nevertheless, a growing body of research shows that SLIT may have a role in immunotherapy. Of 18 double-blind, placebo-controlled clinical trials in the past 15 years, 16 confirmed the effectiveness of SLIT in reducing allergy symptoms triggered by grass pollen, house dust mites, or birch pollen. Other studies found that drops were as effective as shots, that patients liked them better (surprise!), and that they were safer than shots. In November 2003, the World Health Organization supported the use of SLIT for certain patients, particularly those who don't take their meds, refuse injections, and/or have systemic reactions to injection immunotherapy. SLIT is under investigation in the United States and may be available in the near future.

your doctor's office afterward. However, reactions can occur even later, so remain alert to any symptoms.

Overall, immunotherapy is quite safe. A report from the Mayo Clinic on 79,593 immunotherapy injections over a 10-year period showed the incidence of adverse reactions was less than $\frac{2}{10}$ of 1 percent. Most were mild and responded to immediate medical treatment. There were no fatalities during the study.

Going back further, the record isn't pristine, but it is still good. Between 1985 and 1993, when an estimated 52.3 million immunotherapy shots were given, 35 deaths occurred, making the incidence of fatality less than 1 per million.

Medicines for Asthma

The goal in treating asthma is to use the smallest amount of medication necessary to achieve two goals: keeping the airways in your lungs open, both during attacks and over the long term, and reducing the ongoing inflammation that's the cornerstone of the disease.

There are three types of anti-inflammatory drugs that doctors typically prescribe for asthma: inhaled corticosteroids, cromolyn, and leukotriene modifiers. To keep your airways open, they often prescribe short- and long-acting bronchodilators known as beta2-agonists. We'll talk about each of these shortly.

How your doctor chooses to treat your asthma depends on how serious your disease is. There are four categories of asthma: mild intermittent, mild persistent, moderate persistent, and severe persistent. Where your asthma falls along this continuum determines the treatment approach your doctor takes.

Most doctors follow the National Heart, Lung, and Blood Institute's step approach for treating asthma in adults and children.

- **Mild intermittent.** Prescribe only a short-acting beta2-agonist for when attacks occur.
- **Mild persistent.** In addition, prescribe a daily low dosage of an inhaled corticosteroid, or cromolyn or nedocromil. Also consider a leukotriene modifier.
- **Moderate persistent.** Change the daily inhaled corticosteroid to a medium dosage. Also prescribe a daily inhaled long-acting beta2-agonist. Continue to consider a leukotriene modifier, and continue prescribing a short-acting beta2-agonist for when attacks occur.
- **Severe persistent.** Same as above, but change the daily inhaled corticosteroid to a high dosage, and prescribe oral steroids as needed for disease control.

Once your symptoms are under control, the goal is to gradually reduce the amount of medication you're taking to the lowest possible level necessary to control your asthma.

Conversely, you want to be sure you're taking medication if you need it. The Dallas Asthma Consortium has come up with what it calls the Rules of Two. If you use a short-acting beta2-agonist (known as rescue therapy and used during asthma attacks) more than twice a week, wake up with asthma attacks more than twice a month, or refill your quick-relief inhaler (which contains the short-acting beta2-agonist) more than twice a year, you probably need at least two medicines for your asthma. If you're not taking any or are taking only one, see your doctor.

steroids

- **PRESCRIPTION (nasal):** Flonase (fluticasone), Nasacort (triamcinolone), Nasalide (flunisolide), Nasonex (mometasone), Pulmicort and Rhinocort (budesonide), Qvar, Vancenase DS, Vancenase pocket inhaler, Vanceril, and Vanceril DS (beclomethasone)
- **PRESCRIPTION (nebulized):** Pulmicort Respules (budesonide)
- **PRESCRIPTION (systemic—injected and oral):** Celestone (betamethasone), Decadron (dexamethasone), Medrol and Solu-Medrol (methylprednisolone), Orapred and Pediapred (prednisolone), Prednisone and Prelone Syrup (prednisone)

Since allergies and asthma are first and foremost inflammatory diseases, the world of medicine's best anti-inflammatories—corticosteroids, also called glucocorticoids or steroids—are the most important class of drugs for treatment of serious cases.

Steroid Nasal Sprays

If you have only allergies, you're likely to be prescribed topical nasal steroids, which you sniff into your nose rather than inhale into your lungs. Several nasal steroids are also approved for nonallergic rhinitis, including fluticasone (Flonase) and budesonide (Rhinocort AQ).

Steroid nasal sprays work by preventing mast cells and basophils from releasing chemicals that call in the cavalry, i.e., eosinophils and other inflammation-triggering cells, in response to the mast cell reaction. Thus, they slam the brakes on an allergic reaction. In fact, a study published in the journal *Archives of Internal Medicine* in November 2001 found that steroid nasal sprays were more effective in treating seasonal allergies on an as-needed basis than antihistamines. Most likely, however, your doctor will recommend a combination of antihistamines and nasal steroids for allergic rhinitis, particularly if you have severe

insider information: To reduce the risk of septal perforation when using nasal corticosteroids, aim the spray toward your ear and away from the septum, the wall of cartilage that divides the nose. This works best if you hold the inhaler in one hand and spray the medicine into the opposite nostril; this way, the inhaler is turned slightly to the outside, so there's less irritation of the septum and less potential for bleeding.

How Dangerous are Inhaled and Nasal Steroids?

Steroids have a bad name because they can cause significant side effects, including osteoporosis and cataracts. The steroid nasal sprays and inhaled corticosteroids used to treat allergies and asthma, however, have far fewer side effects because they affect only a small part of your body (your respiratory system), unless they're used excessively. While they're definitely safer than oral steroids, they do carry some slight risks and may have some side effects. That's why your doctor will put you on the lowest possible dose to treat your symptoms and control your asthma. Among the potential side effects:

Headaches and nosebleeds. These are rare but should be reported to your healthcare provider immediately.

Impaired growth. The major concern for children is whether inhaled steroids adversely affect growth. While they may have some slight, temporary effect, studies find that children on inhaled corticosteroids ultimately reach their predicted adult height.

Eye diseases. One possible side effect of inhaled steroids is glaucoma, a known side effect of oral steroids. Also, some ophthalmologists have observed higher pressure in the eyes (a risk factor for glaucoma) of some people who use nasal steroid sprays. Some studies also sug-

gest a higher risk of cataracts in patients over 40 who use steroids, although no increased risk has been found in younger patients. Regardless, if you're using any form of steroids, be sure to see an ophthalmologist annually for a complete eye exam.

Nasal injury. Steroid sprays may injure the nasal septum (the cartilage that separates the nasal passages) if the spray is directed onto it and can lead to septal perforation (a hole in the septum). This complication is very rare.

Decreased bone density. There's better news here. While oral steroids can have a negative effect on bone density, a large study published in the January 2003 issue of the *Journal of Allergy and Clinical Immunology* found that inhaled steroids did not reduce bone mineral density in postmenopausal women with asthma, the group at highest risk for such a side effect.

Oral yeast infections. Topical corticosteroids may lead to an overgrowth of yeast in the mouth and throat, so rinse your mouth and gargle after each inhalation. Be sure to spit out the water.

Other side effects. Other rare, short-term effects may include euphoria, depression, water retention, increased appetite, hyperactivity, and weight gain.

allergies or allergic asthma. Be patient, though; corticosteroids take a few hours to work. Among their benefits:

■ **They reduce the number of mast cells** in your nose, thus significantly reducing mucus secretion and nasal swelling.

■ **They may help you sleep** and keep you more alert during the day if you have perennial allergic rhinitis.

■ **They may be useful** for treating nasal polyps.

Six nasal corticosteroids are approved for use in the United States in patients 6 and older, with two approved for even younger children. Studies find that all work just about equally well; what your doctor prescribes may depend on what your insurance covers, the dosing frequency, and side effects. If cost is a problem, talk to your doctor. Some steroids are less expensive than second-generation antihistamines, so perhaps you could use one and not the other. These sprays may also be a safer choice if you're already taking several other medications, as many elderly people do.

Inhaled Corticosteroids

This class of steroids is used to treat asthma. It may take up to a month of daily doses to see any difference in your symptoms and derive the drugs' full benefits, however. The good news is that numerous studies show that people with mild asthma who take daily steroids can reduce their dose after a time without compromising the drugs' effectiveness. Be sure to ask your doctor if you're taking the lowest possible dose. Inhaled corticosteroids are typically prescribed in either a metered-dose inhaler (MDI), a dry-powder inhaler, or a compressor-driven nebulizer, depending on the brand (see page 112 for more on these delivery systems).

Oral Steroids

Very rarely, and only as a last resort, your doctor may prescribe oral steroids, such as prednisone and methylprednisolone. They're very good at reducing inflammation, but because of their side effects, including cataracts, glaucoma, osteoporosis, and diabetes, they're used only in the short term, most often to treat a severe asthma attack.

bronchodilators

- **PRESCRIPTION (short-acting inhaled beta2-agonists):** Alupent and Metaprel (metaproterenol), Brethaire, Brethine, and Bricanyl (terbutaline), Isuprel, Norisodrine, and Medihaler (isoproterenol), Maxair Autohaler (pirbuterol), Proventil and Ventolin (albuterol), Tornalate (bitolterol mesylate), Xopenex (levalbuterol)
- **PRESCRIPTION (short-acting nebulized beta2-agonists)**: Bronkometer and Bronkosol (isoetharine)
- **PRESCRIPTION (long-acting inhaled beta2-agonists)**: Foradil (formoterol), Serevent and Serevent Diskus (salmeterol xinafoate)

Bronchodilator medications open (and keep open) the large and small airways in your lungs. They come in two forms: short-acting (also known as rescue medications), which are used when your asthma symptoms are worsening or you're having an attack, and long-acting, used on a daily basis to prevent your asthma from getting worse.

Getting the Medicine to Your Lungs

You'll find that most asthma medications need to be inhaled directly into the lungs. Luckily, people with asthma have far more options today than the cigarettes, pipes, and other rudimentary devices asthma sufferers used until the early twentieth century. Here are the options and how to use them properly to ensure that you get the maximum amount of medication.

Metered-dose inhalers (MDI)

The term *metered dose* means the medication inside the pressurized canister is released in a single, measured, controlled dose every time you use the inhaler. You must shake the canister vigorously so the ingredients mix properly and you get the right amount of medication with each dose. When using this form of inhaler, it's very important to properly time your breathing with the release of the medication; otherwise, the medicine may wind up in your mouth, not your lungs. To use it properly:

1. Shake the inhaler.
2. Breathe out slowly and completely for 3 to 5 seconds.
3. Position the mouthpiece two finger-widths away from your mouth. Press the top of the metal canister down firmly once and breathe in deeply through your mouth until your lungs are full. (You must start inhaling a second before you press down on the canister and release the medication.)
4. Lower the inhaler, press your lips together, and hold your breath while counting slowly to 10. This allows the medication to spread throughout your lungs.
5. Breathe out slowly.

6. Wait the prescribed length of time, then repeat as necessary.

Holding chambers and spacers

These devices can help with the delivery of metered-dose inhaled medication to the airways and are particularly recommended for anti-inflammatory medication. To use them:

1. Insert the inhaler mouthpiece or canister into the holding chamber according to the manufacturer's directions.
2. Shake well.
3. Exhale slowly and completely. Put the mouthpiece of the holding chamber into your mouth.
4. Hold your breath for 10 seconds, then exhale slowly.

These medications have very little effect on inflammation, though, so they won't provide the kind of long-term relief you need for this chronic condition. And they may not work as well if you're taking other drugs, specifically beta-blockers, which are often prescribed for high blood pressure and heart conditions. Be sure to tell your doctor about all medications you're taking. If you have diabetes, heart disease, high blood pressure, hyperthyroidism, an enlarged

5. If you are prescribed two puffs, wait the recommended amount of time, shake, activate the inhaler, and repeat the previous steps.

Dry-powder inhalers

These inhalers come in different shapes and sizes and are set to deliver bronchodilators as well as anti-inflammatory medications. They're easy to use and very effective. Because the particles of medication are so small, they can easily reach the tiniest airways. And, unlike metered-dose inhalers, you're less likely to taste or feel the medication when using it. You also don't need a spacer with dry-powder inhalers. Make sure you follow the manufacturer's directions, since various brands may differ slightly. In general, though:

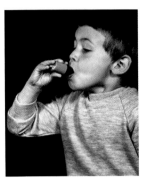

1. Prime your inhaler per the manufacturer's instructions, then load the prescribed dose.
2. Breathe out slowly and completely for 3 to 5 seconds.
3. Put your mouth on the mouthpiece, then inhale deeply and forcefully.
4. Hold your breath for 10 seconds, then exhale slowly.
5. Repeat until you've taken the prescribed number of doses.

Nebulizer therapy

A nebulizer is a special device used to deliver liquid medicines to the lungs. It's composed of an air compressor (which turns the liquid into a mist), tubing, and a container for the medication. The force of the compressor helps you receive the medicine without having to take a deep breath, which is why they're particularly beneficial for infants and small children. (Kids use a mask that fits snugly around their nose and mouth instead of a mouthpiece.) Nebulizers are most often used in a doctor's office, emergency room, or hospital, but if your (or your child's) asthma is frequently out of control, you may have one at home. Here's how to use it:

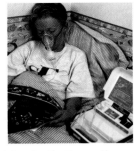

1. Put the liquid medication in the nebulizer cup.
2. Attach the nebulizer unit to the compressor with the tubing, making sure all connections are tight. Check the mouthpiece for foreign objects.
3. Place the mouthpiece in your mouth and close your lips around it to make a seal (or fit the mask snugly over your nose and mouth), then turn on the compressor.
4. Breathe in and out as you normally would (don't take any extra breaths). With each fifth breath, hold the medicine in your lungs for 5 to 10 seconds, then exhale. Continue until all the medicine is gone.

prostate, or a history of seizures, discuss these conditions with your doctor and find out if bronchodilators are right for you.

While many bronchodilators are prescription drugs, some, such as Primatene Mist and Bronchaid, are available over the counter. They pose the same risks as their stronger prescription counterparts, so again, don't self-prescribe them. Ask your doctor first, particularly if you have the health issues just mentioned.

Short-Acting Beta2-Agonists

Beta2-agonists relax and open constricted airways during an asthma attack. They're inhaled (via a nebulizer or other delivery system) and work for 3 to 6 hours. While they relieve the symptoms of acute attacks, they don't control the underlying inflammation. If your asthma continues to get worse while you're taking these drugs, talk to your doctor about the possible need for anti-inflammatory agents.

Albuterol (Proventil, Ventolin) is the standard short-acting beta2-agonist used in the United States. Similar drugs include isoproterenol (Isuprel, Norisodrine, Medihaler-Iso), metaproterenol (Alupent, Metaprel), pirbuterol (Maxair), terbutaline (Brethine, Brethaire, Bricanyl), and bitolterol (Tornalate). Another drug, isoetharine (Bronkometer, Bronkosol) comes in nebulizers.

Some newer beta2-agonists, including levalbuterol (Xopenex), have more specific actions than the older types. Studies find they're as effective as albuterol at lower doses, resulting in fewer side effects. Xopenex is presently available for use with a nebulizer and is available without preservatives. Studies are under way on a metered-dose inhaler for Xopenex, which will make it much easier to take.

Long-Acting Beta2-Agonists

Long-acting beta2-agonists such as salmeterol (Serevent) and formoterol (Foradil) help prevent asthma attacks. They're typically not used as rescue medication, but since Foradil works within 3 to 5 minutes, some physicians think it could be used during an attack. It has not been approved for this use in the United States.

Taking Serevent during an attack could actually be dangerous because it takes so long to work that, in your desperation, you could inadvertently take too much or stop breathing before it kicks in.

In mid-2003, the FDA added new safety information and warnings to the labeling on drugs containing salmeterol, as well as a boxed warning

revealing **research**

Hormones May Improve Lung Function and Asthma

A study published in the March 2003 issue of the journal *Annals of Allergy, Asthma & Immunology* found that progesterone and estrogen may improve lung function and asthma across women's life spans.

It seems that the hormones play a role in strengthening respiratory muscles and increasing the relaxation of bronchial smooth muscle, reducing airway constriction. They also have some anti-inflammatory properties. That may partly explain why some women have increased asthma episodes and are hospitalized more often for asthma during their premenstrual and menstrual phases, when these hormone levels are low. It also provides a possible explanation for why some women have improved lung function and a decrease in asthma problems when they take oral contraceptives and hormone replacement therapy.

If you're susceptible to the effects of hormonal cycles (i.e., you have PMS), let your doctor know. It could help him or her fine-tune your asthma treatment to avoid symptom spikes throughout the month and provide a clue as to how to control your asthma during pregnancy.

about a small but significant increased risk of life-threatening asthma episodes or asthma-related deaths observed in patients taking salmeterol in a large U.S. safety study. The increased risk was particularly apparent in people who weren't using inhaled corticosteroids concurrently and in African-Americans, who seem to have a different response to beta2-agonists.

One dose of long-acting beta2-agonists lasts about 12 hours, so they're particularly effective when used at night and to prevent exercise-induced asthma. If this is the only type of drug you're taking, though, talk to your doctor. Since beta2-agonists have very little effect on inflammation, you're missing treatment for half of the asthma equation. In fact, combining a long-acting beta2-agonist with a corticosteroid or other anti-inflammatory drug may let you reduce the dose of steroids you're taking. These days, you can even get both in one medicine with fluticasone and salmeterol (Advair).

Side effects of long-acting beta2-agonists are similar to those of the short-acting forms.

revealing **research**

Considering Genetics Along with Prescriptions

One of the most commonly prescribed drugs for asthma is albuterol, which is sold as Ventolin and Proventil, but it isn't equally effective in all people with asthma. It turns out that your genetic makeup may determine how well albuterol and quite possibly other asthma medications work. In a study published in September 2000 in the journal *Proceedings of the National Academy of Sciences*, researchers determined the genetic fingerprints of 121 asthma patients. The patients later underwent spirometry, a test to measure their lung function, before inhaling albuterol and again 30 minutes later. Those with a certain genetic code for the beta-2 receptor responded best. Those with a different type responded worst.

While it's unlikely that your doctor is going to start doing genetic tests before writing a prescription, if you find albuterol isn't working for you, sticking with it may be simply a waste of time. Talk to your doctor about other options.

theophylline

- **PRESCRIPTION:** Constant-T, Resbid, Slo-bid Elixophyllin, Slo-phyllin

Theophylline isn't used very much any more to treat asthma, even though it was once one of the primary asthma drugs. It works by relaxing the muscles around the airways and stimulating breathing. One study reported that it may also have anti-inflammatory qualities even in low doses. The problem is that it can be dangerous.

The main concern about theophylline is that it could build up to toxic levels in your blood. This risk increases if you have liver problems, such as hepatitis, or are taking drugs, such as erythromycin and systemic antifungal medications, that can interfere with your liver's ability to break down theophylline.

Monitoring Asthma Drugs

Just because you've filled your prescriptions and are using the medications according to your doctor's instructions doesn't mean you're done worrying about drug treatment. Now it's up to you to monitor how well the regimen is working so you can fine-tune your medications whenever necessary.

For those with asthma, one of the most important tools for monitoring the condition is a peak flow meter, described in chapter 6. You should use it daily, tracking the results on a chart like the one adjacent. As with a race, you're always trying to match or beat your "personal best"—in this case, the highest peak flow number you can reach over a two- to three-week period when your asthma is under control. Your doctor will help you determine your personal best (in children, it increases as a child grows). Once you determine your personal best, aim to maintain a peak flow reading within 80 percent of that number. The following three zones tell you how well you're doing at controlling your asthma.

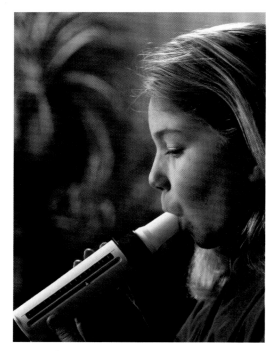

• **Green zone.** Peak expiratory flow rate (PEFR) 80 to 100 percent of personal best. You are relatively symptom-free and can continue your current asthma-management program.

• **Yellow zone.** PEFR 50 to 80 percent of personal best. Your asthma is getting worse. You need a temporary increase in your asthma medication, and, if you're on chronic medications, you may need to increase your maintenance therapy. Call your doctor for some fine-tuning.

• **Red zone.** PEFR below 50 percent of personal best. This is the danger zone. Use your inhaled bronchodilator to open your airways. If your peak flow readings don't return to at least the yellow zone after using your bronchodilator, call your doctor.

Chronic smokers absorb the drug much more quickly than nonsmokers, so they require higher doses. Theophylline also interacts with other drugs for a variety of medical conditions, including, ironically, asthma. For instance, you probably shouldn't use beta2-agonists and theophylline together. Theophylline should also not be used as a rescue medication if you have an asthma attack, and it shouldn't be taken by people with peptic ulcers. If you're elderly or have heart or liver disease, hypertension, seizure disorders, gastroesophageal reflux, or congestive heart failure, you should use extreme caution in taking this drug; you should probably talk to your doctor about alternatives.

So why use it at all, then? Well, believe it or not, some people get their

My Asthma Symptom and Peak Flow Diary

1. Start-of-the-Week Readings

My personal best peak flow reading is _____   Last week, my best reading was _____

2. Daily Readings

	MON		TUES		WED		THU		FRI		SAT		SUN	
	A.M.	P.M.	A.M.	P.M.	A.M.	P.M.	A.M.	P.M.	A.M.	P.M.	A.M.	P.M.	A.M.	P.M.
My peak flow reading was:														
Enter the number from your meter														
My peak flow ranking was:														
more than 80% of personal best														
50%–80% of personal best														
less than 50% of personal best														
The severity of my symptoms was:														
None														
Mild*														
Moderate**														
Serious***														
I used a medicine for my symptoms:														
(y/n)														
My activities were curtailed:														
(y/n)														

3. End-of-the-Week Readings

This week's best reading was _____   The general peak flow direction was ($\uparrow$ $\downarrow$ $\longleftrightarrow$)_____

4. Notes

_____

_____

_____

_____

*only during physical activity; **also at rest, affecting sleep or activity level; ***serious while at rest, affecting ability to breathe or talk

greatest relief with theophylline. If their blood levels are closely monitored while they're taking the drug, they seem to do very well on it.

leukotriene modifiers

- **PRESCRIPTION (nonsteroidal anti-inflammatories):** Accolate (zafirlukast), Singulair (montelukast), Zyflo (zileuton)

Leukotrienes are among the molecules that mast cells, eosinophils, and macrophages release when they encounter asthma triggers. They are partly to blame for the increased mucus production, airway constriction, and inflammation of asthma and for the runny and stuffy nose of allergies. That's why leukotriene modifiers such as montelukast (Singulair)—which stem the tide of leukotrienes, can be taken orally once a day, and have minimal side effects—were eagerly welcomed when they were first approved in 1997.

Allergy and Asthma Medications during Pregnancy

Pregnant women often think that as soon as the stick turns pink, they have to dump all medications—prescription and OTC—down the sink, lest taking them harm the developing baby. Well, that may be true with certain drugs, but there are also numerous medications considered to be safe during pregnancy. Here's what we know for sure (or as surely as one can ever know such things, since it's unethical to test medications on pregnant women, and most of the information we have comes from long-term use). The American College of Allergy, Asthma, and Immunology and the American College of Obstetricians and Gynecologists suggests the following guidelines regarding asthma and allergy medications. Still, try to hold off on taking any medication during your first trimester if possible.

• **Inhaled cromolyn.** This should be the first-line therapy for pregnant women with asthma.

• **Inhaled budesonide.** If cromolyn doesn't control symptoms, follow with inhaled budesonide (Pulmicort), the only inhaled steroid that's approved as a category B drug, meaning it's generally safe for use during pregnancy. A Swedish study that evaluated 99 percent of the births in Sweden from 1995 to 1998 found that mothers who took budesonide had babies that were born on time and at normal weights and lengths, with no increase in stillbirths or multiple births.

• **Serevent, leukotriene modifiers, and newer inhaled corticosteroids.** If you had a good response to these agents before you became pregnant, you and your doctor may consider continuing them during pregnancy.

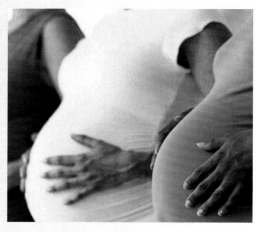

• **Allergy shots.** You can continue allergy shots at a constant dose, but don't start them for the first time while pregnant.

• **Short-acting bronchodilators.** Short-acting bronchodilators such as Albuterol (Ventolin, Proventil) may be used during pregnancy, while ipatropium (Atrovent) may be used if necessary. Another option, terbutaline (Brethaire) is particularly safe during pregnancy, since it's often used intravenously to halt premature labor.

• **Antihistamines.** Chlorpheniramine (Chlor-Trimeton), tripelennamine (Pyribenzamine), loratadine (Claritin), and cetirizine (Zyrtec) are all safe.

• **Decongestants.** Although pregnant women have used the decongestant pseudoephedrine (Sudafed) for years, reports suggest a slight increase in abdominal wall defects in newborns, so it's suggested that women avoid oral decongestants during the first trimester. One of the best treatments for congestion may be simple saline irrigation—washing out your nose with saltwater.

They are particularly useful for preventing exercise-induced asthma and asthma triggered by allergens. In patients with aspirin-induced asthma, leukotriene modifiers seem to be especially effective at blocking the effects of aspirin exposure. They also have some bronchodilating effects, opening up airways within 2 hours of taking them.

Leukotriene inhibitors aren't just for asthma, however; in late 2002, the FDA approved the use of Singulair for treating allergic rhinitis.

Medicines of the Future

With the number of people with allergies and asthma continuing to increase, pharmaceutical researchers are scurrying to discover the next great breakthrough in treatment for these conditions, and possibly even a cure.

Research into other anti-IgE medications continues to be a hotbed of activity, but scientists are exploring the following potential treatments as well.

Immunotherapy and Vaccines

- To turbocharge immunotherapy, researchers are adding immune-boosting molecules called oligonucleotides to the allergen mix. One such compound already in clinical trials goes by the name A1C (Amb a1-SS Conjugate). Early studies found that a single six-week series of weekly shots not only significantly reduced symptoms in people who were allergic to ragweed but also continued working for two years with no maintenance shots required. That sounds much better than the 100 or more shots required in traditional immunotherapy.

- Investigators are studying so-called rush immunotherapy, in which patients achieve the full maintenance dose with several shots a day over a period of three to five days instead of the three to six months it usually takes.

- Scientists are using recombinant biotechnology to create synthetic allergen solutions for immunotherapy, producing purer substances that be can mixed together and resulting in the need for fewer shots that are both safer and more efficient.

- Researchers planned to begin clinical trials of a vaccine against peanut allergies in 2004 or 2005. Studies in mice have found that the vaccine, made from bacteria genetically engineered to produce modified peanut proteins that are then killed with heat treatment, prevents mice with peanut allergies from having reactions.

- In a totally new approach, in early 2003, a Danish pharmaceutical company began conducting clinical trials of a gel-cap, tablet-based immunotherapy for allergies to grass, dust mites, ragweed, and birch.

Anti-IgE Drugs: New Hope for the Future

The summer of 2003 marked one of the most exciting times ever in the treatment of allergies and asthma. That's when the FDA approved omalizumab (Xolair), the first in a new class of drugs for the treatment of allergic asthma. Eventually, this class of drugs—called anti-IgE drugs—is expected to revolutionize the treatment of allergies in a way no other has done.

Xolair is a genetically engineered drug called a monoclonal antibody. It works by stopping an allergic reaction before it starts by blocking the IgE antibody that causes the reaction. Everything else in our allergy arsenal treats only the symptoms of allergies or blocks your reaction to specific allergens.

Xolair came about as a result of the discovery in 1998 of the precise shape of the receptor molecule that triggers the allergic response in your immune system. These receptors, with the tongue-twisting name of high-affinity immunoglobulin-E receptors, sit on the surface of mast cells and serve as "docking stations" for IgE. Once scientists found the docking stations, the race was on to figure out how to prevent IgE from getting to them in the first place. If the IgE antibodies couldn't "park" on mast cells, they couldn't flip the switch to start the cells' release of histamine and other inflammatory chemicals. Basically, then, the molecules that make up Xolair grab IgE antibodies and keep them from ever reaching the mast cells.

Currently, Xolair is approved only for moderate to severe allergic asthma in people 12 and older whose asthma has not responded well to other treatments. It's given by subcutaneous (under-the-skin) injection once or twice a month. Its use can really change your life. People taking Xolair are often able to live very normally for the first time ever, being able to visit a friend with a pet, for instance, or sleep with the windows open in the spring—the kinds of things those of us without allergic asthma take for granted.

Many people are also able to significantly reduce their use of other medications, if not discontinue them altogether. For instance, in studies of Xolair in adults and children, some of those taking the drug were able to cut back on or even stop using inhaled corticosteroids. Eventually, Xolair will probably be approved to treat allergic asthma in children as well.

One problem with Xolair is the cost: A year's supply costs between $5,000 and $10,000, depending on the dose. It's so expensive because it requires a very sophisticated manufacturing

Anti-Inflammatories

A new class of anti-inflammatory compounds currently under investigation works to inhibit phosphodiesterase-4, a chemical that's involved in the inflammatory reaction. These drugs are related to the old asthma standby theophylline, but they have far fewer side effects. Among the drugs that were in late-stage clinical trials in late 2003 was a compound called roflumilast, which is also being investigated for future use in treating chronic obstructive pulmonary disease.

Inhaled Corticosteroids

Look for new drugs to enter the market in 2004 and 2005, including ciclesonide (Alvesco). One advantage of this drug is that it isn't activated until it

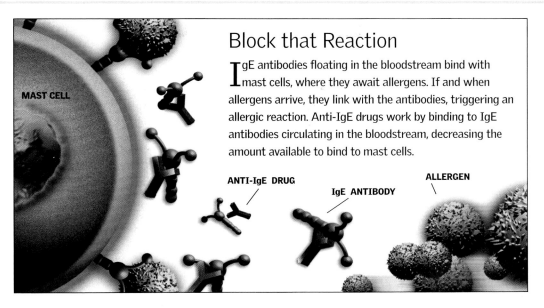

Block that Reaction

IgE antibodies floating in the bloodstream bind with mast cells, where they await allergens. If and when allergens arrive, they link with the antibodies, triggering an allergic reaction. Anti-IgE drugs work by binding to IgE antibodies circulating in the bloodstream, decreasing the amount available to bind to mast cells.

MAST CELL

ANTI-IgE DRUG

IgE ANTIBODY

ALLERGEN

method. Also, it's given by injection once every two to four weeks, a regimen you may have to maintain indefinitely. Studies find that once you stop using Xolair, your IgE levels gradually return over several months to where they were before you began using it.

Ideally, as more drugs in this class are approved and are used more widely, the price should come down. Additionally, there's some thought that a short course of Xolair for those with allergic rhinitis who haven't developed asthma may prevent asthma from developing at all. Anti-IgE medications may also prove effective for people who don't follow their daily medication regimens very well, and possibly for those with difficult-to-manage atopic dermatitis, allergies to hard-to-avoid foods, and latex allergies. Studies using another anti-IgE formulation on people with peanut allergies found that it significantly reduced their reactions to peanut proteins.

So keep an eye out for more news about Xolair and other anti-IgE medications; they may very well change the way you and your doctor treat your asthma and allergies.

comes into contact with the surface of airways in your lungs, thus minimizing any effects on your throat or the rest of your system.

Nasal Sprays

Olopatadine (Patanol), the best-selling prescription eyedrops for allergic conjunctivitis, is being developed into a nonsteroidal nasal spray that's expected to be called Patanase.

Immunomodulators

These drugs, originally used to prevent organ transplant rejection, work to suppress the immune system. Applied to the skin, immunomodulators tacrolimus (Protopic) and Elidel (pimecrolimus) have already been approved to treat atopic

Asthma Meds Raise Risk to Dental Health

Antihistamines and possibly corticosteroids may dry your mouth out so badly that it puts your teeth at risk. That's because you need a steady saliva flow to wash away sticky food particles, which adhere to your teeth, become a breeding ground for bacteria, and lead to cavities and gum disease. The solution is obvious: Drink plenty of water to keep your mouth moist, and brush and floss more frequently than usual, since water isn't as effective as saliva in keeping your mouth clean.

dermatitis (eczema), an allergic skin condition. An inhaled form of tacrolimus is now being tested for asthma. It would be ideal for those who don't respond to or don't want to take steroids but still need an anti-inflammatory.

Novel Compounds

■ **Heterocyclic thiourea (HCT) compounds.** This new class of drugs works to prevent the release of leukotrienes from mast cells. Work on them is still quite preliminary, however, and it will probably be 10 years or more before actual drugs in this class come to market.

■ **GE2 molecule.** This genetically engineered molecule, called a fusion protein, works to prevent both mast cells and basophils from releasing histamine. It binds to two receptor molecules on mast cells. One acts as a kind of gas pedal, starting the allergic response, and the other as a brake, stemming the allergic response. By binding to both receptors simultaneously, GE2 halts the allergic reaction altogether. This compound is also several years away from testing in humans.

■ **Interleukin-4 and -5 inhibitors.** Interleukin-4 and -5 are cytokines that play a role in the inflammatory process. Drugs to prevent the production of interleukin-5 are under investigation as a long-term treatment for asthma.

■ **R112.** This experimental drug, the first in its class, is being tested for treating allergic rhinitis. Unlike current allergy drugs, such as antihistamines and anti-leukotrienes that target only a single chemical involved in activating mast cells, R112 is thought to work by blocking all major chemicals from the mast cell response that contribute to inflammation. If it proves effective for allergic rhinitis, it may also be tested for asthma.

Genetic Treatments

The genetic revolution is alive and well when it comes to allergies and asthma. So far, researchers have identified more than 291 genes associated with asthma, paving the way for numerous new targets for drugs. One that has researchers quite excited is the gene responsible for the enzyme arginase, previously thought to be involved only in the liver. Today, researchers know that arginase plays a major role in asthma, appearing to be the molecule that "kicks off" the chain of actions that leads to asthma symptoms.

More Individualized Treatments

Rather than lumping asthma patients together into broad categories such as moderate persistent or severe persistent and designing treatment strategies by category (as is currently done), researchers have begun considering individualized asthma treatments, depending on the form of asthma you have. For instance, some people have asthma attacks predominantly when mast cells infiltrate the smooth muscle of the airways, while others are more affected by the inflammatory effects of eosinophils. Each requires a different treatment approach. Look for doctors to spend more time determining the specific cause of your asthma attacks and exacerbations before prescribing medications.

More Combination Drugs

Look for more combination therapies such as Advair that bring beta2-agonists and corticosteroids together in some combination. The fewer drugs people have to take, the more likely they are to take them, improving overall asthma control. For instance, Symbicort HFAMDI, still under development (although currently available as a turbohaler in other countries), combines the steroid budesonide and the long-acting beta2-agonist formoterol. Similar to Advair, it will be available in three different strengths.

into the future: beyond drugs

Researchers don't stop their allergy/asthma efforts with drugs. They're also working on other novel approaches, including:

■ **Genetically modified forms of grass, peanuts, and soybeans.** For instance, researchers at the Plant Biotechnology Center in Melbourne, Australia, genetically modified ryegrasses, used in lawns all over the world and the main hay fever culprit in Europe and Australia, to eliminate two common hay fever allergens. Additionally, soybeans currently growing in Hawaii have been genetically modified to eliminate a gene believed to trigger most allergic reactions.

■ **Nasal plugs for allergic rhinitis.** These plugs, developed by Australian researchers, come with sticky filters that catch pollen grains before they can enter the nasal cavity and trigger an allergic reaction. The idea is that you'd use them when you go outside on days with high pollen counts.

■ **Preventing allergy sensitization.** Rather than treat allergies and asthma, what if you could prevent them in the first place, much like preventing measles or chickenpox? That's the thinking behind preliminary studies in Finland in which pregnant women, breastfeeding mothers, and newborns are given probiotics—a type of bacteria normally found in the gut that affects the immune system—to try to prevent allergy development in at-risk infants. In a study published in the

Can Asthma Drugs Make My Asthma Worse?

While this seems like a silly question, it's not. And the answer is that yes, in some instances, certain drugs, particularly when overused, can have a boomerang effect, making your condition worse. Several studies have found that people who use short-acting bronchodilating beta2-agonist medications such as albuterol several times a day can ultimately develop increased symptoms of airway constriction, which worsens asthma. If you're using rescue medication this often, your disease is not well controlled. It's time for a visit with your doctor.

British medical journal *Lancet* in May 2003, researchers gave a group of pregnant women either probiotic capsules or placebos every day beginning a few weeks before their due dates; those who breastfed continued to receive either placebos or probiotics for six months, while bottle-fed babies received placebos or bacteria in their formula. By age 4, those in the probiotic group were significantly less likely to have developed the allergic skin condition known as atopic dermatitis, often a precursor of allergic rhinitis and/or asthma.

Future preventive efforts may be more bold, says Harold S. Nelson, M.D., professor of medicine at the National Jewish Medical and Research Center in Denver. For instance, someday doctors may give infants endotoxin or killed bacterial DNA to counteract the cleanliness believed to be related to the increasing incidence of allergies (the so-called hygiene hypothesis).

beyond medications

Still with us? If you are, we hope you feel awed and amazed at the intense scientific investigations that are going on to treat and prevent allergies and asthma. The investments are huge; the stakes are high; and the number of doctors, researchers, and laboratories working worldwide on asthma and allergy cures is probably in the thousands.

Let's be grateful . . . and then let's get back to reality. The best thing you can do for yourself is to not need any medicine at all, and the best way to do that is to keep allergens at bay. So let's leave the labs behind and enter a more toxic place: your home. In the next chapter, we'll show you all the ways you can improve your personal spaces to reduce your chances of allergies and asthma.

chapter **eight**

the right
environment

Back in the sixteenth century, the Archbishop of St. Andrew in Scotland invited the acclaimed Italian physician Gerolamo Cardano to his country for advice on treating his asthma. Cardano's diagnosis was simple and astute: The problem was the bed, and he recommended that the Archbishop get rid of his feather bedding. The result? A "miraculous" recovery.

Some 400 years later, in 1927, Storm van Leeuwen created a "climate" chamber in the Netherlands to make a similar point. He successfully showed that asthmatic patients improved when moved from their homes into the chamber. Van Leeuwen wrote: "In our endeavours to find the cause of the attack...we utilised the known fact that the environment of the asthmatic patient is, as a rule, of primary importance in determining the intensity and frequency of his attacks."

Cardano and Van Leeuwen came upon truths that even the most amazing medical advances of recent years haven't changed: If you want relief from allergies or asthma, you need to get rid of the triggers in your home.

It may not seem logical, but the cozy indoors is often worse for your allergies and asthma than the great outdoors. Your home—with its fabric-covered furniture and pillows; its carpeting; tightly sealed windows; and warm, damp spaces—is like a field strewn with allergy land mines. Research shows that indoor air pollution can be up to 10 times greater than outdoor pollution and its effects much more intense, since we generally spend more than 90 percent of our time indoors.

To be clear, people are rarely sensitive to the things that make up the house itself—that is, the paint, wood, steel, plastic, and such. Instead, it's the microscopic things that grow and accumulate in the house that cause allergies and asthma attacks.

These unwanted occupants come in several forms, but the most prevalent in-home allergens are dust and its components (primarily dust mite and cockroach droppings), molds, fungi, and pet hair and dander. We'll discuss each in this chapter, as well as the places where they accumulate most: bedding, carpets, damp areas, and air filters. Most important, we'll show you how to make your home as allergen-free and fresh as possible.

One caveat: All the cleaning tips in the world won't make a bit of difference if someone in your home smokes. We're not even going to begin to tell you what smoking does to the lungs of someone who has allergies or asthma, but second-hand smoke is just as detrimental for a child or spouse who has them. If someone in your household must smoke, outside is the only place to do it.

dust: the dirty truth

One of the biggest culprits in your home is often invisible: It's dust. Studies have found that the average six-room home in the United States collects 40 pounds of dust each year. "Wait!" you wail. "I'm a great housekeeper. I dust every few days and wash the floors, scrub the bathrooms, and change the linens weekly. I even wipe the baseboards at least once a year. How could I have that much dust?"

Relax. The dust in your home is inevitable and would be there even if you scrubbed daily. It's composed of flakes of dead skin, pet hair and dander (even if you don't have pets, you may track hair and dander into the house), breakdown of fabrics, debris blown in from outside, and so on. As if that weren't bad enough, that layer of dust coating your coffee table or television screen or lying behind the sofa may also contain cockroach droppings, another potent allergy trigger. There *is* a correlation between cleaning and dust levels, however, and as you've undoubtedly figured out by now, the more you clean, the less dust you'll have.

The problem with dust stems not just from an aesthetic perspective but also from the fact that it provides a regular supply of food for dust mites. As we said in chapter 3, these microscopic bugs are literally everywhere in your home, happily munching away on teeny flakes of your skin that have sloughed off in the course of normal living. They're a major source of allergies, with about 10 percent of the population and 90 percent of people with allergic asthma having positive skin tests to dust mites. Those figures are even higher in children, with recent studies suggesting that at least 45 percent of kids are allergic to dust mites.

Dust Mites Unveiled

Picture this: There may as many as 19,000 dust mites in 1 gram of dust, about the weight of a paper clip. And each female can add another 25 to 30 mites to the population before she dies. It's enough to send you running for a super-size can of Lemon Pledge.

Mites aren't ubiquitous, however, and if you live in the desert, you may be in luck. That's because these tiny creatures thrive in warm, humid conditions, when the relative humidity is 75 to 80 percent and the temperature at least 70°F. Reduce the humidity and you reduce the mites, since they can't survive in humidity of less than 40 to 50 percent.

If you have mites, they're most prevalent in the room where you spend the most time. No, not the bathroom—the bedroom, where we inhabit the bed for about one-third of our lives. To a dust mite, your bed is an all-you-can-eat buffet and a five-star hotel rolled into one.

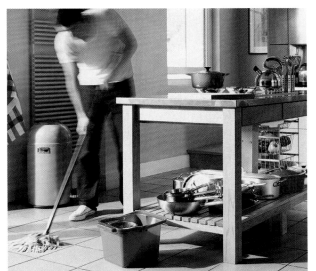

Forget insecticides; they generally don't work, and those touted for mites, called acaricides, can cause skin or lung irritation. Still, there are ways to reduce your exposure to mites in your home, and it's a goal that's definitely worth pursuing. One study found that reducing levels of dust mites in children's beds by one-third cut the number of days they wheezed and missed school by nearly a quarter (22 percent).

As part of the Breathe Easy Plan, we're going to give you a step-by-step, room-by-room guide to making your home as allergy-free as possible. In the meantime, however, here are some ways to reduce the levels of dust mites (and dust) throughout your house.

The problem with dust isn't just aesthetic—it provides *a regular supply of food for dust mites,* and they are a major source of allergies.

■ **Wrap your mattress and pillows.** In years past, your only option for mattress and pillow covers was slippery, hot vinyl. Today, however, for a few more dollars you can get covers made of tightly woven fabric or semipermeable polyurethane, both of which are as comfortable as regular covers. But forget so-called hypoallergenic covers and pillows; they still attract dust mites. Also, your problem isn't solved once your bedding is

What Does Hypoallergenic Mean?

It just means that something is *unlikely* to cause an allergic reaction. What it doesn't mean, however, is that the item *won't* cause an allergic reaction. Use hypoallergenic products with care, particularly if you're highly allergic.

safely covered. You still need to vacuum the mattress cover or wipe it off with a damp cloth every month. Otherwise, mites will just begin multiplying on top of the cover as you shed skin flakes.

Unfortunately, just one-third of people with allergies use these covers, even though numerous studies find they're effective in reducing medication use and asthma attacks in adults and children.

■ **Wash with hot water.** Forget babying your sheets and blankets with cool or warm water. The best way to kill those mites is washing in very hot water (at least 130°F) at least once a week. No time to do laundry? An hour in a hot dryer will also kill most mites, or you can put items in a plastic bag and stick it in the freezer overnight (but neither will get rid of mite by-products, i.e., eggs and feces).

■ **Dry out the air.** This isn't much of a problem in the winter, when central heating tends to dry the air and reduce humidity. In the summer, though, running your air conditioner even on cooler days can keep humidity levels, and thus dust mite levels, lower. Make sure the fan in the air conditioner is running at all times so air constantly goes through the filter. You can purchase an inexpensive instrument called a hygrometer to measure the level of indoor humidity. Be sure it remains under 50 percent, particularly in your bedroom. If the humidity is still high despite air conditioning, or if you don't have air conditioning, try using a dehumidifier in any rooms that retain dampness, such as the bathroom and basement, or put one in your bedroom to ensure extra-dry air.

■ **Dust with damp cloths.** Using a dry cloth just stirs up mite allergens. And dust *everything*. Dust lurks in miniblinds and on the tops of ceiling fan blades, both of which can easily scatter dust everywhere. If you're particularly sensitive to dust, ask a nonallergic friend or family member to do the job. Each month, put your houseplants in the bathtub and treat them to a de-dusting shower.

■ **Bag it right.** Use a vacuum cleaner with either a double-layered microfiltration bag or a HEPA filter to trap allergens that pass through the vacuum's exhaust. If you have your house professionally cleaned, be sure the cleaners use your vacuum; otherwise, they could release allergens from other people's homes.

■ **Go unnatural.** Replace wool or feather-stuffed bedding materials with synthetic materials. Select stuffed animals and other toys that are washable.

■ **Nix foam mattresses.** Although they're popular, they're also more likely to harbor dust mites and mold. A study found that the risk of finding mite feces (a sign of dust mites) was four times higher in foam mattresses with covers and eight times higher in foam mattresses without covers than in spring mattresses.

■ **Change your filters.** It seems like a simple thing to do, but according to a 2002 survey commissioned by the American Lung Association Health House program and 3M Corporation, 4 out of 10 Americans didn't know that regularly changing the filter in a forced-air heating/cooling system could help improve air quality inside their homes. This explains the fact that more than half of all Americans with forced-air heating/cooling systems fail to change their filters every two to three months as recommended.

■ **Use steam.** Dry steam, available now in home carpet and floor cleaners, is most effective at getting dust mites and other allergens out of carpets and upholstery. Use it on mattresses and pillows, too. And if you have your carpets professionally cleaned, make sure the cleaner uses dry steam, not a wet shampoo method. The shampoo just provides a more tasty meal for mites, and the dampness can bring on molds and fungi.

cockroaches: vanquishing the invincible

You might call cockroaches eternal. They've been around since before the dinosaurs, existing on Earth for some 350 million years and making it through various ice ages, meteor hits, and evolutionary landslides, not to mention every chemical poison we can throw at them. But their droppings are one of the top two causes of perennial allergies, plus they carry mites and diseases, such as dysentery, hepatitis, salmonella, and typhus. Also, they're just disgusting, so eliminating them from your home is critical to breathing easy—but not easy to do.

Part of the problem is that cockroaches eat anything. And we mean *anything*—from vegetables and meat to starch, grease, paper, soap, cardboard, book bindings, ink, shoe polish, and even dirty clothes. They've been known to gnaw on fingernails while people sleep, and they're especially fond of beer. And, in a habit that ranks as a 10 on the truly disgusting scale, they even eat one another's feces.

No food around? No problem. They can go three months without food and one month without water.

Forget about poisoning their food, though; they know what you're up to. Cockroaches carefully taste their

Breathe Easy Tip: Eucalyptus Oil Kills Mites

A study published in the *Journal of Allergy and Clinical Immunology* found that when eucalyptus oil was used to presoak loads of bedclothes, it killed 95 percent of mites that survived high-temperature water. The researchers mixed 1 part liquid detergent and 4 parts eucalyptus oil in a small container, then added 1 teaspoon of the mixture to an 8-ounce glass of water. They filled the washer with water, added the diluted detergent and eucalyptus mixture, and let the bedding soak for an hour before washing. You can buy eucalyptus oil at healthfood stores or wherever healing oils are sold.

food before eating it. If it tastes "off," they'll go scavenging elsewhere. Interestingly, they seem to despise okra, raw or stewed, so putting a dish of the green pods in cabinets that have roach problems may send them quickly scurrying for sweeter pastures.

Like dust, cockroaches are not necessarily a sign of bad housekeeping. For instance, millions of New York City residents have them because the subterranean networks that bring utilities into apartment buildings are all connected, and they're teeming with the nasty bugs.

You could call an exterminator. You could also take the following, more natural steps.

■ **Take away their favorite foods.** This includes putting all open foods in your pantry into the refrigerator, freezer, or tightly sealed containers. Don't forget to clear out under the bathroom sink, too. Roaches just love dark, dampish places.

■ **Spray naturally.** Try eucalyptus oil or peppermint soap (2 ounces per 1 gallon of water), rosemary oil (3 ounces per gallon of water), or insecticidal soap (follow the label directions and add 5 drops of citrus oil per gallon before spraying). You can use these sprays alone or together. Spray indoors and out, and be sure to coat the water pipes.

■ **Dust the problem spots.** Sprinkle a thin layer of boric acid in trouble spots or try a dust made of 1 part natural pyrethrins (from chrysanthemums) and 2 parts diatomaceous earth. Well-stocked garden-supply stores should carry these.

■ **Get them drunk.** Soak a cloth in stale beer and place it on the kitchen floor at night; the roaches will drink the beer and get so drunk they'll pass out—in the middle of the floor. Next morning, give them a good stomping, then sweep them away.

■ **Try bait.** For every cockroach you kill with poisoned bait, another 20 or 30 will die (recall that feces-eating thing they do). Try a concoction of flour, cocoa, oatmeal, boric acid, and plaster of Paris, mixed well.

■ **Freeze them.** A shot of hairspray will immobilize them so you can dispose of them.

■ **Entice them.** Put about an inch of Gatorade or other yummy food in a quart jar, then put masking tape on the outside of the jar so they can climb up it. In the morning, put the cap back on the cockroach-filled jar and toss it.

It's also important to cut off the roaches' access to your house in the first place, which is where caulking your home comes in. Be sure to use a 100 percent inorganic brand of caulk, then seal up all the cracks in every wall and ceiling, around doors and windows, and around the wiring entrances to all electrical outlets and light switches and fixtures. If the cavities are too large to caulk, stuff them with roach- and mouse-repelling steel wool.

carpet: put your foot down on allergens

People with allergies are in luck these days; after decades of wall-to-wall, thick pile carpeting representing the ultimate in home flooring, today's homes are more likely than ever to have flooring made of hardwood, laminate, tile, or vinyl.

Why is that good? Well, carpeting can act as a veritable SuperGlue for indoor air pollutants, trapping dust mites, molds, fungi, pet hair and dander, and other irritants in its fibers. In fact, one study found that carpeting collects allergens at 100 times the rate of bare floors.

If you must have carpeting, select a type with low pile; shag carpeting is the worst for people with allergies. And always use a vacuum with a HEPA filter; otherwise, you'll just scatter the dust mites around the room.

What's the Best Vacuum Cleaner for Allergies?

Well, that depends. The basic fact is that vacuuming often releases just as much dust *into* the air as it picks up out of the carpeting. For instance, one 2003 study compared five brand-new HEPA filter vacuum cleaners with an old, non-HEPA filter vacuum. Researchers tested the machines in five homes that had cats and then in an experimental (dust-free) chamber. Then they measured the amount of cat allergens (the Holy Grail when it comes to airborne allergens) in the home's air. Rather than clearing the air, both types of vacuums significantly *increased* the amount of airborne cat allergens when used in the home. The HEPA vacuums worked better, however, in the experimental chamber. It seems that the force of vacuuming in the home increases levels of airborne cat hair by pulling it from clothes, skin, and other surfaces.

The good news is that vacuums are improving. A 1999 study found that year's models released far fewer allergens into the air than models from 1993, the last time the researchers conducted the study. Chances are, today's vacuums are even better, so if you've been wielding a vacuum that's more than three years old, consider replacing it with a new one.

On your must-have list is a vacuum with a HEPA filter. It helps with leaking, keeping fewer allergens from exiting the vacuum. If you get a vacuum that uses bags, buy high-quality, triple-thick types called microfiltration bags, which studies find are best at keeping dust where it belongs. And consider an upright vacuum over a canister, since a 1999 study found that uprights leaked fewer particles into the air. Another study found that whole-house central vacuums, the kind that vent to the outside, were much better than canister types at sucking up cat allergens and left fewer such allergens in the air. If you're building a house, think about installing such a system.

As for brands, well, it's nearly impossible to tell you which work best; even *Consumer Reports* hasn't tested vacuum cleaners for their ability to suck up (and more important, keep down) allergens. Only one study compared brands, and that was conducted in 1999. It found that the Eureka Excalibur and the Hoover Dimension picked up the greatest amount of cat allergens, with the Hoover Micro vacuum bag doing the best job at collecting them.

Bottom line: There is no impartial evidence that says high-end, high-priced vacuums do a better job of corralling allergy-causing dust. Find yourself a good upright with a HEPA filter and triple-filtration bags, and you've got the best that the limited research reveals.

Sneezing? Blame the Fish

Quite often, the only pets children and adults with asthma or allergies have are fish. Believe it or not, though, your fish tank could be contributing to your allergies, since the fish-food residue that accumulates on the inside of the tank above the water line is a magnet for dust mites. Make sure you wipe the inside of the tank once a week and check for leaking filters, which could be a potential source of mold.

Also, don't lay your carpeting directly over concrete; this just encourages dust mite growth. Instead, make sure you lay carpet and padding over a subfloor, usually made of plywood. Plus, steam clean your carpets at least every three to six months. Several studies in which carpeting and furniture were steam cleaned found significant improvements in levels of allergens and allergy symptoms. In one study, people with asthma whose homes were steam cleaned had a fourfold reduction in bronchial hyperreactivity nine months after the cleaning, compared with no change in a group whose homes received "fake" treatment. Another approach might be to treat carpets with tannic acid, which kills dust mites but has some side effects.

If your basement is finished or you're considering finishing it, try using Pergo or another type of laminated flooring instead of carpet. With just a bit of dampness, that carpet could become a breeding ground for molds and fungi.

pets: the most loving allergen source

As we discussed in chapter 3, if you're allergic to your pet, don't blame the hair. You're really allergic to proteins secreted by oil glands in the animal's skin, as well as proteins in saliva, which sticks to the fur when the animal licks itself. Another source of allergy-causing proteins is animal urine. When the substance carrying the proteins dries, they're free to float into the air.

Obviously, if you're allergic to animal dander, you know the best thing to do is find a new home for the pet, be it a gerbil or a German shepherd. Unfortunately, about one-third of the estimated 6 million people who are allergic to cats have cats in their homes, and we suspect the figures are just as high when it comes to dogs. This is a situation in which allergy shots are a good idea, but there are also some steps you can take to minimize the dander as much as possible.

■ **Keep pets out of your bedroom.** Not just at night, but every single minute of every single day. Keep your bedroom door closed during the day as well to prevent pets from wandering in and napping on your bed.

■ **Have someone else do the grooming.** Pets should be brushed regularly, but not in the house and not by you. Even cleaning a litter box is a chore best left to your nonallergic spouse or child.

■ **Treat dander like dust.** Many of the recommendations for managing dust mites and such hold true for pet-generated allergens. Use HEPA filters in your vacuum. Dust regularly with a damp cloth. Emphasize smoother, harder surfaces in your floors and furniture so they're less likely to harbor animal hair or pet dander.

■ **Wash your hands every time you touch your pet.** And invest in some heavy-duty moisturizing lotion to balance the washing.

■ **Have your pet bathed regularly.** Some studies find a significant reduction in the amount of pet allergens when dogs are bathed weekly. There's little evidence that bathing works for cats, however.

■ **Change your pet's diet.** The right diet can minimize hair loss, reducing dander indoors. Talk to your vet about what kind of food will work best for your pet.

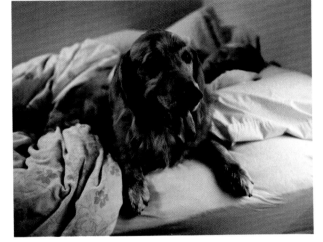

■ **Consider using a product like Allerpet.** This is a special treatment that purports to reduce dander when you wipe or spray it on your pet. The clinical evidence is mixed, however: One study found no difference in levels of cat allergens when the product was used, while two others found fewer cat allergens in the dust from carpeting in the homes where the cats lived. Allerpet comes in formulations for both cats and dogs.

Keep your pets out of your bedroom, *not just at night*, but every single minute of every single day.

■ **Make extra-sure your pets are housebroken.** If Tabby is peeing in the corner of the living room or Fido has accidents when you're at work, you probably have mold and fungus growing on your carpet, not to mention the allergens in the urine.

filters: making a clean sweep

If your home was built after World War II, chances are it has the type of heating or air-conditioning system that blows air directly into a room. If this is true of your residence, you can be certain that the furnace (or air-conditioning unit) has an air filter to either protect the machinery, keep the blown air clean, or both. That sounds wonderful, except that filters get dirty—and when that happens, they can substantially add to indoor air pollution.

The filters for most home systems don't help much with dust mites in furniture or carpets, but if they're clean and functioning properly, they can help contain other airborne allergens. The primary types of air filters include:

■ **Panel filters.** These 1-inch fiberglass filters are the typical furnace filters installed in most home heating and/or air-conditioning systems. Although panel filters are used in 85 percent of American homes with forced-air heating and central air conditioning, they do little to remove contaminants from the air. Their primary function is to protect the fan and minimize the amount of dust on the heating and cooling coil.

■ **Washable/reusable filters.** These are designed to be washed and reused, but they never get completely clean and can therefore restrict air-flow. These filters are generally ineffective at capturing small particles.

■ **Pleated filters.** These have been pleated or folded to provide more surface area and are typically more efficient than panel filters. Increasing the surface area for collecting particles reduces the velocity of the airflow through the filter, thus reducing airflow resistance. It's important to change these filters regularly, however, so they don't restrict airflow.

■ **High-efficiency particulate air (HEPA) filters.** These filters, touted for minimizing allergies and asthma, remove submicron particles with high efficiency. They consist of a core filter that's folded back and forth over corrugated separators, thus adding strength to the core and forming air passages between the pleats. The filter is composed of very fine submicron glass fibers in a matrix of larger fibers. HEPA filters won't fit most

Natural Cleaning Products

Irritants such as the chemicals found in most residential cleaners can worsen airborne allergy symptoms, so avoid them as much as possible. That's easier to do these days, given the movement toward more natural cleaning products that come in beautiful packaging, with names such as Method and Caldrea (rosemary/mint-scented window cleaner, anyone?). They don't come cheap, however: A 16-ounce bottle of Caldrea window spray costs about $8, compared with about $1.99 for the same-size bottle of store-brand window cleaner. For just pennies, though, you can make your own natural cleaning products, ensuring that you're protecting not only your own health but also the long-term health of the environment.

Grease cutter: Mix 1 cup lemon juice and 1 cup water.

Scouring powder: Mix 1 cup baking soda with enough water to form a paste.

Laundry stain remover: Use 1 teaspoon white vinegar or baking soda per machine load.

Toilet bowl cleaner: Pour 1 cup vinegar into the toilet, leave overnight, and scrub with a toilet brush the following day.

Floor and furniture polish: Mix 2 parts vegetable oil and 1 part lemon juice. For leather furniture, use 1 cup vinegar mixed with 1 cup linseed oil.

Metal cleaners (brass and copper): Mix lemon juice and salt until it forms a paste, use a lemon wedge dipped in baking soda, or mix hot white vinegar with salt to make a paste. Believe it or not, hot ketchup applied with a rag will also clean these metals.

Glass cleaner: Mix 1 part vinegar and 1 part water.

Rug and carpet cleaner: Try rubbing a bit of baking soda on wet stains or baking soda dissolved in water on dry stains.

standard furnaces in homes with forced-air heating and central air conditioning, however. In those cases, you'll need a separate filter system with a fan. You can find vacuum cleaners as well as heating and air-conditioning units with these filters.

■ **Ultra low penetration air (ULPA) filters.** These are even more effective than HEPA filters, trapping 99.9 percent of all particles larger than 0.12 micron (for comparison, a human hair is about 50 microns thick) at a minimum of 99.97 percent efficiency.

■ **Electronic air cleaners.** These use an electrical field to trap charged particles. Like mechanical filters, they can be installed in central heating and/or cooling system ducts. They're very effective but can also be quite expensive, costing up to $800 to install. Also, they may produce ozone, which may exacerbate asthma, and may require frequent (weekly to monthly) cleaning to maintain their effectiveness. In fact, they often don't work well because they're not cleaned often enough.

Check Products for Allergen Safety

Wondering whether that new laundry detergent could be making your allergies worse? Or if the wax you used to shine up your car might be the reason for that asthma attack you had soon after you finished the job? The Specialized Information Services of the National Library of Medicine have developed a vast database of common household products that includes the potential health effects and other safety and handling information for each. Just go to http://hpd.nlm.nih.gov/ and click on the category of product you're interested in. For instance, did you know that X14 toilet bowl cleaner may be irritating to the upper respiratory tract?

Another smart move for allergy sufferers is to hold off on trying brand-new products that promise relief. For instance, S.C. Johnson's AllerCare Dust Mite Carpet Powder and Dust Mite Allergen Spray, which claimed to rid homes of dust mites, were recalled when it turned out that their strong fragrance could cause—what else?—asthma attacks.

When selecting a filter, it's important to keep in mind that efficiency changes over time. As filters become loaded with particles, the available openings for air to flow through become smaller. The result is better filtration but less air movement, which makes your furnace work harder to move air through the system and can cause costly damage. That's why filters need to be replaced on a regular basis (follow the manufacturer's instructions) to ensure proper airflow.

As for electronic air cleaners, they are most efficient when first installed and lose their efficiency as they get dirty. Regular maintenance and monthly cleaning is required to keep them operating at peak efficiency. Before buying filters, always ask:

■ **What size particles will it trap?** You want to trap those smaller than 5 microns.
■ **Does it meet FDA ozone standards?** If not, don't buy it.

You can also use a vent filter kit over room outflow vents to form a final filter before air is released into the room.

air purifiers: the real deal

If you're allergic, you're no doubt inundated with information about air purifiers. Pick up any Sharper Image catalog these days, and you might think the company has the cure for allergies in their room-size ionic air purifiers—just buy one for every room and say goodbye to your allergies!

No wonder consumers are gobbling them up like jelly beans. According to *Consumer Reports*, 3.4 million of the units were sold in 2002, 70 percent more than in 2000. But are they worth the cost, which can run to several thousand dollars? Probably not

First of all, regardless of what the advertisements say, air purifiers do nothing to curtail that greatest of all indoor allergens, dust mites. Remember: Dust mites aren't airborne. They're snuggled up in your furniture, draperies, carpets, and mattress.

Second, the machines don't help much with either asthma or allergies. A January 2000 study of asthma and indoor air exposure by the Institute of Medicine found that air cleaning "is not consistently and highly effective in reducing [asthma and allergy] symptoms."

Other scientific studies have found the same results. When researchers evaluated 10 studies on air-filtration devices and people with asthma, they found that the systems had no effect on medication use or morning PEFR values, although they were associated with fewer asthma symptoms. And the systems aren't much better for allergies. While some studies do find they're pretty good

Put the Hot Tub Outside

Hot tubs and spas are hot in this country, with more than 5 million installed in residential homes in the United States. But if you buy a hot tub, particularly if you have asthma, install it outside. Several physicians around the country have reported cases of what they're calling hot tub lung disease, a form of lung inflammation caused by a bacterium called Mycobacterium avium complex (MAC), which thrives in the warm, moist environment of an indoor spa. MAC that accumulates inside a tub hitches a ride on the air-jet bubbles, which are the perfect size to be inhaled into the lungs. Chlorine doesn't work on it, since the disinfectant loses much of its punch at temperatures higher than 84°F. Outdoor spas aren't affected, because sunshine kills MAC, and fresh air harmlessly dissipates it.

The condition doesn't affect everyone, just those who are hypersensitive to MAC, almost like an allergy. Also like an allergy, it appears that the more people use their indoor hot tubs, the more likely they are to develop the condition.

Can't give up your spa room? Try disinfecting with bromine, a chemical that seems to do a better job of eliminating MAC. Also, follow the manufacturer's directions for maintaining your hot tub, including changing filters and chemicals frequently. One other tip: Watch out for mold growth underneath the cover.

at removing animal hair and dander, they show minimal, if any, effectiveness in relieving allergic respiratory diseases.

When *Consumer Reports* evaluated the top-selling Sharper Image Ionic Breeze in 2002 and 2003, it concluded that the machine "proved unimpressive," and its tests "found almost no measurable reduction in airborne particles."

Also, some ionic room purifiers emit ozone, which is known to exacerbate asthma. Some (called ozone generators) even use an electrical charge to generate ozone, which may be called trivalent oxygen or saturated oxygen. The FDA has set a limit of 0.05 part per million of ozone in indoor air, so make sure that any electronic air cleaner you buy has been tested for ozone production, and stay away from ozone generators. You'll know yours is putting ozone into the air if the room begins to smell like a swimming pool.

allergy **sufferers ask**

Should I Have My Air Ducts Cleaned Every Year?

Not unless you can see stuff in them. Regardless of what duct-cleaning services may tell you, there's no medical evidence that cleaning ducts prevents health problems, such as asthma and allergies, or that dust levels in homes increase because of dirty air ducts. The U.S. Environmental Protection Agency does not recommend that you clean your air ducts routinely but only as needed, meaning when, upon visual inspection (take the panel off the duct in a room and peek inside), you see large deposits of dust or mold. Don't worry if your return registers are dusty; that happens normally as dust-laden air is pulled through the grate. Just vacuum or wipe away the dust as necessary.

If you do have your ducts cleaned, contact the National Air Duct Cleaners Association, a nonprofit trade association that certifies its members, at (202) 737-2926 or www.nadca.com. Also get written estimates from at least three different service providers before deciding whether to have your ducts cleaned. Then, when the providers come to your home, ask them to show you the contamination that would justify having the cleaning done.

One thing you might consider is an air purifier that blows fresh air over your bed while you're sleeping. Three studies involving people with perennial allergy or asthma symptoms found improvements in symptoms and measurable outcomes from machines that blew the filtered air over the bed.

Expect to pay between $80 and $500 for a room-size filtration device and up to $1,000 for a whole-house system. The overall effectiveness of an air-cleaning device depends on the efficiency of the unit and the amount of air drawn through it. Although no industry-wide performance standards exist to help consumers compare units, the Association of Home Appliance Manufacturers has developed a standard for portable air cleaners called the clean air delivery rate (CADR). The CADR expresses the number of cubic feet of clean air a unit delivers each minute. If whole-house air cleaners and filters are labeled at all, they carry a minimum efficiency reporting value (MERV) instead of a CADR number. The higher the MERV, the better the system is at trapping small particles.

mold: minimizing the growth

Checked your shower curtain lately? Unless you take it down and dunk it in bleach and hot water every couple of weeks, chances are it's incubating mold spores. At least 60 species of molds have spores thought to be allergenic, and 30 percent of people with respiratory allergies seem to be particularly sensitive to molds, with children appearing the most sensitive. There's also a strong link between molds and asthma.

The problem with mold is that it's often hidden—behind walls, in dark closets, under your refrigerator. As you'll see when you work through the Breathe Easy Plan, nearly every room in your house can contain mold. But doing battle isn't that hard. The best mold remover is merely 1 part bleach and 10 parts water, or about 1½ cups of bleach to 1 gallon of water.

What about the mold on those month-old leftovers in the refrigerator? Well, it's a legitimate problem. In fact, if you're allergic to molds, even cheese can be a trigger, for what is cheese but moldy milk? Stay away from fermented cheeses such as blue cheese, Brie, and Camembert, and trash any moldy food, even if the mold is on only one tiny corner.

preparing for the breathe easy plan

In this chapter, we've given you a lot of advice on reducing allergens in your home. In step 3 of the Breathe Easy Plan, beginning on page 197, we'll put it into a simple, room-by-room program for you, complete with a checklist.

chapter **nine**

the right
foods

We think highly of you, and we would never dare to call you an "average" person, so we hope the following description of the average American's diet seems as horrifying to you as it does to us. He (or she) subsists primarily on prepared and processed foods, eats hardly any fresh fruits and vegetables, and consumes unnaturally high amounts of sugar and salt. Nearly one-third of the liquid he drinks comes from carbonated soft drinks, and overall, one-third of his diet is composed of junk food. Chances are two in three that he is overweight.

While unappealing, this is a very accurate portrait of the collective American diet. Interestingly enough, the decline in the quality and nutritional healthfulness of our eating patterns closely parallels the rise in allergies and asthma in this country. Coincidence? An increasing body of evidence suggests not.

It's only been within the past decade or so, with the increase in allergy and asthma rates, that researchers have begun examining a possible connection with diet. What they're finding is downright intriguing. For instance, who knew that whole milk could protect you against asthma? Or that eating margarine could increase your risk of developing asthma? Or that apples might as well be called "asthma-protective round fruits"?

In this chapter, we'll not only explore the possible nutritional contributors to asthma and allergies, we'll also let you know about dietary changes that can help with your condition. Then, in step 4 of the Breathe Easy Plan, we'll put it all together for you in an easy-to-follow "Eat to Beat Allergies & Asthma" nutritional program.

watch your weight

Obesity and overweight have been linked with everything from heart disease to increased rates of cancer. Now you can add asthma to the list. Not only can being overweight (defined as having a body mass index, or BMI, of 25 or higher) increase your risk of developing asthma in the first place, it can also make existing asthma much, much worse.

First, the asthma development connection. When researchers in southern California looked at information on 3,792 children who were asthma-free when they first enrolled in the study, they found that those who were overweight or obese, particularly boys, were much more likely to develop asthma than those who remained at healthy weights. Similar studies have found that the risk of developing adult-onset asthma also increases with obesity.

Researchers don't know for sure why this is true, but they have lots of theories. When it comes to children, they suspect it may have something to do with the fact that overweight kids are less likely to be outdoors on the soccer field and more likely to be inside playing video games and watching television. All that indoor time may lead to a greater propensity for allergies because indoor air is significantly more polluted than outdoor air. And allergies, of course, are a strong trigger for asthma.

BMI Defined

Body mass index, or BMI, is a popular, well-established tool for indicating weight status in adults. It measures your weight in relation to your height. You will find your BMI in step 4 of the Breathe Easy Plan (the chart is on page 209). For now, you should know that for adults over 20 years old, BMI places people into one of these categories:

BMI	Weight Status
Below 18.5	Underweight
18.5–24.9	Normal
25.0–29.9	Overweight
30.0 and above	Obese

There are also physiological changes that occur when you're overweight. For instance, the more fat cells you have, the more inflammation you have, because fat cells are important sources of the chemicals that encourage inflammation. There's also some evidence that increasing weight contributes to bronchial hypersensitivity, a hallmark of asthma in which the bronchial openings spasm with very little provocation.

Then there are the effects of excess weight on existing asthma.

Banish the Milk Myth

So you've cut out all dairy products in the hope of improving your allergies or asthma. Well, grab a quart of ice cream, because the whole idea that milk contributes to the production of mucus is nothing more than an old wives' tale, an urban myth that has taken on truly mythic proportions. The worst milk does is temporarily thicken your saliva.

Need proof? Well, consider this study in which researchers recruited 20 people with asthma, half of whom believed their symptoms got worse when they consumed dairy products. When researchers had them drink either about 10 ounces of milk or a placebo beverage, they found no statistically significant differences between the groups when comparing lung function tests.

In fact, consumption of milk products is actually associated with a *reduced* risk of asthma. That's what Dutch researchers learned when they studied 3,000 children in the Netherlands. Those who consumed full-fat milk and butter daily had far lower rates of asthma than those who didn't. Other studies confirm those findings. The researchers hypothesize that various substances, including certain fatty acids, in dairy foods could play a role, as could antioxidants and other beneficial chemicals. It's also possible that by drinking whole milk and eating butter, the children got fewer omega-6 fatty acids (which contribute to inflammation) in their diets than those who drank low-fat milk and used margarine. In fact, a German study found a strong correlation between consumption of margarine (which contains high levels of omega-6's) and asthma in boys.

So, unless you have a true dairy allergy or are lactose intolerant and can't drink milk, there's no reason to give it up.

When researchers in Australia compared medical data on 1,971 adults with asthma, they found that those who were severely obese (with BMIs above 40, about 100 pounds overweight for men and 80 pounds for women) were significantly more likely to wheeze, have shortness of breath when they exerted themselves, and use much more medication to treat their asthma than those with lower BMIs.

The reasons are numerous. More fat around your abdomen prevents your lungs from fully expanding and your diaphragm from moving downward because they have to fight all that fat. In other words, you just can't get a good, deep breath. Plus, if you weigh more than you should for your body frame and height, you require more oxygen just for everyday living. Getting enough oxygen is hard enough when you have asthma and aren't overweight; adding the extra pounds is like tying a set of barbells to a marathon runner.

The good news? While being overweight may increase your risk of asthma or make your asthma worse, there's compelling evidence that losing weight can improve the situation. Researchers in Finland had 38 overweight or obese adults with asthma either enter a 14-week weight-loss program or do nothing. Those in the weight-loss group slimmed down an average of 31.2 pounds; the other half, predictably, remained the same or even gained a couple of pounds. Those who lost weight found that their lung function tests significantly improved compared with those of the control group. Better yet, the changes held for an entire year, during which the thinner participants radically reduced their use of steroid medications and experienced far fewer asthma flare-ups.

What's the connection? Well, researchers speculate that losing weight reduces the incidence of early airway closing, especially while lying down. It also improves the ability to exercise, lowering the likelihood of asthma symptoms during exertion. And it's likely that reducing the amount of fat around the abdomen reduces symptoms of gastroesophageal reflux disease (GERD), which, as discussed in chapter 4, can make asthma much worse.

As part of the Breathe Easy Plan, we'll give you some easy-to-follow tips to lose some weight, thus relieving some of the worst aspects of your asthma.

the heartburn-asthma connection

So you tackled the all-you-can-eat buffet at the Chinese restaurant down the road, and later that evening, you had a pretty severe asthma attack. You blamed it on your sensitivity to MSG, a common flavoring ingredient in Chinese dishes. Instead, it could be that you overate, exacerbating your heartburn, or gastric reflux, which in turn made your asthma worse.

The link between the two conditions—GERD and asthma—is pretty clear, with as many as 70 percent of people with asthma also suffering from GERD. Now, as promised, we're going to tell you how to control it. And controlling it is critical, since studies find that treating GERD symptoms often improves asthma symptoms.

You could go the medication route with antacids and proton pump inhibitors such as omeprazole (Prilosec) and esomeprazole (Nexium), but you can also go the smarter-eating route, an approach you should try first.

Essentially, small meals that are rich in vegetables and include modest servings of complex carbs and lean protein are—as usual—the order of the day. Meals like this are not only healthy for your heart and body but also the easiest on your digestive system.

When it comes to specifics, it's easiest to detail the foods to avoid. The following foods aggravate the acid reflux effect, in which stomach acid spurts up into your lower esophagus. Some are otherwise healthy—particularly tea, onions, and garlic—so avoid them only if they irritate your stomach.

■ **Fatty or fried foods.** Instead of high-fat hamburger, for instance, opt for low-fat chicken, fish, and turkey. Bake chicken instead of frying it, and eat potatoes mashed, not fried.

■ **Peppermint or spearmint.** Stay away from peppermint herbal remedies for asthma, as described on page 167, if you have GERD.

■ **Whole milk.** Substitute low-fat or fat-free milk and other dairy products.

■ **Oils.** Foods cooked in oil or butter tend to linger in the stomach and are likely to cause digestive problems.

■ **Chocolate.** Chocolate interferes with the ability of the lower esophageal sphincter to prevent stomach acids from creeping back up the esophagus.

■ **Tomatoes.** The acid in tomatoes can aggravate heartburn.

■ **Creamed foods or soups.** Too rich and fatty.

■ **Most fast foods.** Ditto.

Next, try to at least limit the following foods, if not eliminate them altogether. They irritate an already inflamed lower esophagus.

■ **Citrus fruits and juices** (nix the orange juice or grapefruit and reach for an apple or a banana)

■ **Coffee,** regular and decaffeinated

■ **Soft drinks,** caffeinated and noncaffeinated (just imagine how much you burp after downing a can of soda)

■ **Tea**

■ **Alcoholic beverages**

■ **Garlic and onions**

■ **Vinegar**

■ **Spicy foods**

■ **Junk food,** particularly oily types such as potato chips

Foods to Focus On

Several studies show links between individual foods, such as salt and sugar, and asthma or allergies. Based on the research, here's what we suggest.

Stick to brown bread. A large Dutch study evaluating 3,000 children in the Netherlands found a significantly reduced risk of asthma in those who ate brown (whole grain) bread instead of white bread. Whole grain bread (look for "whole grains" on the label) is chock-full of valuable antioxidants.

Limit salt. Americans get far too much sodium, primarily because of all the processed foods we eat. Now, several studies point to an association between asthma symptoms and salt intake. For instance, in one well-designed study, 37 people with mild to moderate asthma stayed on either a low-sodium diet (1.92 grams a day) for five weeks or a high-sodium diet (4.8 grams a day) for one week. While on the high-sodium diet, their asthma symptoms and use of medications increased, while their lung function test results dropped.

Load up on fruit. Apples, pears, and citrus fruits come up winners in terms of reducing the risk of asthma, as well as wheezing, in children.

Watch your sugar and fat. An Australian study found that children who showed signs of airway hyper-responsiveness (an early sign of asthma) ate 23 percent more refined sugar and 25 percent more high-fat foods than children who did not have such symptoms.

Drink coffee or tea. It seems these beverages contain substances called methylxanthines, which act as natural bronchodilators. Several studies have found a reduction in asthma incidence and symptoms with consumption of black or green tea or of coffee. For instance, in one study, subjects who regularly drank coffee were nearly one-third less likely to have asthma than non-coffee drinkers, and the more they drank, the less likely they were to have it.

GERD is a product not only of what you eat but also of how you eat. Here are some additional recommendations to avoid heartburn and, by extension, asthma attacks.

- Eat several small meals throughout the day rather than just a few big meals. This alone can make a huge difference by keeping your digestive system from being overloaded at any one time.
- Start every meal with a glass of water or a bowl of healthy soup. The liquid not only dilutes stomach acid, it also helps fill you up so you eat less.
- Eat slowly and calmly. Put your fork or spoon down after each bite. Sip water between bites. Intersperse eating with telling your dining partner about the amusing things that happened during your day. Heartburn can be caused by overloading your system with food faster than it can handle it. Plus, your brain follows your stomach by about 20 minutes when it comes to hunger signals. If you eat slowly enough, your brain can catch up to tell you that you are no longer in need of food.

Making Restaurants Agreeable

If you're eating out, follow these guidelines from the National Heartburn Alliance at www.heartburnalliance.org to avoid an after-dinner bout of heartburn and asthma.

Italian Restaurants

Avoid:	Go for:
• Heavy tomato or cream sauces	• Dishes with little or no cheese
• Pizza toppings such as double cheese, sausage, and pepperoni	• Pasta "en brodo," which is a light, broth-type sauce
• Lots of garlic	• Minestrone (vegetable) or pasta fagioli (macaroni and bean) soup
• Oil-based salad dressings	• Veal or chicken in a light mushroom sauce
• Rich, heavy desserts such as cheesecake or tiramisu	• Biscotti—crunchy Italian cookies—for dessert

Mexican Restaurants

Avoid:	Go for:
• Hot salsa	• Guacamole on a flour tortilla
• Fried tortilla chips	• Fajitas or other grilled items
• Condiments such as jalapeño peppers, onions, and hot sauces	• Dishes flavored with herbs such as cumin and cilantro, which tend to be heartburn-friendly
• Mole (chocolate) sauce	• Low-fat refried beans and rice
• Flan or other rich desserts	
• Sangría and margaritas	

Chinese Restaurants

Avoid:	Go for:
• Egg rolls, ribs, shrimp toast, and other high-fat dishes	• Dishes made with vegetables in a light sauce
• Breaded and fried entrées	• Brown rice
• Sauces thickened with eggs and butter	• Sauces thickened with broth and cornstarch
• Overly spicy dishes	• Entrées such as beef with broccoli, velvet chicken, or shrimp with mushrooms and bamboo shoots

choose the right fats

What more can we tell you about dietary fats? After all, you know that low fat is good and high fat is bad, right? Well, that's not exactly right, and despite Americans' love affair with low-fat diets over the past 15 years and the vilification of all things fat, low fat isn't necessarily the way to go. Instead, especially if you have asthma and allergies, you want to worry about the *kind* of fat you eat. A growing body of research suggests that it's the type of fat—not the amount—that may play a role in the rise in and severity of asthma and allergies.

The culprits appear to be the large amounts of polyunsaturated fats in the diets of Americans (and people in other Westernized countries). Not that polyunsaturated fats are bad; for years, nutritionists have been telling us that these fats, found in vegetable oils and some nuts and grains, are good for us—or at least much better than the heart disease–promoting saturated fats found in animal protein and dairy products.

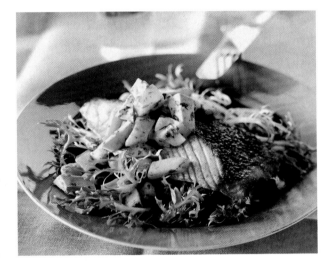

The problem comes in balancing the types of polyunsaturated fats we get. There are two main types of polyunsaturated fatty acids: omega-6 fatty acids, which are abundant in vegetable oils, margarine, and baked goods, and omega-3 fatty acids, found in high amounts in cold-water fish such as mackerel, salmon, and swordfish; in flaxseed; and in some dark green vegetables.

Salmon and other cold-water fish are rich in omega-3 fatty acids, which *reduce inflammation and lower the risk* of developing asthma.

If we consumed equal amounts of omega-3's and omega-6's, everything would be great. But the American diet—heavy on processed foods and vegetable oils and light on fish—is also heavy on omega-6's. And those fatty acids, it turns out, increase inflammatory reactions that lead to asthma and allergies. Omega-3 fatty acids, on the other hand, *reduce* inflammation, so you can see why a 1:1 ratio, instead of the 6:1 ratio in the typical American diet, would be most beneficial.

In fact, researchers attribute lower rates of cancer, heart disease, asthma, and autoimmune diseases in parts of the world where people eat far more omega-3's—such as Greece and Greenland—to consumption of these beneficial fats.

In studies, researchers have found that children who eat fish more than once a week have one-third the risk of developing asthma compared with children who eat no fish. And that's not just any fish, but oily fish rich in omega-3's (in actuality, the fish is about as "oily" as a piece of toast). Other studies find that adults with asthma who regularly eat oily fish have better lung function, less wheezing and breathlessness, and fewer episodes of waking up with chest tightness.

Additionally, when 29 children with bronchial asthma received either fish-oil capsules containing 84 milligrams of EPA and 36 milligrams of DHA (both forms of omega-3 fatty acids) or placebos (dummy pills), those receiving the fish oil had fewer asthma symptoms and responded better to beta2-agonist medications such as albuterol (Proventil and Ventolin) than those who got the placebos. Similar results have been found in adults, where a study of people with allergic asthma who took daily fish-oil supplements for a month found that participants had reduced levels of leukotrienes. Those are the nasty molecules, remember, that are released by mast cells and are to blame, in part, for the increased mucus production, airway constriction, and inflammation of asthma and the runny, stuffy nose of allergies.

For the record, olive oil and macadamia oil, considered monounsaturated fats, have very few omega-6's (they're composed mainly of omega-9 fatty acids), making them an ideal choice for cooking. Stay away from canola oil unless you use it cold; when heated, it turns into that most unhealthy of all fats, trans fatty acids, which are linked to heart disease and other ills.

Another polyunsaturated fat that you want to watch out for is arachidonic acid, found in relatively high amounts in beef, pork, lamb, dairy products, and shellfish. It also contributes to inflammation, giving you yet another reason to get your omega-3's, which counteract the actions of arachidonic acid. This could be why one long-term trial of a vegan diet, in which all animal products were eliminated, found that 92 percent of the 25 asthma patients who completed the study significantly improved. The response didn't happen overnight, however; participants had to stay on the diet for a year before the 92 percent success rate was reached.

You don't have to go that far, though. Instead, as we'll show you in the Breathe Easy Plan, reducing your dependence on red meat and sources of omega-6 fatty acids while upping your intake of omega-3 fatty acids should give you the relief you crave.

probiotics: powerful anti-asthma nutrients

If you've eaten live-culture yogurt, you've eaten probiotics. These healthy bacteria normally spend their lives swimming around in your gut, helping keep the fauna and flora balanced down there. They stimulate your body to produce certain white blood cells and antibodies, as well as various growth factors that are

The Elements of an Anti-Asthma Diet

When researchers in the United Kingdom evaluated the diets of 1,471 people ages 15 to 50 with asthma and 864 people without asthma, they found some interesting correlations.

• The more fruit and vegetables the participants ate, the less likely they were to have asthma.

• People who ate apples (a rich source of important phytochemicals called flavonoids) two or more times a week were 32 percent less likely to have asthma.

• People who ate onions (rich in the antioxidant quercetin) two or more times a week were 18 percent less likely to have asthma.

• People who drank tea (another excellent source of flavonoids) two or three times a day were 17 percent less likely to have asthma than those who didn't drink tea.

• People who drank one to two glasses a day of red wine (also rich in flavonoids) were 18 percent less likely to have asthma; in those who had asthma, it was likely to be less severe.

This study provides a good example of why food is better than food-like supplements as part of your asthma plan. As the researchers themselves note, there are numerous phytochemicals in apples and the other foods that could be responsible for their beneficial effects. The most likely ones are the aforementioned flavonoids. These chemicals, of which there are several (including ones we probably haven't even identified yet), have antioxidant, anti-allergenic, and anti-inflammatory properties; prevent the release of nitric oxide (implicated in asthma) and histamine; and interfere with arachidonic acid metabolism and cytokine production. There's even one flavonoid in apples called khellin, which is known for its antihistamine properties and was historically used to treat asthma.

So here's the menu. How about ratatouille (sautéed eggplant, tomatoes, onions, zucchini, squash, and herbs), served with a glass of good Cabernet and followed by a baked apple and a cup of hot tea?

important for preventing allergies and asthma and keeping your body from overreacting to allergens.

But numerous things, ranging from stress and antibiotics to fluoridated water and chlorine, can kill off these helpful little guys, contributing, it's now thought, to allergies and asthma. For instance, studies suggest that lactobacilli (a form of probiotic) are less common in the intestines of Westerners than in those of people from the Third World and less prevalent in children with allergies than in those who aren't allergic.

It turns out that probiotics are critical in helping stem inflammation and control your immune response to stimulants like allergens, particularly when it comes to food allergies. In fact, probiotics have been found to be beneficial in controlling and preventing food allergies, as well as atopic dermatitis (eczema), an allergy-related skin condition.

And, in the most exciting study to date on the role of probiotics in allergies and asthma, a group of Finnish researchers is following 132 children at high risk of developing allergies or asthma. Their mothers took probiotics during pregnancy and, if they breastfed, for the first six months of breastfeeding. The infants who were bottle-fed received their probiotics in their formula. Four years later, the researchers found that children in the probiotic group had half the rate of atopic eczema, often a first sign of asthma or allergies, when compared with the placebo group.

You can get probiotics (another form is bifidobacteria) in live-culture yogurt (look for "live cultures" or "acidophilus" on the label) or in supplements.

fruit and vegetables: always healthy

Every time you breathe, eat, or run (or walk, watch TV, make love, or sleep), your cells take a hit. Through a process called oxidation, many of the activities of daily living actually have the power to harm cells, leading to disease

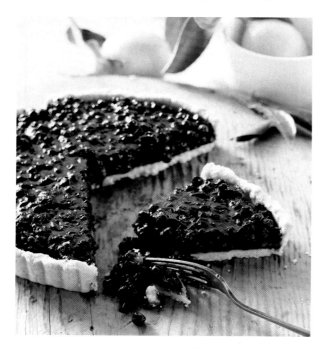

(including asthma) and aging. It happens when rogue molecules called free radicals zoom around trying to snatch electrons from healthy molecules, thus harming cells.

Oxidation is not all gloom and doom, however. Powerful chemicals called antioxidants, found in the foods you eat as well as occurring naturally within your body, act as scavengers, passing on one of their electrons to free radicals and disarming them. This process helps prevent cell and tissue damage that could lead to disease.

As you might have suspected when you started reading this section, oxidation and free radicals play a role in

Antioxidants, found in fruits and vegetables, *help prevent free radical damage*, a suspect in exercise-induced asthma.

asthma. For instance, some researchers suspect that exercise-induced asthma attacks may be due, in part, to the free radical damage that occurs during exertion. To test their theory, Israeli researchers gave 38 people with exercise-induced asthma 64 milligrams per day of natural beta-carotene (a powerful antioxidant supplement) for one week. Fifty-two percent had no exercise-induced asthma.

A Norwegian study found that young adults with asthma who smoked (a major contributor to free radical development) but who also consumed large amounts (at least 395 milligrams) of the antioxidant vitamin C from food had much less wheezing and coughing than smokers who didn't get as much vitamin C. Of course, they'd probably improve much more if they just quit smoking, but you work with what you've got, right?

Other studies have found lower levels of vitamin C in the blood and sputum of people with asthma. In fact, studies show that vitamin C, a natural antihistamine in large doses, is effective in treating asthma and in reducing the severity of asthma symptoms.

The antioxidants coenzyme Q_{10} (CoQ_{10}) and vitamin E may also be important when it comes to asthma. One study of 77,866 women found that those with the highest vitamin E intake from food (whole grains, sunflower seeds, wheat germ, and spinach) had half the risk of asthma compared with those who got the least.

Then there's the antioxidant quercetin. Found in many fruits and vegetables, it controls inflammation by reducing the release of histamine and other chemicals involved in allergic reactions and stabilizing cell membranes so they're less reactive to allergens. Although there have been few clinical trials with people, a Japanese study in which mast cells from the nasal mucus of people with perennial allergic rhinitis were treated with quercetin found that the supplement significantly inhibited the release of histamine, with an effect twice that of cromolyn sodium at the same concentration. You can get quercetin from apples, onions, and green and black tea.

vitamins and minerals

Although a healthy diet is critical, taking a good-quality multivitamin/mineral supplement is also a good idea, and one that's part of the Breathe Easy Plan. That's because, in addition to the benefits of the antioxidants mentioned above, numerous other links between vitamins and minerals and asthma have been found. Specifically:

■ **Magnesium.** This mineral, plentiful in seafood, legumes (especially soybeans), nuts, whole grains, and dark green, leafy vegetables, is often given intravenously in the hospital during an asthma attack. It relaxes the smooth muscles that line your airways, minimizing the spasms characteristic of an attack. Magnesium levels are frequently low in people with asthma, and many doctors recommend that such patients take a daily magnesium supplement of 200 to 400 milligrams.

■ **Selenium.** A trace mineral found in the soil, selenium is absorbed by plants as they grow. But because levels of selenium differ dramatically depending on where plants are grown, it's difficult to estimate the amount of selenium in fruits and vegetables. What *is* known is that selenium is a valuable antioxidant,

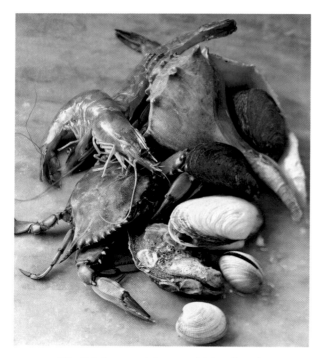

that people with low levels of this vital mineral have an increased risk of asthma, and that people with existing asthma have very low selenium levels.

So what happens when you supplement with selenium (and this is one nutritional component that is best gotten via a single supplement or a daily multivitamin/mineral)? Well, when researchers in Sweden gave 24 adult asthma patients either a placebo or a supplement of 100 micrograms of selenium daily for 14 weeks, the selenium group had significant improvement in their asthma symptoms.

■ **Vitamin B$_6$.** This vitamin is often called the "energy" vitamin,

Shellfish are rich in *asthma-fighting nutrients* such as magnesium and selenium, as well as iron, zinc, and omega-3 fatty acids.

and it's often low in people with asthma. Plus, the asthma drugs theophylline (Respbid) and aminophylline (Phyllocontin) can depress B$_6$ levels. Adding B$_6$-rich foods (bananas, avocados, chicken, beef, fish, brown rice, and peanuts) to your diet or taking a supplement could improve your asthma. At least, that's what researchers found in one study of 76 asthmatic children who received 200 milligrams of B$_6$ daily for five months. Not only did their symptoms improve, but their use of bronchodilators and cortisone decreased. In another study, this one in adults, taking 50 milligrams of vitamin B$_6$ twice daily dramatically decreased the frequency and severity of asthma attacks.

■ **Molybdenum.** You don't hear much about this trace mineral, but if you have asthma, it's one you should study up on. Found primarily in legumes, leafy vegetables, and cauliflower, this tongue-twister nutrient (pronounced *mo-lyb-de-num*) helps the body detoxify sulfites, chemicals added to foods that often provoke asthma symptoms. Although there have been few studies on its use in people with asthma, one 1989 report in a medical journal described how three months of daily molybdenum injections reduced one woman's wheezing and allowed her to cut her use of inhalers from four times daily to twice daily.

In an Australian study of 1,750 asthma patients, 41.5 percent were deficient in molybdenum. When molybdenum was added to their diet, their symptoms improved. Most multivitamin/mineral supplements contain molybdenum.

elimination diets

Many people with allergies and asthma, and particularly parents of asthmatic or allergic children, swear by elimination diets, in which they cut out certain foods they think make their conditions worse, such as dairy products, meat, wheat, and sugar. It's not that they're allergic to these foods but rather that they think they have food sensitivities that trigger asthma or allergy attacks.

It is true that food allergies can trigger or exacerbate bronchial constriction in asthma and that food allergies are often underdiagnosed in children with asthma. But it's also true that food alone will *not* trigger an asthma or allergy attack unless you have a bona fide food allergy, as described in chapter 5.

Nevertheless, people have very strong emotional feelings about foods, and if someone truly believes that a food is problematic, it's very hard to convince them otherwise. For instance, if you eat a piece of chocolate, and an hour later, you have an asthma attack, the two become forever linked in your mind.

So here's the bottom line, then, on elimination diets. If you do try one, eliminate one food at a time, then wait at least two weeks before either putting it back into your diet or eliminating another food. Track your asthma and allergy symptoms before and after the food is eliminated, using the chart in step 4 of the Breathe Easy Plan. If you don't notice any consistent, long-lasting improvement, there's no sense in depriving yourself of that food.

Also, don't try these diets with children. Severely restrictive diets are especially dangerous for children, who need a careful balance of vitamins, minerals, and other nutrients to ensure healthy growth and development.

no way around it

There's simply no way around it: You *are* what you eat. Following a healthy diet can protect you and your children from developing asthma in the first place as well as help keep symptoms of existing asthma under control.

In the next chapter, we'll take a look at some alternative therapies designed to help you both relax and de-stress and target your asthma/allergy symptoms.

the right
alternative
choices

Looking for something new to treat your asthma? How about swallowing live fish stuffed with herbs? That's what a half-million people with asthma do each June in India, arriving on special trains and buses in Hyderabad for the secret concoction a local family provides free of charge.

While the idea of a live fish curing asthma (actually, the fish is just a convenient way to get the herbs into the stomach, clearing phlegm as it goes) may sound ludicrous, it's just one in a long list of alternative remedies that people use to treat allergies and asthma.

Twenty to 60 percent of people with asthma, and more than 42 percent of those with allergies, turn to alternative medicine for their conditions. (Its use has finally become pervasive enough that the mainstream medical world has come up with a formal name for the genre: complementary and alternative medicine, or CAM.) These more open-minded patients are trying everything from herbal remedies such as ephedra and grapeseed extract to yoga, acupuncture, breathing exercises, and homeopathy. Some people with asthma even spend hours a day in subterranean caves or salt mines during a treatment called speleotherapy.

Some of these efforts work, some don't, and some may actually be dangerous. In fact, one study found that people with asthma who self-treated with herbs, coffee, and black tea had higher rates of hospitalization than those who followed more standard medical advice.

The reality is that there's very little scientific evidence to support or disprove many of these alternative therapies. The reasons for this lack of knowledge are many. Not only is it difficult to find funding for well-designed research on alternative remedies, it's often difficult to design such studies. Even the studies that have been conducted often have methodological flaws that limit their interpretation and application to contemporary medical practice.

Obviously, though, people with allergies and asthma aren't waiting for scientific evidence, since they're trying CAM therapies at ever-increasing rates. And while that's probably okay for some things, you need to understand that just because something is natural, that doesn't mean it's safe; in fact, some herbal remedies can have dangerous interactions with prescription or over-the-counter medications you're taking. Others can dangerously exacerbate allergies or asthma.

It's also important that you don't *substitute* alternative remedies for traditional medical therapies, such as medication. If you stop taking your asthma medication, for instance, you could wind up very sick and in the hospital—regardless of any alternative therapy you're trying. Instead, if you want to try

Clinical Trials Defined

Throughout this chapter, you'll see references to clinical trials performed to determine the effectiveness and safety of various alternative treatments. Here's a primer on clinical trial verbiage.

Blind. A randomized trial is blind if the participants don't know whether they are getting the treatment being tested, a placebo, or standard therapy; also called masked.

Single-blind study. A study in which one party, either the investigator or the participant, is unaware of what medication the participant is taking; also called single-masked.

Double-blind study. A clinical trial in which neither the participants nor the study staff know which participants are receiving the experimental drug and which are receiving a placebo (or another therapy). Double-blind trials are thought to produce objective results, since the expectations of the researchers and the participants about the experimental drug don't affect the outcome; also called double-masked.

Controlled trials. Control is a standard against which experimental observations may be evaluated. In clinical trials, one group of participants is given an experimental drug, while another group (i.e., the control group) is given either a standard treatment for the disease or a placebo.

Placebo. A placebo is an inactive pill, liquid, or powder that has no treatment value. In clinical trials, experimental treatments are often compared with placebos to assess the treatment's effectiveness. In some studies, the participants in the control group receive a placebo instead of an active drug or treatment.

Placebo effect. A physical or emotional change occurring after a substance is taken or administered that is not the result of any special property of the substance. The change may be beneficial, reflecting the expectations of the participant and often of the person giving the substance.

alternative remedies, work with your doctor to integrate them into the traditional medical treatment you're following.

Also, don't try *anything* without first talking to your doctor. More and more physicians are making it a point to learn all they can about these options because they know their patients are exploring them.

Our goal with this chapter is to set the record straight. Here's what we do and don't know about alternative therapies and their efficacy for these two diseases, as well as what you need to be especially careful about.

Deciding on a Complementary Health Care Provider

You want to determine four things before handing over your money—and your health—to alternative healthcare providers.

1. Are they licensed, certified, and/or affiliated with the appropriate professional organizations?

Licensing and certification vary widely by healing method. For example, only 30 states have established training standards for certification to practice acupuncture, and not all states require a license to practice. It's different for chiropractors: All states mandate licensing, and the standards to get a license are very high.

2. Do they have a good reputation and track record?

Word of mouth is good; a doctor's recommendation is better. Plus, explore the length of time the practitioner has been in business and whether he has switched practices or locations frequently; stability in this business is a good sign. And don't hesitate to ask for a few names of patients who have similar conditions and might be willing to share their experiences with the treatment.

3. Do they answer your questions well, and are you in agreement with their approach or advice?

An alternative healer should be clear about the specific plan of action, the benefits you can expect, the cost of the treatment, and the possible side effects. The treatment should make sense to you, and you should believe in its value.

4. Does their treatment conflict with your doctor's remedies and prescribed medications?

Both the alternative healer and your doctor should offer you an opinion. Even if your doctor doesn't approve of an alternative healing method on principle, she should be honest about whether it poses a conflict with the medicines and other changes she has prescribed. Of greatest concern is adverse interactions between your presciption medications and any herbs or supplements an alternative practitioner suggests.

Here are a few websites that can help you in your research.

- **Acupuncture**
  www.medicalacupuncture.org
  www.aomalliance.org
  www.aaom.org
- **Chiropractic**
  www.amerchiro.org
  www.chiropractic.org
- **Homeopathy**
  www.homeopathic.org
  www.homeopathicdirectory.com
- **Biofeedback**
  www.bcia.org
- **Hypnosis**
  www.apmha.com
  www.asch.net
- **Massage**
  www.amtamassage.org
- **Alternative healing research**
  www.nccam.nih.gov

■ acupuncture

If there's any CAM therapy that's gained credibility in the past decade, it's acupuncture, which has traditionally been used for asthma treatment in China and is increasingly being used in the United States. In the United Kingdom, a survey found that 7 percent of 3,837 people with asthma had tried acupuncture, with most of those (71 percent) saying they thought it was helpful. Even the National Institutes of Health, in a 1997 consensus statement, said acupuncture may be useful for asthma as an adjunct treatment or acceptable alternative or as part of a comprehensive management program.

You may think of acupuncture as needle therapy, but that's just one very small part of it. The underlying principle of the therapy is that vital energy, or Qi (pronounced *chee*) flows along certain pathways in your body called meridians. When Qi is blocked, pain and illness result. Acupuncturists unblock Qi by inserting hair-thin needles at specific points in the body. In some instances, they use a laser beam that doesn't break the skin or apply very strong pressure with their hands.

Each illness relates to certain acupuncture points that tend to be areas of decreased electrical resistance, which may be part of the scientific basis for acupuncture's effects. Also, acupuncture is believed to release certain brain chemicals such as endogenous endorphins (think runner's high) that reduce pain and discomfort.

What the studies show: One study found that acupuncture during an acute asthma attack increased lung function by 58 percent in one test and 29 percent in a different form of test, both significant improvements. Overall, studies of acupuncture during asthma attacks have found it improves airflow about half as much as an inhaled beta2-agonist, such as the prescription inhaler albuterol (Proventil and Ventolin).

Several small, controlled trials found that a short-term program of acupuncture (1 to 12 weeks) positively affected lung function, enabling patients to reduce their use of medication. One well-designed study, however, in which adults and children with moderate to severe asthma received 4 weeks of biweekly acupuncture or sham acupuncture (the placebo), found no significant effect on symptoms, medication use, or pulmonary function during the treatment period or for several weeks thereafter. Yet another study, which compared the effect of 5 weeks of biweekly electro-acupuncture therapy in adults with moderate to severe asthma, found a significant improvement in lung function and a significant decrease in beta2-agonist use compared with the control group. So the results are mixed. One review of seven well-designed studies concluded that "no recommendation can be made one way or the other to either patients, their physicians, or acupuncturists on the basis of available data." In other words, it's up to you.

Precautions: Although complications from acupuncture are rare, make sure your acupuncturist follows strict sterilization procedures, and inform the practitioner of any medications you're taking or medical problems you have. Also, go to only well-trained, certified acupuncturists.

Cost: It varies depending on the practitioner, but you can figure on $40 to $65 a session.

Bottom line: Acupuncture is safe and won't interact with medications or make your asthma or allergies worse. However, it's still not known conclusively if it makes a significant difference in asthma.

■ chiropractic

You probably think about chiropractic for back pain or other muscle or joint aches, but people are increasingly turning to it for asthma and allergies. Typically, chiropractic includes joint manipulation, use of physical therapy tools such as ultrasound and electrical magnetic stimulation to strengthen muscles and reduce inflammation, and rehabilitative exercises.

What the studies show: As with so many alternative therapies, the studies are few and mixed in their findings. One study, published in the *New England Journal of Medicine*, compared chiropractic spinal manipulation for children with mild or moderate asthma with simulated chiropractic (the placebo). Although symptoms of asthma decreased, use of short-acting beta2-agonists was reduced, and quality of life increased in both groups, there was no significant difference between the two. Another study, conducted on 36 children ages 6 to 17, found that after three months of combining chiropractic therapy with optimal medical treatment, the children rated their quality of life substantially higher and their asthma severity substantially lower—and the benefits were maintained at a one-year follow-up. However, objective lung tests showed little or no change.

Precautions: Serious complications are rare, with some short-term discomfort being the most common side effect. Beware, however, of chiropractors who immediately recommend several visits a week for several weeks or months.

Cost: Chiropractic is the one alternative therapy most likely to be covered by health insurance. Even Medicare and Medicaid cover it. Cost varies per visit, with an average of about $60.

Bottom line: Again, there is no clear answer. There's very little evidence showing any objective physiological improvement in asthma as a result of chiropractic. Most of the improvement was subjective.

■ homeopathy

Homeopathy works on the principle that "like cures like." Thus, homeopathic remedies contain a minute dose of the substance which, in higher doses, would cause symptoms similar to those of the condition being treated. The substance—in the case of allergies, an allergen—is dissolved in alcohol, and a few drops are taken by mouth. The more a substance is diluted, the more potent the remedy is considered to be. Sometimes the dilution is so intense that just a few molecules remain. The idea is that this will stimulate your body's natural powers of defense and recovery.

Today, there are more than 2,000 homeopathic substances on the market, all available without a prescription. Yet the FDA classifies them as drugs: The Homeopathic Pharmacopoeia—the official listing of homeopathic remedies—was incorporated into federal law in 1938. This ensures more oversight of production and quality control of homeopathic remedies than of other supplements. Still, the FDA regulates homeopathic drugs in several significantly different ways than it does other drugs. Manufacturers do not have to submit new drug applications, and their products are exempt from manufacturing practice requirements related to expiration dating and from finished product testing for identity and strength.

What the studies show: A few studies have shown positive effects of homeopathic remedies on allergic rhinitis. In one randomized, double-blind, placebo-controlled study of 28 subjects with moderately severe allergic asthma, treatment with a homeopathic preparation of the diluted allergen for four weeks significantly reduced the severity of symptoms compared with a placebo. However, a large double-blind, controlled trial examining homeopathic immunotherapy in 242 asthmatic adults allergic to house dust mites found no significant differences between those who received the remedy and those who received a placebo. Thus, there's really no evidence it's effective for asthma.

Precautions: Generally, homeopathy is considered safe. Watch out for preparations prepared by practitioners of phytotherapy, a related discipline, in which the allergens are more concentrated in the solutions. These could trigger a potentially dangerous reaction.

Cost: Prices vary depending on whether you buy a remedy in the drugstore (a few dollars) or see a homeopathic practitioner, who mixes it up individually (in which case, you're paying for the office visit as well as the treatment).

Bottom line: There is minimal evidence that homeopathy provides symptom relief for allergic rhinitis. Although the practice is generally safe, as with any alternative therapy, don't turn to it instead of traditional medical treatment. Talk to your doctor about using homeopathy along with your regular treatment.

■ relaxation therapies

Hypnosis, yoga, meditation, visualization, controlled breathing. They all fall under the rubric of relaxation therapies—and relaxation is critical when it comes to asthma. While we no longer think asthma is "all in your mind," your levels of stress and anxiety can trigger attacks or make existing symptoms worse. That's why it's worth exploring the remedies described below. When used in conjunction with your medical treatment, they may result in your using less medicine and having fewer symptoms overall than if you just took your medicine.

Jacobson's Progressive Relaxation

This exercise teaches you to discriminate between states of tension and relaxation by tensing and relaxing each of the 15 muscle groups, paying close attention to the sensation. Also referred to as progressive relaxation, it's often used to help people with insomnia fall asleep by helping them become especially aware of the parts of their bodies that are particularly tense. Eventually, they learn to become more sensitive to rising tension levels before the tension gets so great it causes distress. The method is named after Edmund Jacobson, M.D., who pioneered the technique in the 1920s.

What the studies show: Studies are fairly positive, with one study of 44 children with moderate to severe asthma finding that lung function significantly increased in a group of kids who learned progressive relaxation as compared with others who just sat quietly. Another study of 20 asthmatic boys who received either Jacobson's relaxation training or assertiveness training found that by the end of the training, lung function measurements in the relaxation group improved by 17.7 percent and remained far superior to those in the assertiveness training group even one month after treatment ended.

Strengthen Your Breathing Muscles

Take a deep breath in. Now take another. See how your chest rises and falls? Well, it isn't doing it on its own. There are muscles in there called inspiratory muscles (or intercostal or subcostal muscles). They lie between and under your ribs and work by reflex, expanding as you breathe in and contracting as you breathe out. In other words, you don't even know they exist until you have trouble breathing.

If you have problems inhaling or are never able to completely fill your lungs with air, those muscles, like any that lie unused, grow weak. Taking corticosteroids for asthma can make them even weaker. The idea behind a technique called inspiratory muscle training is that by strengthening those muscles, you can enhance your ability to breathe.

Inspiratory muscle training occurs in two primary ways, either by taking a deep breath and holding it, with your lungs full to bursting, for as long as possible, or by using a device called POWERBreathe. The drug-free device looks like a large inhaler and contains a fan and a valve. As you breathe through the mouthpiece, your respiratory muscles are forced to work harder because air is released through the fan only when you build up enough pressure within the device to open the valve.

In an Israeli study published in 2002, researchers compared 15 patients who received inspiratory training with others who received sham training, evaluating the perception that they were short of breath and their use of beta2-agonists. They found that the stronger the patients' inspiratory muscles became, the less shortness of breath they reported and the less medicine they used.

You can purchase POWERBreathe over the Internet at www.powerbreathe-usa.com for about $70.

Precautions: None; this is a great way to relax and is often used at cardiac rehabilitation centers.

Cost: Most cardiac rehab centers offer training in this technique. Fees vary.

Once you receive the necessary training from a class or audio tape, you can practice the technique on your own wherever and whenever you like.

Bottom line: Who couldn't use some help relaxing? Check out the tapes or sign up for a class.

Biofeedback

Biofeedback is a therapeutic technique that teaches you how to control physical responses, such as breathing, muscle tension, hand temperature, heart rate, and blood pressure, which are not normally controlled voluntarily. You achieve this control by learning how to focus on and modify signals from your body. For instance, in the case of asthma, biofeedback could help you learn to control your breathing and lower your anxiety level when your symptoms act up.

What the studies show: One study of 20 children with non-steroid-dependent asthma who received either biofeedback for facial tension or were in a control group found that the perception of asthma severity decreased significantly in the biofeedback group as compared with the control group, although there was no effect on lung function.

Precautions: None; biofeedback is safe when performed properly.

Cost: Biofeedback can be expensive: Sessions cost $50 to $80, and you may require 20 or more sessions. Insurance may not cover the treatment.

Bottom line: Biofeedback is successful for a variety of stress-related conditions, such as migraines, pain, and anxiety. It's worth a try if your doctor is aware of it and is comfortable with your integrating it into traditional medical treatment.

Breathing Retraining

You already know how to breathe, right? You do it every day without even thinking about it. Chances are, though, you're breathing wrong—too shallowly, without the deep breaths that are to lungs what a cool shower is to the body on a steamy summer day. Breathing correctly can also help with your asthma, with anecdotal evidence finding that asthma responds well when you control the associated hyperventilation. That's where breathing retraining techniques come in—to teach you how to stop hyperventilating.

Breathing retraining takes several different forms, such as Buteyko breathing (named after Konstantin Buteyko, a Russian physician), in which you learn a series of exercises to reduce the frequency of your breaths. Part of the training involves breath-holding exercises, yoga breathing and physical exercises, and deep diaphragmatic breathing that is designed to build up your diaphragm muscles. The idea is to increase the diameter of the thoracic cage, thus increasing your chest capacity for maximum lung efficiency.

In step 7 of the Breathe Easy Plan, we'll show you how to breathe properly to reduce asthma symptoms. For now, here's what research has to say about breathing retraining.

What the studies show: In one study, 67 asthmatic adults participated in a 16-week program in which they received either diaphragmatic breathing training or physical exercise training or were put in a waiting-list control group. Those receiving deep diaphragmatic training significantly reduced their medication use and the intensity of their asthma symptoms. They also found they could spend nearly 300 percent more time in physical activities than before they learned the breathing technique. In another study, 36 adults with asthma were either trained in the Buteyko breathing technique via a video or received a placebo video to watch at home twice a day for four weeks. Those in the Buteyko group significantly improved their quality of life (based on a scientific survey) and significantly reduced the amount of inhaled bronchodilator medication they used.

allergy & asthma **sufferers ask**

Why Do People Turn to Alternative Therapies?

The reasons are numerous, says Esther L. Langmack, M.D., assistant professor of medicine at the National Jewish Medical and Research Center in Denver.

1. They're frustrated with conventional medications. Face it, many medications for asthma and allergies have side effects and take a while to work. They can also be expensive, and natural remedies may provide a cheaper alternative.

2. They want something "natural." Some people are uncomfortable taking medicines that were conceived in laboratories and manufactured on assembly lines. Their mistake, however, is to conclude that "natural" means safe. That's not always the case.

3. They want a cure. Unfortunately, there is no cure for asthma or allergies, whether you try traditional medicine or alternative medicine.

4. They want to be in control. Because alternative remedies don't require prescriptions, patients can decide what to take.

5. They want to address what they perceive as the underlying cause of their illness. Many alternative therapies are designed to reduce stress or bolster a weak immune system.

6. They want to honor cultural beliefs. Many cultures have a long tradition of using natural remedies and other alternative therapies; to them, it's the modern world of pharmaceuticals and scientific research that is "alternative."

Precautions: None; this technique is safe and painless.

Cost: The cost of training varies depending on whether you receive it from a private practitioner or from a video or CD-ROM.

Bottom line: It's breathing; how bad could it be? The studies show improvement, so it's worth trying.

Hypnosis

If you're used to thinking of hypnosis as an entertainment, complete with magicians, think again. Today, hypnosis is used in numerous areas of medicine, from pain management to the treatment of chronic conditions such as irritable bowel syndrome and, of course, asthma. It's even being used to improve wound healing in surgical patients!

This is not new. The use of hypnosis in medical healing dates back nearly 300 years, with published reports noting that patients who were hypnotized before surgery in pre-anesthesia days were not only more likely to survive the operation but also healed faster and with fewer complications.

The core of hypnotherapy lies in the complex connection between the mind and the body. It's not news anymore that illness can affect your emotional state (consider the correlation between heart disease and depression), or that your emotional state can affect your physical state (just think of the dozens of medical conditions caused or made worse by stress). Hypnosis carries that connection to the next logical step: Deliberately harnessing the power of the mind to affect physiological systems in the body.

Ran Anbar, M.D., professor of pediatrics at SUNY Upstate Medical University in Syracuse, began using hypnotherapy in his pulmonology practice about five years ago, when a teenager with very bad food allergies and asthma told him he had an asthma attack every time he smelled cheeseburgers or even *imagined* eating cheeseburgers. Dr. Anbar had the boy close his eyes and begin thinking about cheeseburgers. Sure enough, within seconds, he was

Not Worth Trying

Throughout this chapter, we've told you about remedies and therapies for which there is little concrete evidence of efficacy but which can't hurt to try. The following, however, *can* be harmful, either physically or to your pocketbook, and there is really no evidence as to their efficacy. Skip them.

Ozone therapy. This newest addition to alternative treatments for asthma involves either exposing a person's blood to ozone gas and then reinjecting it or directly introducing ozone either rectally or vaginally. It could have serious adverse effects, since ozone is a well-known trigger for asthma.

Enzyme-potentiated desensitization. This treatment, popular in the United Kingdom, involves mixing an allergen with beta-glucuronidase, a common enzyme in the body, and applying it to the body in very low doses. Studies find no significant benefits to this treatment.

Urine autoinjection. This treatment involves injecting freshly collected, sterilized urine back into the donor. There is no clinical evidence it works, and it may cause kidney problems.

having an asthma attack, serious enough that Dr. Anbar grew concerned and yelled "Stop!"

"That was my introduction to hypnosis," he says. "I thought, if it could bring on an asthma attack, then could I take it away?"

It turns out he could. Once Dr. Anbar trained the teen to use hypnosis, the boy began using it to relax himself whenever he had an asthma attack. Once, in the midst of a serious attack that landed him in the emergency room, he used the technique to relax his lungs. The speed with which his throat relaxed and his breathing eased amazed even the emergency room physicians, who had been preparing to insert a breathing tube.

What the studies show: Results are mixed, with one study of 252 children finding that those who received hypnotherapy had a 4.3 percent improvement in one measure of lung function, a significant increase. Another study, this one over a one-year period, found that those who received training in hypnosis and self-relaxation were able to reduce their use of beta2-agonists.

Precautions: None, if you use a well-credentialed, experienced hypnotherapist.

Cost: Varies widely, based on the practitioner, the type of hypnosis, and where you live.

Bottom line: Hypnotherapy could be a good healing option if integrated into your traditional medical therapy.

Yoga

These days, yoga studios are becoming almost as ubiquitous as McDonald's restaurants. The practice itself, which originated in India, is more than 5,000 years old. It involves a combination of physical and breathing exercises and meditation and is heralded as an excellent stress-reducing technique. There are indications it can improve asthma as well. Any yoga practice includes *pranayama,* or breath-slowing exercises, and meditation. Thus, yoga's benefits may be related to its relaxing effects on those who practice it, reducing stress hormones that can lead to inflammation, the bane of anyone with asthma.

What the studies show: Numerous studies show beneficial effects from yoga, regardless of the type practiced, on asthma symptoms. In one study, 53 people with asthma trained for two weeks in an integrated set of yoga exercises, including breathing exercises and meditation, and then were told to practice the exercises for 65 minutes daily. Compared with a control group that didn't do anything, the yoga group significantly improved in terms of fewer asthma attacks, scores for drug treatment, and peak flow rates.

Another study of 17 adults with asthma—in which 9 were taught yoga and relaxation exercises, including breath-slowing exercises, physical pos-

tures, and meditation, three times a week for 16 weeks, and the rest received no training—found the yoga group used fewer beta2-agonists even though pulmonary function in both groups didn't differ significantly. The yoga group, however, had a greater level of relaxation, a more positive attitude, and better yoga exercise tolerance than the control group, leading the authors to conclude that "yoga techniques seem beneficial as an adjunct to the medical management of asthma." A larger study of 287 subjects found that those who practiced yoga had a statistically significant increase in vital lung capacity over time.

Precautions: Be sure you tell your instructor about your asthma, allergies, or any other medical conditions and about any medication you're taking.

Cost: A yoga class generally costs $8 to $10.

Bottom line: Yoga seems to have some significant benefits for those with asthma. It is safe, is an excellent relaxation therapy, and provides a good workout for flexibility and muscle strength. Go for it—but don't give up your regular treatment.

Massage

Who wouldn't love a massage? Well, far from being simply a self-indulgent luxury reserved for special events and five-star resorts, massage is a centuries-old healing technique whose medical benefits are now being shown in study after study—even for asthma.

What the studies show: In the only study that's been done on the effects of massage on asthma, 32 children ages 4 to 14 received either massage therapy or relaxation therapy from their parents 20 minutes before bed each night. The younger children who received massage showed an immediate decrease in behavioral anxiety and levels of cortisol (a stress hormone) afterward. Also, their attitudes toward asthma and using their peak flow meters and other pulmonary function tests improved throughout the study. The older children

But Can You Prove It Works?

Although many complementary therapies have been around for thousands of years, there are often few, if any, solid clinical studies proving they work. One reason is that until fairly recently, it was difficult to get funding for such research. Another is that designing a traditional prospective, double-blind, placebo-based study with therapies such as massage or meditation is difficult at best. After all, how do you "pretend" to give a massage or teach someone to do "fake" meditation? All that is slowly changing, however, with the increasing prominence of and funding for the National Institutes of Health's Center for Complementary and Alternative Medicine.

Keep in mind, though, that we often don't know how traditional therapies and drugs work, either—or even if they really *do* work. For instance, for more than 40 years, doctors have been prescribing hormone replacement therapy (HRT) to women to help prevent heart disease after menopause. It was only in 2001, after a major government-funded study, that we learned HRT not only didn't protect women against heart disease, it actually increased their risk.

Many of the techniques described in this chapter, particularly the relaxation techniques, can benefit anyone, whether or not they have asthma or allergies. We can all use ways to help us better cope with the stress in our lives, and most of these relaxation techniques have been shown to lower levels of stress hormones such as cortisol.

Plus, don't discount the power of the mind. If you take an herb or smooth on an aromatic oil or get a massage and then find you're breathing easier, that's great. The bottom line is that *you feel better*. Never forget that the mind is one of the most powerful medicines.

also reported lower anxiety after the massage and improved attitudes toward asthma, but only one measure of lung function (FEV1) improved.

Precautions: You may feel sore the day after, but there is little risk of other adverse effects.

Cost: From $35 to $75 an hour, typically not covered by insurance.

Bottom line: Massage therapy may be a viable adjunct to traditional asthma treatment, especially for children.

Meditation

The central idea behind mindfulness and meditation is that of staying in the present. It's about showing up for your life and handling what's happening in a graceful way so you have more clarity, more awareness, and more choices. With asthma, learning meditation can be a valuable adjunct to medication in terms of helping you cope with stress in your life that could exacerbate your condition.

What the studies show: Little research has been conducted on meditation and asthma (much more has been done on yoga and asthma), but one six-month study of 21 patients trained in transcendental meditation found the practice was a "useful adjunct" in treating asthma. Though it is not directly relevant, it's noteworthy that many major medical centers and cancer clinics have added meditation and yoga centers in recent years, and urge patients with serious chronic disease to enroll.

Precautions: None; mindful meditation is safe and noninvasive.

Cost: An eight-week, hospital-based Kabat-Zinn program (see below) may cost upwards of $400; other programs may cost significantly less.

Bottom line: As a relaxation therapy for asthma and other conditions you may be coping with, meditation is a good adjunct to traditional medical therapy.

■ herbs and supplements

You don't have to go far to see the explosion in herbal remedies and other supplements that has hit this country. These days, even convenience stores sell pills, powders, and solutions that promise to improve everything from your memory to your sex life, so it's no surprise to find many claiming to improve asthma and allergies, too.

Before you grab your wallet and head to the drugstore, however, you need to learn a bit about the wild world of nutritional supplements. When it comes to regulation and oversight, they're about as far from prescription drugs as candy pills.

Unlike its oversight of prescription and over-the-counter medicines, the FDA doesn't rigorously regulate herbal remedies and other nutritional supplements. These supplements face no extensive tests before they're marketed and don't have to adhere to any standards of quality in manufacturing. So when you buy a bottle of grapeseed extract, for instance, there's really no way to know how much of the active compound the supplement contains. There's also no way to know if the recommended dose is effective, if the supplement contains any contaminants, or if the plants used were grown with pesticides, which could have some adverse effects, particularly in children.

With that in mind, here are steps to follow to make sure you're savvy about supplements.

■ **Talk to your doctor.** We've said it before, and we'll say it again: Tell your doctor about everything you're taking, even if it's just a vitamin.

■ **Talk to a pharmacist.** Registered pharmacists often have more information and knowledge about potential drug interactions than doctors, and many pharmacies

Supplement Warning

There are some supplements you should avoid taking at all if you have asthma, because they may exacerbate your condition.

Glucosamine-chondroitin People with arthritis or aging joints often turn to this dietary supplement combo for pain relief and to strengthen joints and bones. But a report published in late 2002 described the case of a woman whose well-controlled asthma suddenly got much worse when she began taking a glucosamine-chondroitin sulfate compound to treat her arthritis-related pain. Once she stopped taking the supplement, her asthma improved within 24 hours. Doctors suspect that her reaction was related to an allergy or sensitivity to seafood, since chondroitin is made from shark cartilage. People with asthma who work with sharks in biology labs should also be cautious.

Melatonin. A study published in the September 2003 issue of the *Journal of Allergy and Clinical Immunology* found that people whose asthma gets worse at night have higher levels of the sleep hormone melatonin. Melatonin induces the release of inflammatory chemicals, which can make an inflammatory disease like asthma worse. Thus, taking over-the-counter melatonin supplements to help you sleep could exacerbate your condition. Try a cup of warm milk instead.

Bee pollen. Often touted as a treatment for allergies, pollen can actually cause a fairly severe allergic reaction in some people.

Lobelia. Also known as asthma weed, this herb, sometimes used in homeopathic asthma medicines, is poisonous.

Speleotherapy

Talk about working in the salt mines. In Armenia in Eastern Europe, people with asthma travel nearly $\frac{1}{5}$ mile beneath the Earth's surface to—yes—a salt mine to reach Republican Speleotherapeutical Hospital, an underground medical clinic specifically designed for the treatment of asthma and other respiratory illnesses. Practitioners of the treatment, called speleotherapy, believe that the salt environment, with its dry air and consistent temperature, has a healing effect on the respiratory system. They also believe that the low carbon dioxide/oxygen ratio in mines and caves leads to deeper, more intensive breathing. Similar clinics can be found in mines and caves throughout much of Eastern Europe, and there are Internet guides to help you locate speleotherapy caves.

There's even some slight evidence that it may have some benefit. Although available studies are few and far between, at least one scientifically designed study conducted in 1994 found a slight improvement in lung function after three weeks of speleotherapy.

today have databases that warn of potential interactions.

■ **Know the source.** There are thousands of supplements and hundreds of brands on the market. Not all are created equal, and in fact, investigative reports in the media find that some don't even have the quantities they purport to contain. Consumer Laboratories independently tests supplements, providing information on hundreds of brands on its website, www.consumerlab.com. Also look for supplements produced with good manufacturing practices (GMP), which are regulations that describe the methods, equipment, facilities, and controls required for producing quality products.

The National Nutritional Foods Association (NNFA), an industry trade group, operates a GMP certification program that includes inspections of manufacturing facilities to determine whether they meet specific performance standards, including staff training, cleanliness, equipment maintenance, record keeping, and receiving of raw materials. Once certified, manufacturers can use the NNFA's GMP seal on their products.

■ **Remember that supplements are still drugs.** Just because they say "natural" on the label doesn't mean they're any safer than pharmaceutical drugs. They're still chemicals doing something in your body. Don't take higher-than-recommended doses, and don't take supplements for more than the recommended time period.

■ **Be skeptical.** If you hear something about a supplement that sounds too good or too bad to be believed, it probably is. To separate the truth from the fiction, check out websites such as www.quackwatch.com, as well as the American Council on Science and Health (www.acsh.org) and the National Council against Health Fraud (www.ncahf.org) sites.

■ **Do your homework.** If you take supplements, you should keep up with the growing body of scientific research about their effects. A good place to start is the National Institutes of Health's National Center for Complementary and Alternative Medicine at www.nccam.nih.gov.

■ **Proceed with caution.** What works for your next-door neighbor may not work for you. Know why you're taking what you're taking; don't rely on a recommendation alone. If you're pregnant or breastfeeding, eschew herbal remedies unless your doctor recommends them.

The following list is not complete by any means. There are numerous mixtures of herbs, particularly in Chinese, Korean, Japanese, and Indian medicine, that purport to help with asthma and allergies. If you're interested in herbal remedies, work with a licensed naturopathic doctor (N.D.), who is usually trained in herbal therapies, particularly Chinese medicine. Just be sure your regular doctor is aware of what you're doing.

Bromelain

Bromelain is an enzyme derived from the stem of the pineapple plant. It works as a decongestant, drying up mucus and other secretions.

What the studies show: Research shows that bromelain works by reducing swelling and mucus production, but none show its effectiveness in people with allergies. In fact, there are several reports of bromelain-related allergies.

Precautions: Allergic reactions may occur if you're sensitive to pineapple.

Bottom line: Pass on this one.

Butterbur

Extracts of this herbaceous plant have been used to treat asthma and allergic rhinitis.

What the studies show: In one study of 125 people with seasonal allergic rhinitis that compared butterbur with cetirizine (Zyrtec), both groups showed improvements in quality of life assessments. But 12 percent of those receiving Zyrtec reported sedative effects, compared with no such reports from those who received butterbur.

Precautions: The plant's pyrrolizidine alkaloids are thought to cause liver damage and be carcinogenic in animals, so be sure to buy extracts from which these substances have been removed.

Bottom line: Try it only with your doctor's knowledge.

Dried Ivy Leaf Extract

Don't go pulling up ivy from your garden if you choose to try this remedy; buy the extract in a health food store.

What the studies show: In a double-blind, randomized clinical trial, 24 children with asthma received about 35 milligrams of dried ivy extract for three days. Although there was no significant improvement in lung function, there was a significant decrease in airway resistance when compared with a placebo.

Precautions: None.

Bottom line: It may be worth trying with your doctor's knowledge.

Chamomile

Chamomile tea has anti-inflammatory properties, which are helpful when dealing with asthma. Plus, chamazulene, an active ingredient in chamomile, is a leukotriene inhibitor.

What the studies show: German studies have found that chamomile reduces the release of histamine from mast cells (at least in rats) and may slow allergic reactions by increasing the adrenal glands' production of cortisone, which reduces lung inflammation and makes breathing easier.

Precautions: None.

Bottom line: Definitely worth trying. Try a cup of chamomile tea before bed; it's often used to help promote relaxation and sleep.

Echinacea

This herbal remedy is often used to treat upper respiratory tract disorders.

What the studies show: A randomized trial with echinacea showed a significant reduction in the number of upper respiratory infections, a well-known trigger for asthma exacerbations.

Precautions: Be careful if you're allergic to ragweed, as echinacea is a member of the ragweed family. And avoid echinacea/goldenseal combinations, since one of the active ingredients in goldenseal, hydrazine, causes constriction of blood vessels and high blood pressure.

Bottom line: It may have some benefit and is relatively safe.

Ginkgo Biloba

A traditional Chinese herbal treatment for asthma/allergies, ginkgo is believed to work as an anti-inflammatory agent and to reduce airway hyperresponsiveness and bronchial spasms.

What the studies show: In one study, researchers gave 61 asthmatic participants (ages 13 to 48) either 15 grams of concentrated ginkgo leaf liquor three times a day or a placebo. Those getting the herb had a significantly greater improvement in their lung function tests after eight weeks.

Precautions: If you're planning to have any type of surgery or dental work, stop using ginkgo for at least 14 days prior to the procedure. Ginkgo may have anticoagulant effects.

Bottom line: If your doctor agrees, ginkgo is worth a try as part of a traditional medical treatment plan.

Grapeseed Extract

Believed to work as a natural antihistamine, grapeseed extract is often touted as a natural remedy for allergies and asthma.

What the studies show: A study of 54 adults, ages 18 to 75, with diagnosed ragweed allergy recorded their symptoms while they took either 100 milligrams of grapeseed extract or a placebo twice daily. After eight weeks, there was no difference in the reported symptoms or use of medications.

Precautions: Grapeseed may enhance the effect of drugs affecting coagulation or platelet aggregation, such as aspirin, warfarin (Coumadin), and clopidogrel (Plavix).

Bottom line: There's little evidence as to its efficacy, but it is relatively safe. It has some antioxidant and anti-inflammatory effects, so it's probably okay to try with your doctor's knowledge.

Another Reason to Legalize Marijuana?

In what seems incredibly counterintuitive, marijuana was once touted as an asthma remedy. In fact, in the early nineteenth century, pharmaceutical manufacturer Grimault and Sons actually marketed ready-made marijuana cigarettes for use as an asthma remedy, and doctors continued to prescribe it throughout much of the early twentieth century.

It turns out, though, that there's something to the evil weed. It works as an excellent bronchodilator, opening up the large and small airways of the lungs. If you put the active ingredient in cannabis, tetrahydrocannabinol (THC), into a microaerosol form, for instance, it's up to 60 percent as effective as a pharmaceutical bronchodilator—and you don't get high.

One oft-cited study of 10 adult asthma patients found that after they smoked a 2 percent THC preparation for 2 hours, their airway resistance decreased 10 to 13 percent compared with when they used a placebo. In another study, researchers induced acute asthma attacks in eight healthy young men and then had them smoke 500 milligrams of marijuana. With the marijuana, the men's bronchial spasms immediately ceased. With a placebo or saline solution, it took about 30 minutes for their lungs to return to normal.

If you live in a state that has legalized marijuana for medical use, you can talk to your doctor about a prescription for it.

Jimsonweed

Also known as datura, jimsonweed is a common plant found along roadsides and in cornfields and pastures. When smoked, it has mildly hallucinogenic properties, which, in 1968, prompted the United States to ban over-the-counter preparations containing it. Still, it has a long history as an herbal medicine for asthma. In fact, people with asthma smoked cigarettes made from this herb throughout much of the twentieth century, and it's still a common ingredient in many over-the-counter "natural" asthma preparations available from other countries, such as Asthmador, Barter's Powder, Kinsman's Asthmatic Powder, Green Mountain Asthmatic Compound, and Haywood's Powder.

What the studies show: One small study of 12 patients with asthma found that inhaling the smoke of one jimsonweed cigarette substantially decreased airway restriction in 11 patients to the point that even inhaling albuterol afterward caused no further improvement for most of them.

Precautions: Don't use this herb if you have glaucoma, a blockage in your gastrointestinal tract, or myasthenia gravis. Also avoid it if you're using anticoagulant (blood-thinning), diabetes, or anti-anxiety medication.

Bottom line: Skip this one. It's too risky.

Ma Huang (Ephedra)

This Chinese herb has been used for thousands of years to treat asthma and other respiratory conditions, including allergic rhinitis. It contains various forms of ephedrine, used in over-the-counter and prescription decongestants, which is why it's so good at drying up symptoms such as a runny nose and leaky eyes. It's often the primary ingredient in Chinese herbal mixtures for asthma, including Minor Blue Dragon (xiao-qing-long-tang, or XQLT). **Ephedra was recently banned for over-the-counter sale by the FDA.**

What the studies show: Of all the herbal remedies used for allergies and asthma, ma huang actually has the strongest basis of scientific support behind it, which isn't surprising when you consider that its active ingredient is the same one used in most decongestants.

Precautions: Taken in large amounts or by people with high blood pressure or certain heart conditions, ephedra can be quite dangerous, causing strokes or heart attacks and even resulting in death. Don't take it for more than a week at a time, and follow the package directions carefully.

Bottom line: You can get the same effects from prescription and over-the-counter preparations, without the worries.

Peppermint

Peppermint has a long history of use in healing and is even an FDA-approved remedy for the common cold. Peppermint oil contains menthol, a powerful therapeutic agent used in numerous over-the-counter and prescription drugs. It acts as a muscle relaxant, particularly in the digestive tract (hence the custom of sucking a peppermint candy after a big dinner), and it can reduce inflammation of the nasal passages, thus making it a common antidote for allergies and colds. It has also been found to prevent the release of histamine from mast cells in allergic rats, decreasing their sneezing and nose rubbing (and no doubt reducing the number of tissues they must need).

What the studies show: No studies have been published on the effect of peppermint on allergies or asthma.

Precautions: People with chronic heartburn problems should avoid peppermint.

Bottom line: A soothing cup of peppermint tea can help relieve congestion from seasonal allergies and may also ease breathing difficulties due to mild asthma. It certainly can't hurt.

Flush Away Your Allergies with a Neti Pot

What if you could just rinse away those annoying allergens so you can enjoy an outdoor picnic with your family? Well, with a small gadget called a neti pot, you can. Resembling a palm-size Aladdin's lamp and found at most health food stores, a neti pot is designed to flush water from one side of your nose to the other. Here's how it works.

- Fill the pot with warm saltwater (about 1 teaspoon of salt per cup of water).
- While leaning over a sink, tilt your head to the left and tip the spout into your right nostril. The liquid should trickle out the opposite nostril, "power washing" your nasal passages on its trip through.
- Continue until the pot is empty, then blow your nose and repeat on the opposite side.

Although it sounds simple, it works! Studies on children and adults who used nasal irrigation (a fancy name for flushing saltwater through your nose) found that those who practiced the technique found that their symptoms significantly improved, and they used considerably fewer antihistamines than those who didn't use irrigation.

Pycnogenol

Pycnogenol is an extract of the bark of pine trees that grow near the sea in France. Studies find that it appears to inhibit the release of histamine. Pycnogenol has some anti-inflammatory effects, inhibiting production of pro-inflammatory chemicals such as leukotrienes, cytokines, and adhesion molecules. It also relieves swelling, supporting easier breathing and reducing hives.

What the studies show: In one study, 22 adults with asthma received either 1 milligram of Pycnogenol per pound of body weight each day (up to 200 grams per day) or a placebo for four weeks. Lung function values in the Pycnogenol group rose significantly, from an average of 60 percent to 71 percent. At the same time, the number of leukotrienes in the participants' blood dropped, as did their ratings on the asthma severity scale.

Precautions: None.

Bottom line: You can try it with your doctor's knowledge.

Saiboku-to (TJ-96)

This herbal preparation has been approved by the Japanese government for the treatment of asthma, contains 10 herbs, including ginger, Korean ginseng, magnolia, Baikal skullcap, and licorice. Studies show it's pretty effective, primarily because it appears to reduce eosinophilic inflammation, a hallmark of asthma, by interfering with production of leukotrienes.

What the studies show: In a double-blind, placebo-controlled study conducted in Tokyo, researchers gave subjects either 2.5 grams of TJ-96 or a placebo three times a day for four weeks. While on the herbal preparation, the participants' symptoms and levels of eosinophils in their blood and sputum significantly decreased. In another study, 40 asthma patients were treated with Saiboku-to for 6 to 24 months, and all were able to greatly reduce their use of steroidal asthma medications.

Precautions: TJ-96 may interact with allergy and asthma medications. It may also increase and prolong effects of steroids when taken with them.

Bottom line: It may be worth trying; be sure your doctor knows so your medication can be adjusted if necessary.

Stinging Nettle

Stinging nettle is a common weed found throughout the world. As its name implies, it can leave you with a nasty stinging sensation if you brush up against its prickly leaves. But those leaves contain a plethora of chemicals and vitamins that give the plant its anti-allergy and anti-asthma properties. For one, they are high in quercetin, the flavonoid we discussed in chapter 9 that helps reduce the release of histamine and blocks inflammation. The leaves are also high in the antioxidant vitamins A and C, and vitamin C also acts as a natural antihistamine. The plant's history as a remedy for asthma dates back to the first century A.D., when Greek physicians used it to treat the disease.

What the studies show: In one randomized, double-blind study, 98 participants with allergies were given either 1,300 milligrams of nettle leaf or a placebo. Overall, 58 percent rated nettle leaf higher than the placebo, reporting a slight reduction in symptoms of hay fever, including sneezing and itchy eyes.

Precautions: None, but don't take it if you're allergic to it.

Bottom line: It doesn't hurt, and it may help.

Tylophora

This plant is indigenous to India and is reputed to provide relief for people with bronchial asthma.

What the studies show: In five double-blind trials on the herb, the results were mixed. Several of the studies showed improvement, while two showed no differences between the herbal group and the placebo group.

Precautions: None.

Bottom line: If you want to give it a try, talk to your doctor.

buyer beware

As you can see, when it comes to alternative therapies, it really is a "buyer beware" world. Unlike pharmaceutical drugs, for which we know we have government oversight as a protection, there is little or no oversight when it comes to these remedies. Be sure to follow these four main rules when using alternative therapies.

1. **Discuss your interests** and plans with your regular doctor.
2. **Integrate them** into your traditional medical treatment. You should never stop taking prescribed medication or seeing a doctor just because you're using alternative therapies.
3. **Avoid remedies** that have been proven useless or dangerous.
4. **Follow directions** carefully.

Up to now, we have been talking mostly about remedies and therapies that require clear thought, expert advice, and good planning and judgment. In the next chapter, we offer advice for those moments—and we hope they're rare—in which you are faced with making an immediate decision about your asthma or allergies.

the right
responses

Choose the right doctor. Use the right medications.

Purge your home of allergens. Improve your diet. Choose the right supplements. Learn to relax. These are all part of sound, intelligent management of an ongoing fight against allergies and asthma; they're also crucial steps in the Breathe Easy Plan.

But we all know there is another side to these diseases: Dealing with an attack. At that moment, all the long-term solutions fade away, and the only thing on your mind is, "What do I do *now* to make this thing pass?"

Welcome to your response guide. In the following pages, we provide all sorts of practical advice for that most unwelcome event—a strong allergy or asthma attack. We've built this chapter as a sequence of scenarios because we know that such reactions take on many forms and intensity levels and occur at many inconvenient times and places.

Of course, if we had wanted to be superficial, we could have written this as a three-word chapter—namely "Take your medicine." As we hope you already know, the best thing you can do is to keep the right rescue medicines with you at all times so when an attack hits, you have the appropriate weapon to halt it. That applies regardless of the form and cause of your allergies or asthma.

In many of the scenarios presented here, we've included something to the effect of "and by accident, your medicine was left at home." It's during such times that knowing what to do is of crucial importance.

As we pulled these examples together, certain themes quickly emerged.

1. **If the reaction is strong,** and you lack the correct rescue medicine, get to a doctor right away. Don't feel guilty, don't feel ashamed, and don't feel you are being overly cautious. A strong asthma attack is serious business.

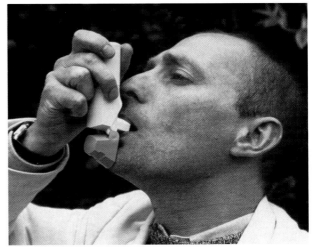

2. **Staying calm always helps.** It not only keeps those around you sane, it also helps mitigate the effect of the attack. Most of all, it helps you focus on the right things to do rather than panicking about the situation.

3. **If possible, immediately move** far away from the allergen or asthma trigger. Continued exposure will only make the attack worse.

The best thing you can do is to *keep the right rescue medicines with you at all times* so when an attack hits, you have the appropriate weapon to halt it.

The following 10 scenarios are all based on actual patient cases. See if you recognize yourself in any of them, and if so, pay close attention to the proper response. If you're lucky, you'll never need to use this wisdom, but if you aren't so fortunate, you'll be glad you had it.

Always check with your doctor before taking any treatment, regardless of whether it's a prescription or nonprescripton preparation.

1 You wake up in the morning with your head stuffed, your nose running, and your eyes streaming and red from allergies. You feel like death warmed over, but you have an important meeting at work in 2 hours at which you have to give a critical presentation. What should you do?

You definitely do not want to turn up half asleep and groggy for your important presentation! Here's what to do.

■ **Take a nonsedating antihistamine.** If you have a prescription medicine, take that; if not, stop at a drugstore and grab a package of loratadine (Claritin or Alavert), the only nonsedating antihistamine sold over the counter.

■ **Try a decongestant spray** such as oxymetazoline (Afrin) for nasal relief.

- **Use a nasal steroid** to help with the congestion. Using the decongestant first helps the steroid get into the nose.
- **Take some acetaminophen** (Tylenol) to ease the death-warmed-over feeling. *Don't* take aspirin or other nonsteroidal anti-inflammatory drugs such as naproxen (Aleve) or ibuprofen (Motrin); they may exacerbate your symptoms if you're allergic to them.
- **Eat the right breakfast** to give you an antioxidant boost for the day. Start with some cut-up fruit or a glass of orange juice for a vitamin C fix. Then choose either a spoonful of peanut butter spread on whole wheat toast or a bowl of high-fiber, fortified cereal for a good dose of vitamin E.
- **Use eyedrops** to reduce the swelling and redness. Another option is to sit with a cold compress on your eyes for a few minutes to relieve the itching and swelling.

2 You have no known food allergies, and you've even had skin tests in an allergist's office that showed no reaction. At a restaurant, you order a shrimp cocktail, which you've eaten dozens of times. Thirty minutes after eating the shrimp, right after finishing your entrée, you develop hives on your abdomen that quickly spread all over your body. At the same time, your face begins to swell and you have difficulty swallowing and severe nausea. What should you do?

We know that certain foods—particularly shrimp—can cause your body to release inflammatory chemicals such as histamine even without an IgE reaction. Thus, an allergy skin test may not indicate an allergy because those tests show only the presence of IgE antibodies.

If your reaction is truly as severe as described above, you are in a life-threatening situation, particularly if you're having trouble swallowing. You need to call (or have your dining companion or the waiter call) the paramedics immediately.

Even if you're experiencing only hives, it's possible that they are just the first part of the reaction. It could get much worse very quickly. Be particularly watchful for difficulty with swallowing. Also, be aware of any tingling in your lips or eyelids. Because the skin is thinnest and has a lot of blood vessels in these two areas, they're likely to swell the most.

If it's clear that your reaction is not progressing past a few hives or itching—and that's the typical case—you should still excuse yourself from the table and quickly find the nearest drugstore or grocery store to buy an over-the-counter antihistamine such as Claritin, Alavert, or diphenhydramine (Benadryl). Take it as directed.

No matter how the severe the reaction, *do not try to vomit.* You've already absorbed part of the food into your bloodstream, and vomiting just increases the risk that that you could inhale, or aspirate, particles of vomited food, which would make a bad situation much, much worse.

3 Your four-year-old has severe atopic dermatitis (eczema), and in the past couple of days, he has had a cold and a slight cough. On the third day of his cold, he suddenly begins breathing very rapidly, coughing, and wheezing in the middle of the night. What should you do?

We know that atopic dermatitis, an allergic skin rash, is very often the first sign of other allergic diseases, such as asthma and allergic rhinitis. What you're seeing with your child is probably infection-induced asthma. Viral infections are the number one triggers of asthma in young children.

Don't waste your time with over-the-counter decongestants and cough syrups. You want to get your child to the emergency room IMMEDIATELY. As you're pulling yourself and your child together for the trip to the hospital, though, there are a few things you can do to provide him with some relief.

- **Keep him hydrated.** The rapid breathing that comes with an asthma attack can be very dehydrating, so try to push liquids, preferably warm ones. Warm tea, which contains caffeine (a bronchodilator), can help. Also try chicken broth. The rich soup contains homocysteine, a chemical that helps break up and thin mucus. If neither of these is available, water will do, as long as it isn't cold.
- **Give acetaminophen for fever.** A high fever can also cause dehydration. Do *not* use aspirin. Not only can it stimulate an allergic reaction, but aspirin given for fever in children can lead to a dangerous condition called Reyes' syndrome.
- **Keep your child sitting quietly.** Read a book together, have him sit in your lap while you rock him, or pop a favorite video into the VCR or a story tape into the tape player. Activity can increase bronchial spasms, making the asthma worse.
- **Do *not* give him a cough suppressant.** It will just make him retain mucus, and you want him to cough. It's a normal physiologic mechanism to get the mucus out of his lungs.
- ***Never* give your child medicine containing codeine** (which many cough syrups contain) if he's breathing rapidly, which is a necessary defense. Codeine will slow his breathing, resulting in retention of more carbon dioxide.
- **Don't give your child any food.** While he is breathing so rapidly, he could aspirate food into his lungs, leading to serious pneumonia or other lung problems.
- **Be a source of calm.** Your child will quickly sense and mirror your emotions, particularly if you show anxiety, fear, or lack of control. Be reassuring and loving and make it seem that you know exactly what you are doing, no matter what's going on inside you.

4 You are scuba diving in Hawaii when you suddenly become short of breath. You didn't bring your asthma medication with you because you haven't had any problems for four years. Now you're underwater and having problems breathing. What should you do?

- **Get to the surface, but don't go any faster** than you're trained to go. You don't want to initiate a bad case of the bends on top of the asthma attack.
- **Get out of the water as quickly as possible,** because the cold water is probably making your breathing worse. Wrap yourself in a warm blanket. If there's hot coffee or tea on board the boat, try sipping that; the caffeine has a bronchodilating effect, and the warmth will relax constricted airways. Also ask the captain if there is any epinephrine aboard; on some boats, it's included in emergency medical kits. Finally, do all you can to calm yourself. It's possible that the excitement and tension of your undersea excursion helped bring on the attack. Close your eyes and relax. It's at times like these that knowing a formal relaxation method, such as those discussed in chapter 10, is most useful.
- **Cut the trip short** if the warming and calming don't curtail the attack within a few minutes. You need to get to a doctor as soon as you reach shore. Gasp out your apologies as best you can so there's no mutiny. And next time, take your inhaler. Asthma is as unpredictable as the weather.

5 You've been diagnosed with allergies and asthma and are on a treatment regimen to control both. You're on a plane home from a wonderful vacation when all of a sudden, you develop chest tightness and shortness of breath. You mistakenly packed your medications in your luggage, which you checked. What should you do?

The bottom line is that you should never, ever check your medication with your luggage, no matter what kind of medication it is or what disease it's for. Having said that, there are a few things you can do if you don't have your medication with you.

- **Let the flight attendant know** what's going on. Some airlines carry emergency medical kits that include epinephrine.
- **Ask the flight attendant** to have the pilot make an announcement to ask if there's a physician on the plane. The doctor may be able to assess the seriousness of the situation better than you can and make an objective determination about whether you should land. She may also have a medical kit along.
- **Have the pilot make an announcement** to ask if anyone has a short-acting

bronchodilator medication available. Given that 5 to 10 percent of the population has asthma, it's quite likely that someone is sitting on the plane with their own rescue medication close at hand.

- **Try sipping hot coffee or tea.** Caffeine acts as a mild bronchodilator, and the warmth itself can often help relax airway spasms. Avoid iced drinks; they will only make the spasms worse.
- **Practice a relaxation exercise.** Close your eyes, visualize yourself in a safe, quiet place, and focus on your breathing, envisioning it gradually becoming slower and deeper.

6 Your asthma has been fairly well controlled for several months, but lately, you've been under a lot of stress at work and at home. Suddenly, you wake up in the middle of the night fighting to breathe. You're having an asthma attack, but you haven't refilled your prescription, and there's no medication in the house. What should you do?

It's really important that you realize that just because your asthma is well controlled, you can't stop taking your medicine. Too many people think that if they're feeling better, they can stop their meds, but the reality is that the medicine is the *reason* they're feeling better. Asthma is a chronic condition like high blood pressure or diabetes, and you wouldn't stop taking insulin just because your diabetes was well controlled, would you? Yet some of the worst cases seen in emergency rooms are people who stopped taking their asthma medication. Obviously, the stress you're under has exacerbated your underlying condition, and boom! There you are in the midst of an asthma attack.

Okay, the lecture's over. Now here's what you do.

- **Make yourself a pot of coffee or a cup of hot tea.** The caffeine and warmth will help open constricted bronchial passages.
- **Don't eat.** Forget that leftover doughnut. Eating when you're in the midst of an asthma attack could result in inhaling particles of food into your lungs.
- **Practice some of the relaxation techniques** you learned about in chapter 10.
- **Don't take a cough suppressant.** That stuff will only keep the mucus in your chest and you *want* to cough it up, no matter how horrible it sounds or feels.
- **If you're still struggling to breathe after 5 minutes, you need to get help—** but make sure you have someone else drive you to the hospital or doctor's office. Carbon dioxide builds up in your lungs and bloodstream during an asthma attack; if the levels got too high, you could pass out at the wheel.

7 You've just moved to Phoenix, where you thought the dry air would be beneficial for your allergies and asthma. Yet here you are, it's your first week in town, the boxes are still packed, and you're wheezing like an 18-wheeler heading up a mountain. You're not about to move again. What should you do?

This is advice that way too many people with asthma and allergies receive: Move to a dry climate, and your condition will improve. Not true. If you're allergic in Minnesota, you're going to be allergic in Phoenix. In fact, dry air exacerbates asthma in some people. Not only that, but transplants to Phoenix have planted so many nonnative trees, such as the mulberry tree, that the city now has one of the highest pollen counts anywhere.

So keep unpacking. Once you find your address book:

■ **Call your allergy/asthma specialist** in your former place of residence and ask for a referral to a new doctor in Phoenix.

■ **Make an appointment** with the new doctor immediately for a complete evaluation and medication check.

■ **Consider having your new home professionally cleaned.** As we've discussed in earlier chapters, cat hair is ubiquitous and nearly impossible to get rid of with just regular vacuuming and cleaning. Plus, all the commotion of moving may be stirring up massive amounts of dust and allergens, be it those left behind in the house or those you just imported in the possessions you're unpacking. A professional cleaning may be what's needed to get your new home ready for living.

■ **Begin making environmental changes** to your surroundings like those described in step 3 of the Breathe Easy Plan in the interim—before the doctor's appointment and before the cleaners turn up.

8 You're visiting your sister in Minneapolis. She has a cat but has given it to a neighbor during your visit because she knows you're severely allergic. Within 10 minutes of sitting down on her couch, you know it doesn't matter; you begin sneezing, coughing, and dripping. What should you do?

Even though the cat is bunking next door, remnants of its presence are everywhere. The antigen that's causing your reaction comes from the cat's saliva, urine, and dander. Because cats lick themselves so much, their hair is very sticky, so all the vacuuming in the world isn't going to get it out of the carpet and upholstery. Here's what to do.

■ **Tell your sister how much you appreciate her** trying to make your visit more comfortable for you. Explain what we just told you about cat allergens and how difficult it is to get rid of them.

- ■ **Ask her to recommend** a nearby hotel.
- ■ **Check in** at the hotel.
- ■ **Buy your sister a really nice dinner** to soothe any remaining hurt feelings.

9 You're doing your Christmas shopping, and the mall is crowded and over-heated. As you walk into Macy's, the strong scent of perfumes from the cosmetics counter at the front of the store hits you like a brick wall. You begin wheezing and feel your chest tightening. What should you do?

- ■ **Get far away from any asthma trigger.** Either leave that part of the store or go to another store. If it's cold outside, don't go out; the cold air will just make your asthma worse.
- ■ **Take your rescue medications or try to enjoy a hot cup of coffee or tea;** relax with the soothing warmth of the liquid as you start to feel the bronchodilating effects of the caffeine.
- ■ **Take the afternoon off if you can,** go home and change into your most comfortable sweats, pop in a DVD or video of *It's a Wonderful Life*, and remember what the season is *really* about while you sip hot chocolate. You were probably also stressed by the pre-holiday commotion and pressure. A crowded, overheated mall can do that. Later that evening, when you're calm and your asthma has subsided, go online and finish your Christmas shopping the dot.com way.

10 It's Thanksgiving weekend, and you're having a pickup football game with some friends when you suddenly feel as if you can't breathe. You've never been diagnosed with asthma. What should you do?

Exercise is a trigger for a majority of people with asthma. That's why you should use your bronchodilator 15 to 30 minutes *before* you exercise, especially if you're exercising in cold outdoor air.

- ■ **If you've never been diagnosed** with asthma, though, you probably don't have an inhaler. In that case, you should try to get inside into warm air as quickly as possible, since the cold air is probably making the exercise-induced asthma worse. At the very least, sit in someone's car with the heater running. Also, ask if anyone in the game has an inhaler you can borrow.
- ■ **If your condition doesn't improve** after you warm up and your body relaxes from the exertion of the game (this should take just 5 to 10 minutes), have someone drive you to the nearest medical center. And first thing Monday morning, make an appointment with an allergy/asthma specialist for a complete evaluation. Even if exercise turns out to be the only trigger for your asthma, you still may need to be on inhaled steroids.

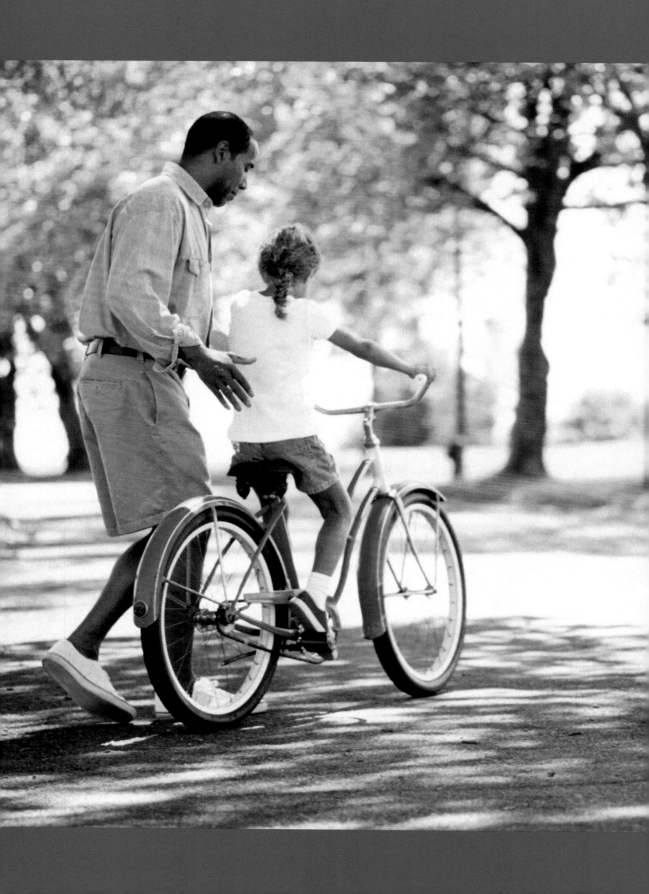

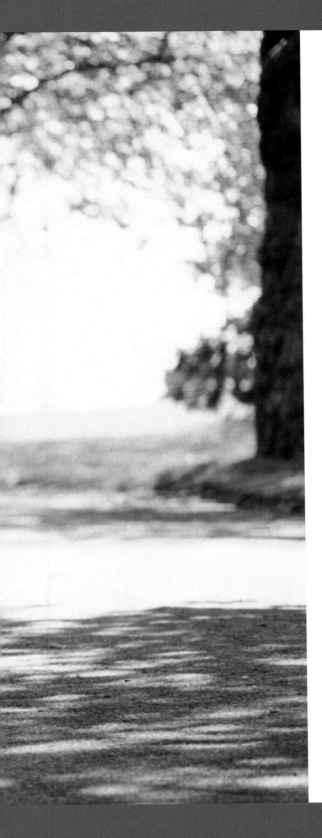

the
breathe
easy plan

Congratulations! By reading this far, you've gained the knowledge you need to control allergies and asthma. Now, with the seven-step Breathe Easy Plan, you'll also have all the specific steps, advice, and wisdom to use that knowledge to end the attacks and fully control your condition.

welcome
to the plan

So now you've come to it: The heart of the book—the Breathe Easy Plan to beat allergies and asthma. We believe we have created the most thorough and effective action plan available for taking control of the allergies or asthma that have been troubling you or your family.

We also know that there is no such thing as a one-size-fits-all plan. Not only do the nature and intensity of allergies and asthma vary with each person, so do schedules, family commitments, financial resources, and levels of motivation. Don't let these issues deter you, though. We've built this plan to be easily adaptable to almost any scenario. In essence, we have taken the seven most important components of allergy and asthma control and given you the tools, tips, and directions to master each, based on your own needs and resources.

here's how we recommend you do the plan

1. Skim all seven steps so you understand what you'll be doing.

2. While we would prefer that you follow the steps in order, it's not mandatory, with the exception of step 1. You definitely need to complete that step first, regardless of where you turn next. It provides a road map to help you understand where your priorities should lie and which steps you should focus on.

3. Think through any issues of timing and effort. Step 2, for example, requires a doctor's visit. Given doctors' schedules today, that will take some advance scheduling, so make the appointment right away. Likewise, step 3 involves some intense housecleaning, reorganization, and a potential financial investment. It may make sense to clear a few days to do the work.

4. Understand that there are no time limits for each step. This is not a weight-loss program that knocks off a few pounds a week for 12 weeks and then is over. Rather, the Breathe Easy Plan is intended for a lifetime of allergy and asthma control. Do each step fully, and you'll have taken control of your condition.

5. In many cases, we give you a menu of tips to consider. Read them all, then pick those that make the most sense for your situation and condition. The trick is to *always take action*. Reading sensible advice is one thing, but the Breathe Easy Plan won't deliver on its promise of better health unless you act on that advice.

6. Enlist your family and your doctor. Don't hide the fact that you're reading this book and following the plan. Announce it proudly and firmly: You have decided that you've had enough with your allergies and asthma and are taking action. Ask for their help. Let them know that the benefits stretch far beyond allergies and asthma; everyone in the household will be much healthier as a result of these steps.

7. If you wish to do the plan for a spouse or child, terrific! Understand, though, that the chances of success are far greater if the other person is actively involved in the process. Their motivation and participation not only make doing the plan easier but also give them the mental edge in making it succeed. Plus, there is only so much you can do for someone else, since some of the steps mandate skills and strategies (such as new breathing techniques) that are entirely personal.

8. Finally, this is not a do-it-once-and-be-done program. You should return to this section of the book every six months or so for fine-tuning, implementing suggestions that may not have worked for you earlier but may fit with your life better now. Make copies of the charts and questions included throughout the section and keep them after you fill them out so you can see your progress.

STEP ONE

determine your situation

If you've read this far, your suspicions about allergies and asthma have probably been confirmed: Both come in many forms, for many reasons, which makes them particularly hard to diagnose.

Our goal in step 1 of the Breathe Easy Plan is to help you come to a clear and correct assessment of your situation. What is it that you're most likely allergic to? How serious is your asthma? When do symptoms tend to hit?

Now, we are not advocates of self-diagnosis. As we have said repeatedly, it takes a trained, experienced doctor to make the official diagnosis of a medical condition. But armed with evidence you'll glean from this part of the plan, you will be able to help your doctor more easily make an accurate diagnosis.

What you will be doing

Filling out five forms to reveal all aspects of your allergies and/or asthma.

How you should prepare

Before starting the forms, talk to people who know you well about their perceptions of your allergies and/or asthma. Good candidates are coworkers, your spouse, your children, and good friends (particularly those with whom you spend time outdoors). They may have noticed certain things of which you aren't aware. For instance, maybe your eyes always water when you visit Aunt Mary (she has a cat). Or perhaps your asthma seems much worse in the spring (a clue that you may have allergic asthma).

What to have on hand

Copies of the forms. You can write in the book, but then you may have to leave the book with your doctor, and you know how that could turn out. It's better to make photocopies. A clipboard or folder to keep them together. And, of course, a couple of no. 2 pencils.

could it be allergies?

Answer these 10 questions will help ascertain whether you do indeed have allergies.

1 My nose often runs with a thin, clear discharge.   YES ☐   NO ☐

2 I regularly have itchy, watery eyes, often with uncontrollable sneezing fits.   YES ☐   NO ☐

3 I am frequently kept awake at night by nasal congestion or an unproductive, hacking cough.   YES ☐   NO ☐

4 I breathe through my mouth because my nose is too stopped up.   YES ☐   NO ☐

5 I often have a tickling or itching feeling in my nose, leading me to rub the bottom of my nose for relief (the so-called allergic salute).   YES ☐   NO ☐

6 I sometimes become weak, irritable, or fatigued or have problems concentrating.   YES ☐   NO ☐

7 I have dark circles under my eyes.   YES ☐   NO ☐

8 Windy days, especially in the spring and fall, cause me to have coldlike symptoms.   YES ☐   NO ☐

9 I get unexplained, itchy skin rashes.   YES ☐   NO ☐

10 Coldlike symptoms emerge or get worse when I do certain activities, like vacuuming, cleaning the cat litter box, or gardening.   YES ☐   NO ☐

THE RESULTS: If you answered *yes* to two or more of these questions, it's likely you have allergies. The more *yes* answers, the more likely that you have the problem. The next form will help determine the nature of your allergies.

seasonal or perennial?

The frequency of your allergic reactions can help determine both the cause and the treatment. If you have symptoms for only a week or two out of the year due to a specific pollen, you may be able to get by with just over-the-counter antihistamines and decongestants. However, if you're like the majority of patients with allergies who have ongoing symptoms that worsen during certain times of the year, you might be a good candidate for a fuller regimen of medicine and preventive care.

Complete this tracking log to determine the timing of your allergies. For each month, check off the symptoms you experience and the time of day when they are most prevalent. If they seem to last all day and night, put a check in each box.

continued »

Month (time of day)	Runny nose	Stuffy nose	Hives or rashes	Red, itchy eyes	Teary eyes	Sneezing fits	Difficulty breathing	Itching	Scratchy throat	Chronic cough	Wheezing
January											
Day (6 A.M. to 6 P.M.)											
Night (6 P.M. to 6 A.M.)											
February											
Day											
Night											
March											
Day											
Night											
April											
Day											
Night											
May											
Day											
Night											
June											
Day											
Night											
July											
Day											
Night											
August											
Day											
Night											
September											
Day											
Night											
October											
Day											
Night											
November											
Day											
Night											
December											
Day											
Night											

THE RESULTS: With this log, your doctor should be able to make some good guesses as to what sorts of allergens are causing you the most trouble. But what can you learn from it? First, if you have five or more boxes marked, or if there's a clear pattern to your marks, you probably do have an allergy that requires medical treatment. If most of the marks are in the "Night" boxes, it's likely that allergens in your house are causing the problem. Daytime symptoms suggest that work or outdoor allergens are responsible.

allergy responses and triggers

Think about where you were, what you ate, and what you were doing when your attacks occurred. Check off each box that applies and list specific items where applicable.

Allergy trigger	Runny nose	Stuffy nose	Hives or rashes	Red, itchy eyes	Teary eyes	Sneezing fits	Difficulty breathing	Swelling of face and throat	Facial flushing	Abdominal pain or cramping	Diarrhea
Foods											
Shellfish (list)											
Peanuts											
Eggs											
Wheat											
Soy											
Nuts											
Dairy products (list)											
Other (list)											
Beverages											
Alcoholic beverages (list)											
Fruit juices with dyes (list)											
Other (list)											
Medications (list specific drugs or types)											
Antibiotics											
Pain medications											
Anesthetics											
Other (list)											
Indoor environment											
Dust											
Mold											
Cleaning products (list)											
Other (list)											
Outdoor environment											
Weeds, trees, or grasses											
Windy days											
Other (list)											
Animals											
Dogs											
Cats											
Insects (list)											
Other (list)											

THE RESULTS: Show this form to your doctor so he can analyze your answers and focus on the right allergens to test for.

could it be asthma?

So far, we've focused mostly on allergies. Now it's time to determine whether your symptoms are related to asthma. Carefully answer these questions, which are adapted from a quiz created by the American College of Allergy, Asthma, and Immunology.

1 When I walk or do simple chores, I often have trouble breathing, or I cough.   YES ☐ NO ☐

2 When I perform heavier work, such as walking up hills and stairs or doing chores that involve lifting, I have trouble breathing, or I cough.   YES ☐ NO ☐

3 Sometimes I avoid exercising or taking part in sports like jogging, swimming, tennis, or aerobics because I have trouble breathing.   YES ☐ NO ☐

4 I am sometimes unable to sleep through the night without coughing attacks or shortness of breath.   YES ☐ NO ☐

5 Sometimes I can't catch a good, deep breath.   YES ☐ NO ☐

6 Sometimes I have wheezing sounds in my chest for no clear reason.   YES ☐ NO ☐

7 Sometimes my chest feels tight for no clear reason.   YES ☐ NO ☐

8 Sometimes I cough a lot for no clear reason.   YES ☐ NO ☐

9 Dust, pollen, and pets make my coughing or breathing troubles worse.   YES ☐ NO ☐

10 My coughing or breathing troubles get worse in cold weather.   YES ☐ NO ☐

11 My coughing or breathing troubles get worse when I'm around tobacco smoke, fumes, or strong odors.   YES ☐ NO ☐

12 When I catch a cold, it often goes to my chest.   YES ☐ NO ☐

13 My breathing problems control my life more than I would like.   YES ☐ NO ☐

14 I feel tension or stress because of my breathing problems. YES ☐ NO ☐

15 I worry that my breathing problems affect my health or may even shorten my life.   YES ☐ NO ☐

THE RESULTS: Each *yes* answer is consistent with symptoms of asthma. The more *yes* answers you have, the greater the need to seek a professional evaluation.

how severe is my asthma?

As first discussed in chapter 4, there are four generally accepted levels of severity with asthma. Often, a doctor will base his medication recommendations on the category in which you fall (more on that in step 2 of the Breathe Easy Plan). The following questions will help you determine your particular level.

Do you...

1. Have symptoms twice a week or less, and nighttime symptoms twice a month or less?   YES ☐   NO ☐
2. Have symptoms that are brief, lasting from a few hours to a few days, with the intensity of the attack varying?   YES ☐   NO ☐
3. Have no symptoms between more severe episodes?   YES ☐   NO ☐

If you answered *yes* to these questions, you probably have **mild intermittent** asthma.

Do you...

1. Have symptoms more than twice a week but less than once a day, and nighttime symptoms more than twice a month?   YES ☐   NO ☐
2. Have more severe episodes that sometimes affect your activity?   YES ☐   NO ☐

If you answered *yes* to these questions, you probably have **mild persistent** asthma.

Do you...

1. Have symptoms daily, and nighttime symptoms more than once a week?   YES ☐   NO ☐
2. Use a quick-relief medication daily?   YES ☐   NO ☐
3. Change your daily activities because of your asthma?   YES ☐   NO ☐
4. Have more severe episodes that occur twice a week or more and may last for days?   YES ☐   NO ☐

If you answered *yes* to 3 or more of these questions, you probably have **moderate persistent** asthma.

Do you...

1. Experience frequent severe episodes?   YES ☐   NO ☐
2. Have continual daytime symptoms and frequent nighttime symptoms?   YES ☐   NO ☐
3. Have symptoms that cause you to limit your activity?   YES ☐   NO ☐

If you answered *yes* to these questions, you probably have **severe persistent** asthma.

concluding step 1

There's a saying that goes, you can't find the right solution if you don't know what the problem is. With these forms filled out, you should have a much better handle on the scope and nature of your allergies and/or asthma.

That's good on many fronts. First, you have the perfect data to help your doctor choose the right tests to do, prescribe the best medicines for your situation, and direct you to the right lifestyle fixes. Second, you now know enough to target your own efforts against allergies or asthma. After all, your doctor is not going to wash your sheets, monitor your food choices, vacuum your carpets, or talk to your boss about the lousy ventilation at work. That's up to you!

If you've never seen a doctor to discuss allergies or asthma, now is the time. In fact, that's the first part of step 2.

What if you've already visited a doctor about your condition and are taking prescription medications? If your findings here surprise you at all or shed new light on your condition, then you should set up a new appointment. Tell the doctor you've been reading this book and that after doing a thorough review of your symptoms and attacks, you realize that you haven't provided the full picture. Explain that you've been learning about allergy and asthma medicines and would like a fuller discussion of what you're taking and whether it should change. Once you do this, you've probably taken the biggest step of all toward breathing easier.

STEP TWO

create your arsenal for relief

Without question, there are many important and effective ways to manage allergies and asthma that don't involve medicine. In fact, the next five steps of the Breathe Easy Plan will detail them clearly. But not even the most extreme alternative healers would say that modern medicine shouldn't be a significant part of your battle against allergies and asthma.

In this step of the Breathe Easy Plan, we are going to achieve three crucial things:

- Get you to the right doctor for your particular situation
- Help you understand the very best medications for your particular situation
- Make sure that you are managing your medicines as smartly as possible

This step is particularly useful if you have not yet seen a doctor about your condition, but even if you have, go through the entire process. With your new knowledge of your condition and how the medicines for it work, along with a renewed commitment to improve your situation, a review of your medicinal arsenal—as well as your effectiveness in deploying it—is extremely valuable.

What you will be doing

First, you'll set up a doctor's appointment. Then you and your doctor will determine the best medicine for your needs. (Do you need preventive medication? Should your prescriptions be changed?) Next, you'll figure out what you need to do to guarantee that you're taking your medicine optimally. Finally, you'll consider using a regimen of supplements that we propose.

How you should prepare

Reread chapters 7 and 10. Be ready for a trip to the doctor's office and then a visit to the drugstore.

What to have on hand

All the forms you filled out in step 1. A list of all the medicines and supplements you're taking, not just for allergies or asthma but for any other conditions as well (we provide the form on page 191).

choosing the right doctor

If you're like many people who have health insurance, you have little choice about whom to see for allergies or asthma: It's your primary care physician. Even if you aren't encumbered by insurance rules, that's the logical first doctor to see. That said, you should know whether seeing a specialist might also be appropriate for your condition. Answer these questions carefully to find out.

1   I have had a life-threatening asthma attack at some time in my life.
YES ☐   NO ☐

2   I am not meeting the goals of my asthma therapy after three to six months of treatment, or my doctor believes I am not responding to current therapy.   YES ☐   NO ☐

3   My symptoms are unusual or difficult to diagnose.   YES ☐   NO ☐

4   I have other conditions such as severe hay fever or sinusitis that complicate my diagnosis. YES ☐   NO ☐

5   My doctor has never run any diagnostic tests to determine the severity of my asthma and what causes my symptoms.   YES ☐   NO ☐

6   I'd like to consider immunotherapy.   YES ☐   NO ☐

7   I have severe persistent asthma.   YES ☐   NO ☐

8   I use continuous oral corticosteroid therapy or high-dose inhaled cortico-steroids and/or have taken more than two bursts of oral corticosteroids in one year.   YES ☐   NO ☐

9   I have made one or more emergency visits to a doctor or emergency room due to asthma or breathing problems in the past year.   YES ☐   NO ☐

10   I have had one or more overnight hospi-talizations due to asthma or breathing problems in the past year. YES ☐   NO ☐

11   I feel that I use my asthma inhaler too often.   YES ☐   NO ☐

12   Sometimes I don't like the way my asthma medicine(s) make me feel.
YES ☐   NO ☐

13   My asthma medicine doesn't control my symptoms.   YES ☐   NO ☐

THE RESULTS: If you answered *yes* to one or more questions, it's time to consider a specialist. Make a strong case to your primary care physician, showing him your answers to these questions. To find a specialist, start with recommendations from your doctor, friends, and relatives or refer to the web-sites of either of the two major professional associations—the American College of Allergy, Asthma, and Immunology (www.acaai.org) or the American Academy of Allergy, Asthma, and Immunology (www.aaaai.org). Both allow you to search for a board-certified allergist by zip code.

Before your appointment, send the doctor the forms from the previous section (step 1). Finally, fill out and take along a copy of the medication log on the next page.

breathe easy medication log

Use this log to inventory all medicines and supplements that you use on a regular basis. We recommend that you keep this updated and post it on your refrigerator or another place where you'll see it every day.

Medication	What's it for?	Date started	Dose	Times per day	Prescribing doctor	Side effects? (yes or no)
Daily vitamins/supplements						
Frequently used over-the-counter (OTC) medicines						
Asthma/allergy medicines						
Other prescription medicines						

allergy medicines

Although only your doctor can prescribe the appropriate medication for allergic rhinitis, this chart gives you the specifics of which medications are best for which symptoms, providing you with the information you need to get the discussion going. Take it with you to the doctor's office if you want a handy reference during your discussion.

Medication class	Brand name (prescription)
Sneezing	
Topical corticosteroid nasal sprays	Beconase AQ, Flonase, Nasacort AQ, Nasalide, Nasarel, Nasonex, Rhinocort AQ, Vancenase DS or Vancenase pocket inhaler
Antihistamines	Allegra, Astelin (nasal), Clarinex, Zyrtec
Mast cell stabilizer	Nasalcrom
Leukotriene modifier	Singulair
Itchy nose and throat	
Topical corticosteroid nasal sprays	Beconase AQ, Flonase, Nasacort AQ, Nasalide, Nasarel, Nasonex, Rhinocort AQ, Vancenase DS or Vancenase pocket inhaler
Antihistamines	Allegra, Astelin (nasal), Clarinex, Zyrtec
Mast cell stabilizer	Nasalcrom
Leukotriene modifier	Singulair
Runny nose	
Topical corticosteroid nasal sprays	Beconase AQ, Flonase, Nasacort AQ, Nasalide, Nasarel, Nasonex, Rhinocort AQ, Vancenase DS or Vancenase pocket inhaler
Antihistamines	Allegra, Astelin (nasal), Clarinex, Zyrtec
Mast cell stabilizer	Nasalcrom
Anticholinergic spray	Atrovent nasal
Leukotriene modifier	Singulair
Nasal congestion	
Topical corticosteroid nasal sprays	Beconase AQ, Flonase, Nasacort AQ, Nasalide, Nasarel, Nasonex, Rhinocort AQ, Vancenase DS or Vancenase pocket inhaler
Decongestants	Allegra-D, Claritin-D, Guaifed PD, Sinuvent, Zyrtec
Mast cell stabilizer	Nasalcrom
Antihistamine nasal spray	Astelin
Allergic conjunctivitis	
Antihistamines	Emadine, Livostin
Combination antihistamine/decongestants	Naphcon-A, Ocuhist, Prefrin, VasoClear, Vasocon-A
Mast cell stabilizers	Alocril, Alomide, Crolom or Opticrom
Nonsteroidal anti-inflammatory	Acular
Combination antihistamine/mast cell stabilizer	Elastat, Optivar, Patanol, Zaditor

Brand name (OTC)	Best way to use
	Daily as a preventive. Make sure your nose is clear enough for the spray to penetrate; you may need to use a decongestant first.
Alavert, Benadryl, Chlor-Trimeton, Claritin, Dimetapp, Tavist-1	Take 2 to 5 hours before exposure to allergens. If you're constantly exposed, take daily.
	Start using 2 to 4 weeks before exposure to allergens.
	Daily as a preventive.
	Daily as a preventive. Make sure your nose is clear enough for the spray to penetrate; you may need to use a decongestant first.
Alavert, Benadryl, Chlor-Trimeton, Claritin, Dimetapp, Tavist-1	Take 2 to 5 hours before exposure to allergens. If you're constantly exposed, take daily.
	Start using 2 to 4 weeks before exposure to allergens.
	Daily as a preventive.
	Daily as a preventive. Make sure your nose is clear enough for the spray to penetrate; you may need to use a decongestant first.
Alavert, Benadryl, Chlor-Trimeton, Claritin, Dimetapp, Tavist-1	Take 2 to 5 hours before exposure to allergens. If you're constantly exposed, take daily.
	Start using 2 to 4 weeks before exposure to allergens.
	Works best preventively.
	Daily as a preventive. Make sure your nose is clear enough for the spray to penetrate; you may need to use a decongestant first.
Oral forms: Phenylephrine (found in numerous OTC products), pseudoephedrine (Sudafed) *Sprays:* Afrin, Allerest, Dristan Long Lasting, Neo-Synephrine, Otrivin, Privine, Vicks Sinex, Vicks Sinex Long Lasting	Be especially careful with nasal decongestants; don't take them longer or more often than the recommended dosage schedule or you may wind up with rebound congestion.
	Start using 2 to 4 weeks before exposure to allergens.
	Can be used preventively and to treat symptoms.
Clear Eyes, Visine	Use during peak pollen season in addition to regular medications.
	Short-acting relief of symptoms
	Start using 2 to 4 weeks before exposure to allergens.
	Symptomatic relief of symptoms
	Can be used preventively and to treat symptoms.

asthma medicines

Here are the standard medication therapies for the four categories of asthma (you should have determined yours in step 1). Talk to your doctor to see if these medicines are appropriate for you.

Daily medication needed?	Daily inhaled cortico-steroid	Leukotriene modifier	Inhaled cromolyn	Theo-phylline	Daily long-lasting beta2-agonist	Oral steroids	Short-acting beta2-agonist
Recommended Medications							
Mild intermittent							
No	Possibly*	No	No	No	No	No	As needed
Mild persistent							
Yes	Low or medium dose	Possibly	Possibly**	Possibly	No	No	As needed
Moderate persistent							
Yes	Medium dose	Possibly	No	Possibly	Yes	No	As needed
Severe persistent							
Yes	High dose	Possibly	No	Possibly	Yes	Possibly	As needed

* low dose and only if symptoms occur more than twice a week
** in lieu of inhaled corticosteroid

managing your rescue medications

Just to remind you, "rescue medications" are the inhalers, pills, or liquids that you use when an asthma or allergy attack occurs. Having them immediately available is essential for controlling the attack. As we're all aware, though, you just never know when the next trigger will trip and you'll wind up gasping for breath. So where to keep it? Here's our plan for ensuring that you always have your rescue medications at hand.

☐ **Keep them everywhere.** If you can afford it, buy a supply of rescue medicines and store one of each wherever you spend significant amounts of time. In addition, place one of each in your most-used purse, briefcase, computer case, or gym bag.

   Let's say you're a businessperson who works out at a gym and occasionally goes on business trips. You may wish to keep five sets of rescue medications:

• At home
• At work
• In your car
• In your gym locker
• In your travel toiletry case

Other places you should consider include:

• With your gardening supplies
• In your home workshop
• In a fanny pack used during walks or exercise
• In a drawer in your bedside table

the breathe easy alternative remedies program

In chapter 10, we provided a thorough review of the many vitamins, minerals, and herbs that are believed to be helpful in managing allergies and asthma. Now's the time to take action. We recommend the following four-part program to complement (not replace!) your medicinal remedies.

- **A daily multivitamin/mineral supplement.** Be sure it includes magnesium, selenium, vitamin C, vitamin E, beta-carotene, and all the B vitamins (thiamin, riboflavin, niacin, B_6, B_{12}, folic acid, biotin, and pantothenic acid).
- A cup of **peppermint or chamomile tea** each night before bed.
- Your choice of one of the following herbal supplements: **butterbur, dried ivy leaf, or Pycnogenol**.
- A daily dose of **echinacea** (follow the package directions) taken two weeks on, two weeks off.

Be sure you check with your doctor before taking these or any other supplements, no matter how innocent they appear, because they may interact with prescription or over-the-counter medications you're taking.

☐ **Stock other supplies, too.** Often during attacks, you need tissues, water, or other personal items. At a minimum, as a courtesy to yourself and others, keep a box of tissues wherever you spend lots of time, be it the car, the office, or the family room. Also keep a supply of bottled water in the pantry, and be sure to have bottles in the car, at work, and in the workshop.

☐ **Create a kit.** If you can't afford to have duplicate sets of medicine, create a single but truly effective kit that goes in a small, attractive carrying case. Make it small enough that it isn't burdensome but large enough that it's not easily lost or forgotten. Think of the kit as you do a cell phone—something you need to keep near you as you go through your day. Probably,

it'll go in a purse or briefcase. Be sure to include your name and phone number in case you happen to leave it somewhere. Also include a set of instructions for exactly what to do when an attack hits: The order in which to use the medicines, the dosages, how fast you should get relief, and any other things to do or watch for.

☐ **Track its use.** Each time you get a new inhaler, stick on a piece of masking tape. Mark the tape whenever you use the inhaler so you have a sense of when it's time to replace it.

☐ **Remember wintertime.** When cold air arrives, keep an inhaler or other rescue medicine in the pocket of your coat or jacket.

the take-your-medicine plan

Of course, all the medicine in the world isn't going to make any difference if you forget to take it or take it at the wrong time. There is no single foolproof system for managing your medicine, so instead, read the following advice and from it, create a personal plan.

☐ **Update the medication log** on page 191 to include your new medicines and supplements. Place a copy somewhere you'll see it every day.

☐ **Associate taking a medication** with an activity. For instance, when you brush your teeth in the morning, use your nasal cortico-steroid. When you eat dinner, take your anti-histamine.

☐ **Use alarms** on clocks, watches, cell phones, and computers to remind you when to take your medications. You can even buy elec-tronic medicine organizers that beep at pre-programmed times. Check in drugstores or at www.domorehealthcare.com.

☐ **Use pill boxes** and other special medication holders to organize your medications by hour, day, and week. Then you can easily see if you've forgotten a dose.

☐ **Keep your medications** in obvious places, such as the bathroom counter, so you see them first thing each morning. If you need to take them with meals, keep them on the kitchen table.

☐ **Use a medication diary,** available in drug-stores or online at numerous websites.

☐ **Take your medications together,** if possible. For example, if you're taking some in the morning and some at night, ask your doctor if you can take them all at one time.

With your medication log in hand and the preceding tips fresh in your mind, answer the following questions, then give yourself 48 hours to put your system in place.

1. Times I need to take my medicines: _____

_____

2. Routines I would like to establish for taking my medicines: _____

_____

_____

3. Reminders I will use to take my medicines: _____

_____

_____

4. Places I will keep my medicines: _____

_____

_____

5. Tools I will use to help manage my medicines: _____

_____

_____

6. A reward I will give myself for doing a good job: _____

_____

_____

STEP THREE

adapt your home

Aren't you glad you've completed the first two steps of the Breathe Easy Plan? You should be, for two big reasons. The first is obvious: knowing that you've gotten the right diagnosis of your condition and the best medicines for your situation. And the second? It's simply that for now, you're done with the world of doctors and health insurance companies. Starting with this step and continuing through the rest of the plan, you are in complete control of the decisions and actions.

Now that we're moving to the lifestyle and nutrition aspects of the plan, it's time to take on what is arguably the greatest challenge to your condition: your home. In this step, you'll systematically examine your home for allergy "hot spots" and do everything in your power to make them go away. Be prepared, though: There's a lot of cleaning involved, and you may wish to set aside a reasonable amount of money for a new vacuum, some better bedding, and other allergen-fighting aids. For those of you with serious allergy or asthma problems, it may be time for some bigger projects as well, such as getting rid of carpet. All of this will take some time and effort, but the payback will be enormous.

What you will be doing

First, you'll do a top-to-bottom inventory of your house to determine where allergens may be congregating. Then you'll tackle a room-by-room cleanup to get rid of the allergens that are there as well as make the rooms less hospitable to allergens in the future.

How you should prepare

Schedule at least one full day to do nothing but a major house inspection and cleaning. Wear comfortable clothes that you won't mind getting dirty. Be prepared to commit to follow-up projects over the next few weekends as well.

What to have on hand

Copies of the logs, questions, and charts in this step of the program. A pen or pencil. Cleaning supplies. A flashlight.

home inventory

Go into each room and use this inventory to mark off which allergen-harboring items and conditions you find there, then use it to determine which rooms to concentrate on and which you should tackle first.

Room	Carpet	Wallpaper	Clutter	Mold	Fabric furniture	Odor	
Bedroom 1							
Bedroom 2							
Bedroom 3							
Bedroom 4							
Bathroom 1							
Bathroom 2							
Bathroom 3							
Living room							
Family room							
Kitchen							
Dining room							
Home office							
Laundry room							
Attic							
Basement							
Other							

get cleaning: our best advice

Your task over the next few days or weeks is to clean out allergens in your house, attacking one room at a time. In general, your tasks include:

- Doing a thorough cleaning to get the room as close to being allergen-free as possible.
- Assessing which items in the room are hotbeds for allergens (use the inventory you just filled out) and taking preventive action to keep the allergens at bay. This could be as simple as changing your sheets more often or as intensive as replacing carpet with wood or linoleum flooring.
- Adding accessories, rearranging furniture, and doing other tasks that can greatly aid you in your fight against allergens.

Each apartment, house, and condo is different, and since we can't honestly say whether this project will take two days or two months, we recommend the following: Read all of our advice on cleaning your rooms, then go back to your inventory and think through what needs to be done in each room.

	Exhaust fan	Ceiling fan	Dust	Dampness	Insects	Wall hanging(s)	Window coverings

Entrance

You probably don't think much about the entrance to your house in relation to allergies, but it's the gateway to your home; whatever is outside gets dragged inside. Here are our instructions.

- ☐ Use a **doormat** made of synthetic material. A doormat made of natural material (such as rope or other fiber) can break down and become a home for mites, mold, and fungus, which then get tracked into the house. Wash all mats weekly.
- ☐ Clean all **dead insects** from porch lights. As they decompose, they can become an allergen source.
- ☐ Put a **shelf or rack** by the front door for footwear and encourage your family and guests to remove their shoes when entering. This will reduce the amount of dust, mold, and other allergens that are tracked in.
- ☐ Keep some **soft slippers** in a basket by the front door for people who don't relish going shoeless, whether it's because they have holes in their socks, they're self-conscious about their feet, or the floors are cold.
- ☐ If you have **carpeting** in your foyer, consider removing it. You want a hard floor for easy cleaning.

continued »

Bedrooms

First, make sure your bedroom is in the right location. If it's in the basement, move it. Any basement, even a finished one, is too damp for the amount of time you spend in the bedroom.

Next, clear out or modify all of the following; they're the worst things to have in your bedroom if you have allergies or asthma.

- **Wall-to-wall carpeting.** If possible, replace it with hard flooring and 100 percent wool area rugs that can be washed or dry-cleaned. If it's not possible to replace it, have it professionally cleaned once a year.
- **Blinds and curtains**, a.k.a. dust magnets.
- **Down-filled comforters**
- **Feather anything** (dust mites love feathers).
- **Stuffed animals**
- **Forced hot-air heating vents.** If you have this kind, use HEPA filter vent covers. You can get them at home improvement stores and some heating/air-conditioning retailers.
- **Pets.** Don't let dogs and cats in the bedroom at any time, and keep your door shut so they can't even cross the threshold.
- **Overstuffed closets.** It's time to give up your packrat ways (see below for tips).
- **Plants.** Ficus trees in particular may cause allergies in previously nonallergic people.
- **Upholstered headboard.** Switch to a metal or wooden bedstead.
- **Piles of pillows.** They look pretty, but they're dust-mite magnets.

Now, start cleaning

- ☐ **Tackle the dust** behind the bed and dressers, under the bed, and on top of the ceiling fan. Always use a damp cloth; dry cloths just spread the dust around.
- ☐ **Wipe every item** in your room, including books, knickknacks, perfume bottles, and jewelry boxes, with a damp cloth.
- ☐ **Wipe down the walls** and woodwork.
- ☐ If you're keeping the **curtains**, wash them in 130°F water.
- ☐ **Strip the bed** and wash everything, including the comforter or blankets, in 130°F water.
- ☐ **Vacuum the bed** with a vacuum equipped with a HEPA filter and wipe down the mattress with a damp rag.

And don't forget to…

- ☐ **Ventilate** your bedroom on a regular basis to minimize mold growth.
- ☐ Use **dust mite barrier** covers on mattresses and pillows in *all* bedrooms, even those whose occupants aren't allergic, to keep down the dust mite population in your house.

Closets

If you're embarrassed to open your closet doors in front of guests, it's likely that you're harboring not just a truckload of junk but also a plethora of allergens.

- ☐ Put clothing in **zippered plastic bags** and shoes in boxes off the floor
- ☐ **Declutter.** Give away coats and other clothing you haven't worn in the past year. Put sports equipment where it belongs. Slip shoes into hanging shoe bags, shoeboxes, or a shoe rack. When you finish, you should be able to clearly see the closet's floor and back wall.
- ☐ **Nix mothballs** in favor of cedar chips, or store clean woolens in sealed plastic bags or

airtight containers. You can also place garments in the freezer for several days to kill adult moths and larvae.

- ☐ Check **corners and walls** for mold; you may have a leak you've never noticed because it's in the back of a dark closet.
- ☐ Check for mold on any **boxes** and other containers stored in the closet.

- ☐ Before switching your clothes each season, **wash or dry-clean** the new season's clothing to get rid of any dust mites that have taken up residence.
- ☐ If dampness is a problem, put **a 75-watt bulb** in the light fixture and leave it on for long stretches to battle mold and mildew.

Bathrooms

Hot steam, flushing toilets, soggy toothbrushes—bathrooms are persistently warm and wet, making them the perfect home to mold and mildew.

- ☐ Check under and **behind toilets** to make sure there's no mold growing as a result of condensation. Make sure toilets are installed properly so water doesn't leak into the walls or floors, which could encourage mold.
- ☐ Check **under the vanity** for any leaks and mold. Throw out any damp items.
- ☐ Wash the **shower curtain** in hot water once a month or use a shower curtain liner that you can replace every couple of months for just a few bucks.
- ☐ Watch out for the slime that can grow in **shower door tracks;** make sure they're cleaned every week.
- ☐ Check **window sashes** for mold.

- ☐ Wash the **bath mat** every week in hot water. The dampness from stepping onto it wet from a shower can attract dust mites and cause mold growth.
- ☐ Always run the **exhaust fan** and/or leave the window and door open when taking a shower or bath. Another option is to use a small portable fan (away from water sources) during and after showers. Also check to see if the duct from the exhaust fan is clear.
- ☐ **Check the ceiling.** If you see mold, you may not have enough ceiling insulation.
- ☐ Regrout as necessary to **prevent leaks** that could lead to mold growth.

Living Room and Family Room

Your everyday spaces are often filled with fabrics, rugs, curtains, and pillows, all of which attract dust. Piles of newspapers, magazines, catalogs, books, and toys are also dust and dirt magnets.

- ☐ If you have a **wood-burning fireplace** and you have asthma, you're better off converting to gas or using it for decoration only. Regardless of how well your chimney works, some smoke enters the house, irritating your lungs. Plus, the wood you're using could have mold on it. When it's burned, millions of spores are free to enter the house. Make sure

any gas fireplaces are vented and burning properly to avoid a buildup of soot.
- ☐ **Watch out for candles.** Although they're romantic and lovely, they can also irritate supersensitive airways (this is especially true of scented types). If you must have candlelight, try electric window candles that use low-wattage bulbs instead of wax and wicks.

continued »

Or stick with natural, unscented beeswax candles, and be sure they have lead-free wicks. Also, avoid candles in jars, which tend to burn unevenly, leaving more soot deposits on walls and floors and thus more potential allergens in the air.

☐ Get rid of your **overstuffed, comfy couch** and replace it with leather or vinyl. Other-wise, all those hours spent lying on the couch playing video games, watching TV, reading, or dozing will be like pouring gasoline on the fire of your allergies.

☐ **Follow the advice** for cleaning the bedroom, including cleaning under the furniture, dusting the knickknacks, wiping down the walls, and cleaning the window treatments.

Kitchen and Dining Room

The problem with these rooms is that there are so many places for allergens to make a home: under-neath appliances, inside cabinets and drawers, in the nooks and crannies of the floor and sink, and in the garbage can. Work hard to keep your kitchen clean and dry.

☐ Put the contents of all **open boxes of food** in your pantry into airtight containers to dis-courage insects.

☐ Clean the tray **under the refrigerator** with a bleach solution; it's a veritable mold magnet. Add salt to the drip tray to help reduce future growth. Also, clean under the refrigerator; food trapped there can become moldy. Each time the refrigerator's com-pressor goes on, the mold spores are blown into the kitchen.

☐ Check **under the sink**. Quite often, a sink sprayer leaks around the fittings, and water drips under the sink, soaking everything down there and creating a perfect environ-ment for mold.

☐ If you have any **evidence of cockroaches,** follow the instructions for cockroach control on page 130.

☐ Clean the sides of the **doors of your oven, dishwasher, and refrigerator** with a bleach solution. It's surprising how mold and grime

In Every Room...

☐ Use a **bright light and a mirror** to check under furniture and in the corners of closets.

☐ Wipe around **air-conditioning and heating vents** with a damp cloth.

☐ Do away with **air fresheners and other fragrances**, which can exacerbate asthma symptoms. If you have odors in your home, try placing bowls of vinegar in out-of-the-way spots; opening the windows on cool, windless days; or leaving a cotton ball soaked in vanilla extract in a saucer to absorb odors.

☐ **Check your houseplants.** If you're overwatering them, you may be contributing to the growth of mold. Often, water leaks through a pot onto the carpet, creating a perfect environment for mold. Also, put pebbles on top of the dirt to prevent mold spores from getting into the air too easily.

☐ **Consider replacing any carpet** with solid-surface flooring such as laminate, vinyl, or wood.

☐ Seriously **consider replacing any blinds or curtains** with simple fabric cellular shades.

can accumulate unseen around the edges of your appliances.

☐ If you leave a **tablecloth** on your dining room table, replace it weekly, even if you haven't used the table. It gathers loads of dust, even if you can't see it.

☐ Be particularly mindful of dust in the dining room, especially if it doesn't get used often.

Dust inside the **china cabinet** as well as outside and underneath.

☐ **Wash your sponge, kitchen towels, and rags.** Their perpetual moistness makes them allergen magnets. Kitchen towels should be changed every two days and washed in hot water. Sponges should be bleached or put through the dishwasher every three days.

Laundry Room

Washers generate lots of moisture, and dryers generate lots of steam, dust, and heat. Together, they make laundry rooms dirty fast, even if you work hard at neatness.

☐ Tear out any carpet **under the washer.** Any leaking can lead to mold that can irritate allergies and asthma. Check and tighten plumbing fittings if necessary.

☐ Use **unscented laundry products.**

☐ Make sure your **dryer is vented** to the outside. For every load of laundry you dry, 20 pounds of moisture has to go somewhere! If your dryer is vented to the garage or basement, you're just asking for mold.

Basement

Every time you enter your basement, basement air enters your house, particularly warm air, which rises. If the basement is rife with mold, those spores are coming into the rest of your house. The goal, then, is to get rid of any dampness that could lead to mold and mildew growth.

☐ **Carefully inspect** every inch of your basement, including crawlspaces, for signs of dampness or mold. If you find any, clean the area with a bleach solution. Also track down the source of the water.

☐ Check under the **forced hot-air furnace** or air-conditioning unit for mold and fungus, not to mention dust.

☐ Consider changing **your landscaping** so water doesn't flow toward the house.

☐ Check all **fittings around pipes** to make sure none leak, and insulate any that show condensation.

☐ Make sure your **sump pump** is clean and working properly.

☐ Check any **visible insulation.** Is it wet or damp? If so, tear it out, find the cause of the dampness, repair it, and install new insulation. Exposed insulation is also a magnet for pet dander and dust mites. If possible, cover it with foil-covered sheet foam insulation, which absorbs less moisture.

☐ At least three times a year, **clean the walls** and baseboards with damp cloths. Dust can accumulate on basement walls just as in any other part of your house and be sucked up through the heating system.

☐ Check all **belongings stored in the basement.** Anything stored directly on a concrete floor—such as boxes, newspapers, clothing, or wood—is subject to mold and rot from condensation.

continued »

» *Task 2 (continued)*

- [ ] **Don't store any clothing** in an unfinished basement, even in a cedar closet, if the basement is damp.
- [ ] If you have **dehumidifiers**, make sure you periodically vacuum and clean off the coils, which can become dust traps.
- [ ] **Measure the humidity** with an instrument called a hygrometer, available in most hard-

ware stores. You want a reading below 50 percent.
- [ ] Make sure there is a **vapor barrier** over all dirt floors in crawlspaces to prevent moisture (and mold) from forming. Crawlspaces can also harbor animal dander and old urine and feces.

Attic

Don't ignore the attic in your whole-house inspection.

- [ ] **Check for animals** such as squirrels, bats, and mice and their droppings, which could contribute to allergies.
- [ ] Check for any **roof leaks** that could soak the inside of interior walls.
- [ ] Make sure there's **adequate ventilation.** It's best to have a professional check this using smoke tube testing.
- [ ] Look for any **ice buildup** in the winter. As it melts, it can result in mold.

Heating and air-conditioning units

They can be your greatest ally…or your worst foe. Work particularly hard to make sure the systems that move and treat the air in your home are clean and efficient.

- [ ] **Disconnect any humidifiers,** They're perfect breeding grounds for mold and mites that can easily become airborne in the microscopic droplets of water from the humidifier.
- [ ] Install a **HEPA filter** in your heating unit and be sure to change it regularly.
- [ ] Have your c**entral air-conditioning** unit inspected and cleaned. These units are perfect breeding grounds for mold and fungus.
- [ ] **Vacuum and clean** the interior of the air-handling unit completely to keep it dust-free.
- [ ] Check the **condensate line,** the drain that removes water that has condensed from the indoor air-conditioner coil, for the bacterial slime that tends to grow there. If you find some, call a service company and ask them to flush it with a bleach solution.
- [ ] Try to **keep the thermostat at 65°F** or higher in winter. Although you probably want to keep the temperature low during the day to save on heating costs, heat prevents mold growth. If you turn the thermostat too far down, you may encourage the growth of mold in the damper air.
- [ ] Clean **electrostatic filters**. To avoid getting dirt in your face or on the floor, hold a trash bag over the filter while removing it and carrying it through your home, then rinse the filter with running water. When you reinstall it, be certain the "airflow" arrow is pointing in the right direction (the same as the air movement).
- [ ] If your air handler is in the attic, the air conditioner's **evaporator coils** operate below

the dewpoint in summer, causing humidity in the air to condense or turn from a vapor to a liquid. Each evaporator coil has a pan under it to collect the condensate that the coils produce. The condensate drains into a drain tube or condensate pump, which then channels it outside the house. Make sure it's draining properly.

Outside Your Home

Finally, you want to make sure the outside of your house isn't contributing to allergies. Below are two tips; also check for mold, rotted wood, perpetually wet spots, and holes and cracks in the foundation.

- ☐ Make sure all **gutters have downspouts** and that drain trays are pointing outward.
- ☐ Make sure your **gutters are clear** so water can't seep into the house through leaking gutters and encourage mold growth in the walls. **Check them when it rains;** you shouldn't see water leaking out of end caps, flowing on the outside, or dripping behind them.

De-Allergizing Your Home: A Planning Guide

Use this log to help you plan and organize your tasks. "Projects" refers to major efforts such as removing carpet, reupholstering furniture, or hiring an expert to leakproof your basement. "Purchases" could range from new bedding or cellular blinds to a shoe rack for your front entry. "When?" is the column in which to target when you intend to start the work.

Room	Cleaning time needed	Project(s)	Purchases(s)	When?
Bedroom 1				
Bedroom 2				
Bedroom 3				
Bedroom 4				
Bathroom 1				
Bathroom 2				
Bathroom 3				
Living room				
Family room				
Kitchen				
Dining room				
Home office				
Laundry room				
Attic				
Basement				
Other				

STEP FOUR

eat to beat allergies & asthma

Is there any health issue that isn't linked to nutrition? We can't think of any.

The relationship is both negative and positive: Improper eating habits can cause health problems or make most health problems worse. Perhaps more important, eating the right foods can help heal nearly any health problem, including asthma and allergies.

As promised in chapter 9, we're going to tell you how to revamp your diet to include more of the foods that can improve your condition, either directly or indirectly. Likewise, we'll help you consume fewer foods that studies suggest may exacerbate allergies and asthma. *Note:* This is not an eating plan for anyone with food allergies. If you have food allergies, or even sensitivities, as described in chapter 5, you need to completely eliminate the problem food from your diet.

What you will be doing

First, you'll assess whether your diet is helping or hurting your condition. Next, you'll take on the issue of weight: Do you need to lose a few pounds? If so, we'll get you started down the path to weight loss. Then, you'll clean your pantry and refrigerator, restocking them with allergy- and asthma-friendly foods. Finally, you'll learn the basic tenets of healthy eating and how to integrate them into your daily habits.

How you should prepare

Rereading chapter 9 would certainly help. As noted, you'll be cleaning out unhealthy foods from your kitchen and replacing them with better alternatives, so be prepared for a pantry cleanup day. Most of all, you need an open mind and a positive attitude. Food habits are tough to change, and the results aren't always tangible or measurable. You need to be committed—the benefits are real!

What to have on hand

Copies of the questions and lists in this chapter. A pen or pencil. A garbage can and a box for cleaning your pantry. A budget for buying new, healthier staples.

assess your eating habits

Back in chapter 9, we discussed five primary ways that food and dietary habits can hurt or help allergies or asthma. They include:

1. **Weight.** Studies have found that carrying extra pounds may trigger asthma symptoms and make asthma worse.
2. **Heartburn.** Studies have also shown a clear link between asthma and gastroesophageal reflux disease (GERD).
3. **The right fats.** Certain polyunsaturated fats (omega-6's) promote inflammation; others (omega-3's) fight inflammation. Inflammation is a major problem in both allergies and asthma.
4. **Probiotics.** Research suggests that having the proper level of digestive bacteria can help your body create cells important in the battle against asthma.
5. **Antioxidants.** Finally, studies show that antioxidants help battle inflammation inside your body, which as we've said, is important in controlling allergies and asthma.

So how does your diet fare in these five categories? The answer, for most people, is hardly obvious: Not many of us can say which foods contain probiotics or which cooking oils have omega-3 fats, not omega-6 fats. The following questions will help you sort it out.

Is my diet hurting or helping my allergies or asthma?

Answer each of these true-false questions, then look at the end of the quiz for the better answers and the reasons they're better.

1 You ate yogurt at least three times last week.   **TRUE** ☐ **FALSE** ☐

2 You ate at least two servings of red or purple foods yesterday.   **TRUE** ☐ **FALSE** ☐

3 You've eaten salmon at least once in the past week.   **TRUE** ☐ **FALSE** ☐

4 The last three times you sautéed food, you used olive oil or broth.   **TRUE** ☐ **FALSE** ☐

5 You can't remember the last time you bought a bottle of antacids.   **TRUE** ☐ **FALSE** ☐

6 You can no longer wear a favorite old belt because it has become too small.   **TRUE** ☐ **FALSE** ☐

7 Your idea of a balanced meal is one item from the fried group, one item from the chip group, and one item from the cake group.   **TRUE** ☐ **FALSE** ☐

8 You count bloomin' onions and French fries as vegetables.   **TRUE** ☐ **FALSE** ☐

9 You drink more soda than water on a daily basis.   **TRUE** ☐ **FALSE** ☐

10 You can count on one hand the number of green vegetables you enjoy eating.   **TRUE** ☐ **FALSE** ☐

continued »

11 Part of your afternoon routine at work is a trip to the vending machine for a snack. TRUE □ FALSE □

12 Your breakfast is usually built around a bagel, Danish, doughnut, or croissant. TRUE □ FALSE □

THE RESULTS: Hopefully, your answers match ours below. If not, you have some work to do, and you should read this chapter very carefully!

1. True. Studies suggest that live bacterial cultures in yogurt may have a beneficial effect on asthma.

2. True. Red peppers, tomatoes, radishes, red onions, and other colorful produce are particularly rich in the antioxidants you need to battle the inflammation so common with asthma and allergies.

3. True. Omega-3 fatty acids (the ones with strong anti-inflammatory properties) are particularly abundant in fatty fish like salmon.

4. True. If you used other oils, such as vegetable and canola oil, they're rich in omega-6 fats, which spark inflammation.

5. True. If you're popping antacids like candy, you may have GERD, which is known to exacerbate asthma. Pay special attention to the section on heartburn-free eating.

6. False. If you're replacing belts and other clothing because you've gained weight lately, pay special attention to the section on weight loss. Studies have found that being overweight can significantly exacerbate asthma.

7. False. If you're eating like this, you're consuming way too many omega-6 fatty acids, known to increase inflammation. A nutritionally balanced diet with plenty of fruits and vegetables has been shown to improve asthma symptoms.

8. False. If you think these are vegetables, we have a bridge to sell you in Brooklyn. To get the most from the vegetables you eat, they should be as close to their natural state as possible. That means staying away from frying, which typically uses oils high in omega-6 fatty acids.

9. False. Regular sodas are filled with sugar, making them super-high in calories, and carbonation (even in diet sodas) can upset your stomach. Plus, they cost a lot. Water is the perfect liquid for health—and from a tap, it's all but free.

10. False. This is a tough one. The popular American diet includes only a few green vegetables: broccoli, green beans, iceberg lettuce, and perhaps some slices of green pepper. From artichokes to zucchini, from Asian greens to southern greens, there are too many vegetables that most of us don't eat, and they're among the most healthful foods on the planet.

11. False. As we'll discuss later, too many of us eat out of habit or boredom, not hunger. Habitual eating is one of the big contributors to America's weight troubles. There are better ways to take an afternoon break than eating a candy bar. Try taking a brief walk outside, for example.

12. False. Another tough one. While any breakfast should include a carbohydrate food, it should be whole grain and high fiber. The popular breakfast foods listed in this question are made with refined wheat, and many are filled with inflammatory omega-6 fatty acids, dangerous trans fatty acids, and calorie-boosting sweeteners.

address your weight

The next phase in this step of the Breathe Easy Plan is to determine if you need to lose weight. You'll use the popular body mass index measurement, or BMI, which we talked about in chapter 9, to determine your current situation.

The BMI assigns a number based on a combination of height and weight. Essentially, the number indicates whether you are carrying a healthy or unhealthy level of body fat. It is a far more useful and accurate measure than weight alone.

To find your BMI on the chart below, locate your height in inches in the column on the left. Then scan the horizontal row of numbers to find your weight (or the number closest to it). Finally, move down to the bottom of the column to the row marked "BMI" to learn your BMI measure.

A BMI of 25 to 29 means you are probably overweight, and a BMI over 30, indicates medical obesity, which is considered a disease that should be treated by a doctor. Your goal should be to have a BMI below 25.

The BMI isn't foolproof. It gives you a very wide target range for your weight, since it doesn't factor in body types.

HEIGHT (inches)	BODY WEIGHT (pounds)																		
58	91	96	100	105	110	115	119	124	129	134	138	143	148	153	158	162	167	172	177	181
59	94	99	104	109	114	119	124	128	133	138	143	148	153	158	163	168	173	178	183	188
60	97	102	107	112	118	123	128	133	138	143	148	153	158	163	168	174	179	184	189	194
61	100	106	111	116	122	127	132	137	143	148	153	158	164	169	174	180	185	190	195	201
62	104	109	115	120	126	131	136	142	147	153	158	164	169	175	180	186	191	196	202	207
63	107	113	118	124	130	135	141	146	152	158	163	169	175	180	186	191	197	203	208	214
64	110	116	122	128	134	140	145	151	157	163	169	174	180	186	192	197	204	209	215	221
65	114	120	126	132	138	144	150	156	162	168	174	180	186	192	198	204	210	216	222	228
66	118	124	130	136	142	148	155	161	167	173	179	186	192	198	204	210	216	223	229	235
67	121	127	134	140	146	153	159	166	172	178	185	191	198	204	211	217	223	230	236	242
68	125	131	138	144	151	158	164	171	177	184	190	197	203	210	216	223	230	236	243	249
69	128	135	142	149	155	162	169	176	182	189	196	203	209	216	223	230	236	243	250	257
70	132	139	146	153	160	167	174	181	188	195	202	209	216	222	229	236	243	250	257	264
71	136	143	150	157	165	172	179	186	193	200	208	215	222	229	236	243	250	257	265	272
72	140	147	154	162	169	177	184	191	199	206	213	221	228	235	242	250	258	265	272	279
73	144	151	159	166	174	182	189	197	204	212	219	227	235	242	250	257	265	272	280	288
74	148	155	163	171	179	186	194	202	210	218	225	233	241	249	256	264	272	280	287	295
75	152	160	168	176	184	192	200	208	216	224	232	240	248	256	264	272	279	287	295	303
76	156	164	172	180	189	197	205	213	221	230	238	246	254	263	271	279	287	295	304	312
BMI	19	20	21	22	23	24	25	26	27	28	29	30	31	32	33	34	35	36	37	38
	NORMAL						OVERWEIGHT					OBESE							

REMEMBER: Losing even a few pounds when you're overweight will make you healthier. Not only can it improve your asthma or allergies, it can also reduce your risk of heart disease and diabetes. If you have a long way to go to get to "24," set some milestones for the road ahead. Reward yourself along the way. Every lost pound is significant!

the golden rules of weight loss

Weight loss boils down to a very simple formula: Burn more calories in a day than you consume. One pound of fat equals about 3,500 calories, so for every 3,500 calories you eat above the amount you burn, you gain a pound. The reverse is also true: If you burn 3,500 more calories than you eat, you lose a pound.

Popular diet programs such as Atkins and South Beach tend to be based on the deeper science of how the body digests, burns, and stores different nutrients. At the end of the day, however, they all get back to the fundamental truth: Burn more calories than you eat. There are two main ways to do that—by increasing your activity levels and by eating fewer calories. The best weight-loss efforts use a combination.

With that preamble, here are 10 rules to start you down the path to permanent weight loss.

1. Increase physical activity

For most people, it is easier to cut calories than to burn calories. And in truth, it takes a lot of exercise to lose a pound. Rigorous exercise burns about 500 calories an hour. Cut out a few snacks, and you've achieved the same calorie deficit as you would if you spent an hour on a bicycle. Having noted that, it's almost impossible to say too many good things about the benefits of exercise. It reduces appetite. It builds muscle that burns more calories around the clock. It strengthens your heart and lungs. It makes you proud. It makes you look and feel better. It's fun. It makes you more energetic. It lifts your mood. And yes, it very definitely helps you lose weight. Look at it this way: If you put away the cookies and go for a walk instead, you not only skip hundreds of calories of unneeded food, you burn off a few hundred calories as well. That's a double win.

2. Halve all portions

Whether you eat at home or in a restaurant, immediately halve the amount on your plate, in the takeout bag, and so on. Arguably, the worst food trend of the past few decades has been the explosion in portion sizes on America's dinner plates (and breakfast and lunch plates, too). We eat far, far more today than our bodies need. Indeed, studies have found that if you serve people more food, they'll eat more food, regardless of their hunger levels. This is another reason to eschew buffets. And forget about going by the portion sizes on the labels. Portion sizes in this country are a mess, and they often don't mean anything.

3. Stick to water

The average American consumes an extra 245 calories a day from soft drinks. That's nearly 90,000 calories a year. Divide that by the 3,500 calories it takes to gain or lose a pound of fat, and you could lose 25 pounds a year just by switching from Coke to water or fat-free milk.

4. Eat at home

You're more likely to eat more—and eat more high-fat, high-calorie foods—when you eat out than when you eat at home. Restaurants today serve such large portions that many have switched to larger plates and tables!

5. Feast on fiber

High-fiber foods—beans, vegetables, fruits, and whole grains—fill you up faster and keep you full longer than simple carbohydrates such as dough-nuts, ice cream, and potato chips. Make them the centerpiece of your meals and save the sugary snacks for infrequent special occasions.

6. Avoid white foods

There is some scientific legitimacy to today's lower-carb diets: Large amounts of simple carbo-hydrates in your diet can wreak havoc on your blood sugar levels and lead to weight gain. But you needn't go to the extremes that some pro-tein-based weight-loss systems call for. Instead, follow a simple rule: Avoid the most popular "white" starches—refined sugar, white rice, and refined flour—and eat whole grain breads, brown rice, and, in general, fewer sweet foods.

7. Plan, plan, plan

If you plan your meals, you're less likely to tear open a package of chips an hour before dinner. This goes for when you're out and about as well. Stock your desk at work with healthy snacks and carry a small cooler in your car with cut-up fruit and vegetables and low-fat cheese sticks so you won't be tempted by the drive-thru when hunger pains hit.

8. Eat when you're hungry

It's stunning how much we all eat out of boredom, nervousness, habit, frustration, or even celebration. Likewise, we eat (and drink) as a social activity, as a way to show love, and as a social custom. What these situations too rarely involve, however, is hunger. Arguably, the best thing you can do to consume fewer calories is to eat for fuel and health and skip all those other eating opportunities. After all, you don't need food to calm yourself, enjoy a party, show your love, or make a problem go away. You're strong enough to do all that on your own.

9. Track what you eat

Studies have found that people who keep food diaries are more likely to lose weight and keep it off than those who don't. Just remember, if you cheat and don't write down what you're eating, the only one who loses (or actually, doesn't lose), is you.

10. Think life, not diet

The best weight-loss efforts are those that are sustainable for a lifetime. They include things like eating more vegetables, developing an exercise habit, and eliminating habitual snacking. The problem with radical 12-week crash diets is the 13th week. If you haven't learned sustainable, sensible long-term habits, you're almost certain to gain back your weight.

the breathe easy eating plan

By now, you've probably figured out that eating well for allergies and asthma isn't much different from eating well, period. The Breathe Easy eating plan is essentially about eating reasonable portions of whole grain foods, lean proteins, and fruits and vegetables. The primary addition to a standard healthy diet is an emphasis on probiotic foods, as well as foods containing omega-3 fatty acids.

We've broken our plan into three parts: A pantry and refrigerator cleanup, a restocking, and 12 guidelines for making food decisions. We've kept this as easy as possible, but there's one final matter to deal with before you begin.

Chances are, you aren't the only person eating in your home. You and your family need to decide whether your change to a healthier diet is a solo effort or one that involves everyone. Don't make presumptions: This should be discussed with everyone who's affected. Tonight at the dinner table, say, "Everybody, I have a very important matter to discuss. I've decided to make significant improvements in the way I eat as part of my battle against my allergies and asthma. I'm also planning to lose some weight as a result. I'm going to be eating less junk food, more vegetables, and so on. I would love for all of you to join me. What do you think?" Then let the conversation develop.

Once that's decided, apply the following steps to either the whole household's food supply or just yours.

1. Clean out your kitchen

Bring a garbage can with a strong trash bag inside into the kitchen for food you're going to trash, along with a sturdy box to hold unopened cans and packages you can give away.

Start with your pantry, then move to the refrigerator and freezer. Throw out or give away:

- [ ] **High-salt processed foods.** This could include canned soups and stews, prepackaged rice dishes, frozen vegetables in sauce, and so on.
- [ ] **Packaged snacks and sweets.** This includes cookies, chips, candy, cheese crackers, and other such foods.
- [ ] **White breads** and other baked goods made with bleached flour.
- [ ] **Margarine**

- [ ] **Large containers of vegetable oil.** You will be using olive oil as your primary cooking oil, so keep only enough vegetable oil on hand for those few recipes in which it's really necessary.
- [ ] **Any and all food** that has been in your pantry, refrigerator, or freezer for more than six months.
- [ ] **Sodas and other sweetened drinks,** such as bottled juice and iced tea.

When you're done, tie up the garbage bag and get it outside, load the giveaways in your trunk (we assume you'll know where to take them), and consider spending an hour or two thoroughly cleaning your pantry and refrigerator now that they've been purged.

2. Go shopping

It's time to refill that space you cleared out. Here's a chance to not only stock up on better foods but also to begin a meal-planning effort. Before you head out, take a pencil and paper and answer the following questions, then add your own items to our recommendations.

☐ How many dinners do you need to buy supplies for on this shopping trip? Be sure to pick up a lean protein food and at least one vegetable for each dinner.

☐ What raw vegetables will my family eat? One of the best tricks for healthier meals is to put a plate of them on the table at every meal. Stock up on cucumbers, carrots, peppers, celery, tomatoes, and other finger foods your family likes. Add a bowl of low-fat ranch dressing for dipping, and you'll be amazed at how fast those carrot sticks and pepper strips disappear.

☐ If each person in your household eats two servings of fruit per day, how many apples, pears, cantaloupes, bananas, and grapes do you need to buy?

☐ If you've banned junk food from the house, but everyone gets hungry at 8:00 P.M., what do you want them to eat? Remember: Snacking is healthy; it's the junk food we often snack on that's problematic. Consider granola bars, extra fruit, low-fat microwave popcorn, or frozen yogurt.

Your shopping list

MEAL FOODS

☐ Fresh salmon (enough for one dinner)
☐ Mackerel or another type of fatty fish, such as bluefish, fresh tuna, or herring (enough for one dinner)
☐ Five different cooking vegetables (be sure two of them are dark green, leafy veggies)
☐ Five different nibbling vegetables
☐ Salad greens
☐ Whole grain breads
☐ _____
☐ _____

PANTRY STAPLES

☐ Olive oil
☐ Canned tuna
☐ Anchovies
☐ Flaxseed
☐ Onions

☐ Garlic
☐ Canned and dried beans
☐ Black or green tea
☐ Low-sodium or sodium-free soups, sauces, and other processed or canned foods
☐ _____
☐ _____

REFRIGERATOR STAPLES

☐ Six different fruits (make one of them apples)
☐ Live-culture yogurt (any flavor)
☐ Bags of frozen vegetables
☐ Bags of frozen shrimp (if no one is allergic to shellfish)
☐ 2 percent or other low-fat milk
☐ Butter
☐ A bottle of red wine
☐ _____
☐ _____

continued »

3. Eat according to the breathe easy plan

Without further ado, here are the basic rules of eating smart. These apply for promoting general health, weight loss, and relief from allergies and asthma.

1. Cook only with **olive oil and other monounsaturated fats.**

2. Use **real butter,** not margarine, when you need a spread.

3. Have one meal every day that's comprised primarily of **vegetables,** with a small side of lean protein. This could be canned chicken mixed into dark salad greens, ratatouille over whole wheat pasta with grated parmesan cheese, or vegetable lasagna.

4. Include **beans or legumes** at least three times a week.

5. **Have fish** at least three times a week. Canned tuna counts, as does spaghetti sauce with plenty of omega-3–rich anchovies. If shellfish isn't a problem allergy-wise, make shrimp a weekly dinner staple. If you simply can't stomach fish, begin taking daily fish-oil supplements to get at least 1 gram of omega-3 fatty acids a day.

6. **Avoid any food that lists sugar** among the first four ingredients on the label. You can get sugar-free varieties of foods such as ketchup, mayonnaise, and salad dressing in the diabetic foods section of supermarkets.

7. Choose foods that are as **close to their natural state** as possible: fresh vegetables and fruits; fresh meat, fish, chicken, and eggs; raw nuts and seeds; and fresh salad greens. You can assume that the more preparation and packaging that were done at a factory, the more healthy ingredients have been removed and unhealthy ingredients added.

8. Choose **whole grain breads and pasta.** Make sure the first ingredient listed on the label is whole grain flour or whole wheat flour. You'll know it's really whole grain bread if it has at least 3 or 4 grams of fiber per slice. Don't be fooled by color, either: Some companies use molasses or artificial colorings to make their breads look like "whole wheat" even if they aren't.

9. Snack on raw **nuts,** fresh **vegetables** and **fruit,** hard and soft **cheeses,** and other "real" foods.

10. **Cut your salt intake** by using "lite" salt and substituting herbs and other spices for salt.

11. At least three times a week, eat a cup of **live-culture yogurt** for its beneficial acidophilus bacteria. If yogurt turns your stomach, take acidophilus supplements, available in drugstores and health food stores everywhere.

12. At breakfast, go ahead and drink natural fruit juice, low-fat milk, tea, or coffee, but for the rest of the day, **focus on water.** For a treat, have a glass of wine with dinner.

STEP FIVE

increase **your resistance**

In simplest terms, allergies—and in many cases, asthma—are caused by flawed responses by your immune system. It would make sense, then, to infer that taking good care of your immune system can have a beneficial effect on your condition.

In fact, that's true. Research is showing that having a weakened immune system increases your chances of allergic reactions or asthma attacks. While it's impossible to boost your immunity enough make your allergies or asthma go away, you can certainly reduce the chances of attacks if you have a stronger immune system.

There are many ways to strengthen your immune system. The supplements suggested in step 2 can do it, as can the foods in step 4. But here in step 5, we'll focus on a few other key strategies, namely reducing stress, increasing physical activity, and bolstering your attitude.

Wait, come back here! We know that stress reduction is one of those topics that get us all, well, stressed. Who has time to relax in this crazy world? But we're sure that after doing the worksheets and absorbing the tips we offer in the following pages, you'll be pleasantly surprised at how easy it can be to defuse the stress that is harming your body.

What you will be doing

There are eight phases to this step. The first is easy: It's just a lesson you need to read and absorb. The rest require you to fill out a form or take at least one action. We suggest you take a week or two to really, truly give each phase an honest effort. Habits require about three weeks to take hold, so keep up with your chosen actions as best you can.

How you should prepare

Reread the section in chapter 10 on relaxation techniques. Make note of any that appeal to you more than others.

What to have on hand

A blank journal, copies of the questions and logs in this step, and writing implements.

lesson: the stress-immunity connection

Have you ever caught a cold right after meeting a tight deadline at work? At the end of a week in which the kids were especially trying, have you ever been struck with the flu or digestive trouble?

If you answered yes to either, you've experienced firsthand the effects of stress on your immune system and your health. Overall, an estimated 43 percent of adults experience adverse health effects from stress, and 75 to 90 percent of all physician's office visits have stress-related components, notes the American Psychological Association.

Numerous studies have also found that chronic stress can exacerbate both allergies and asthma. The more stress you're exposed to, the harder it is to control your asthma and the more likely you are to have allergy-caused eczema.

Now, when we say stress, we're not talking about the kind of acute stress that comes when you're in a car accident. Rather, it's the kind of grinding, daily stress that may have become so much a part of your life that you barely even notice it anymore. Things like living from paycheck to paycheck, coping with a chronic health condition (such as asthma), dealing with challenging children, arguing regularly with your spouse, starting a new job, or continuing in one you hate.

Each time you're confronted with a stressor, your body releases a cascade of stress hormones such as adrenaline and cortisol. They in turn send a volley of signals to various parts of your body to prepare it for action. For instance, your liver releases glucose to provide instant energy to muscle cells. Your lungs expand to take in more oxygen, your heart beats faster, your blood pressure rises to send more oxygen-rich blood throughout your body, and your bowel and intestinal muscles contract. It is a strong reaction, based on ancient wiring that says your response to stress should be physical: fighting, running, or threatening. If this reaction happens day in and day out without physical release, it leads to common stress-related conditions ranging from chronic high blood pressure, angina, and gastric reflux to constipation.

Chronic stress also damages the very system that's supposed to guard your health—your immune system. It turns out that like most systems in the body, the immune system has a feedback loop. After it finishes attacking foreign invaders with inflammatory chemicals, the brain sends out cortisol—the stress hormone—to shut down this inflammatory response and send the immune system back into a quiet, or homeostatic, state. If your body is releasing cortisol all the time—as it does when it's under chronic stress—your immune system is constantly being suppressed, increasing your risk of illness. This has even greater repercussions when you talk about asthma. It means your body isn't getting the message it needs to suppress its inflammatory response, so your asthma worsens.

identify your main stressors

A. How stressful is your life?

Before you can begin reducing the stressors in your life or moderating how you react to them, you need to identify them. Take a few minutes to work through the following questions.

1. The worst part of my day is:
- ☐ a. None; I love all parts of my day
- ☐ b. Daytime, dealing with work
- ☐ c. Morning or evening, dealing with home and family

2. I can feel the muscles in the back of my neck and shoulders tense up:
- ☐ a. Rarely
- ☐ b. Whenever something goes wrong
- ☐ c. When I'm feeling lots of pressure

3. I would describe our financial situation as:
- ☐ a. Comfortable
- ☐ b. Tenuous
- ☐ c. Frightening

4. I find myself yelling at my children:
- ☐ a. Never
- ☐ b. At least once a week
- ☐ c. Several times a day

5. My spouse and I:
- ☐ a. Have a solid, close relationship
- ☐ b. Coexist, with little in common any more besides the kids and bills
- ☐ c. Fight nearly every day

6. Every day when I walk into work, I:
- ☐ a. Am happy to be there
- ☐ b. Get a sinking feeling in my stomach
- ☐ c. Inevitably get a headache or stomachache

7. When it comes to my job, I:
- ☐ a. Feel as if I have a good amount of control over what I do and when I do it
- ☐ b. Feel as if I'm constantly battling one deadline after another
- ☐ c. Feel that I'm entirely at the mercy of others' needs and wants

8. When I look at myself in the mirror, I feel:
- ☐ a. Pretty good; I'm not doing too bad for someone my age
- ☐ b. That I could lose about 15 pounds
- ☐ c. As if I'm looking at a stranger

9. I am caring for:
- ☐ a. Just myself
- ☐ b. My spouse and children
- ☐ c. My spouse, children, and aging parents or other relatives, not to mention the neighborhood kids and several needy friends

10. My weekends are spent:
- ☐ a. Relaxing and doing things I enjoy
- ☐ b. Running errands, cleaning the house, and schlepping the children
- ☐ c. Catching up on all the work I didn't get done during the week, plus entertaining, cleaning, and shopping

THE RESULTS: The more "b" and "c" answers you have, the more likely it is that stress is having an effect on your health, including your asthma or allergies. Optimally, you should have at least seven "a" answers.

continued »

B. And how is the stress affecting you?

We all have challenges in our lives. The question is, how are we dealing with them? The American Medical Women's Association lists the following psychological and physical signs of stress. How many do you have? Answer truthfully.

Psychological signs of stress

1. Are you often nervous or anxious?

    YES ☐ NO ☐

2. Do you often feel depressed or sad?

    YES ☐ NO ☐

3. Are you often irritable or moody?

    YES ☐ NO ☐

4. Do you often become frustrated?

    YES ☐ NO ☐

5. Are you forgetful? YES ☐ NO ☐

6. Do you have trouble thinking clearly?

    YES ☐ NO ☐

7. Can you make decisions without agonizing?

    YES ☐ NO ☐

8. Is it difficult to learn new information?

    YES ☐ NO ☐

9. Do you have insomnia? YES ☐ NO ☐

10. Are you often plagued by negative

    thoughts? YES ☐ NO ☐

11. Are you fidgety? YES ☐ NO ☐

12. Are you accident-prone? YES ☐ NO ☐

13. Do you bite your fingernails or cuticles?

    YES ☐ NO ☐

THE RESULTS: Again, there is no rigorous scale here. Generally, the more *yes* answers, the more likely it is that stress is having a bad effect on your life. You should be concerned if you had more than three *yes* answers.

Physical signs of stress

The following symptoms, if chronic, may be signs of ongoing anxiety or stress problems. If the previous quizzes show that stress is a big issue in your life, and you're experiencing any of the following, it may be time to ask your doctor if the two are indeed related.

☐ Back pain

☐ Muscle tension

☐ Headaches

☐ Tremor of hands

☐ Diarrhea

☐ Constipation

☐ Pounding heart

☐ Chest pain

☐ Sweaty, cold hands

☐ Shortness of breath

☐ Indigestion or gas pains ,

☐ Constant burping

☐ A burning sensation
   in your chest

☐ Feeling faint or dizzy

☐ A lingering head cold

☐ Ringing in the ears

☐ Grinding your teeth

☐ Hives or skin rashes

☐ Loss of appetite

☐ Feeling nauseated
   or vomiting

☐ Stomach pain

identify your stress busters

So what do you do when you're stressed? Reach for a cigarette or a glass of wine? Go for a jog? Take a nap? Do you get depressed or find yourself energized to get twice as much done? How you react to your stress is an important clue to whether you're handling the stress or the stress is handling you. For the next week or two, complete this log to get a sense of what you're doing to cope with the stress in your life.

Date	Stressor	Drink alcohol or take drugs	Smoke cigarettes	Eat	Go shopping	Watch TV	Call a friend	Go to sleep	Try deep breathing or other relaxation	Exercise	Do a hobby	Read	Other

THE RESULTS: If there are more checkmarks in the first five coping technique columns, your stress is handling you. These are not constructive ways to deal with stress; instead, they are unhealthy masking techniques. Read on to discover better ways to handle stress, as well as some simple steps you can take to reduce the most common stressors in your life.

exercise

Your task: Integrate at least 10 minutes of high-energy movement into your day. Every day. Without exception.

Why? Study after study has proven the health benefits of moderate physical activity, including increased resistance to infectious disease. Even if exercise triggers your asthma, there's no reason you can't find ways to get your body moving without causing attacks.

Now, if you read health books at all, you know that the health establishment advocates getting 30 minutes of exercise a day if you want measurable improvements in muscle tone and cardiovascular function. And you know what? They are absolutely correct. But to get to 30 minutes a day, you must first be active for 10 minutes—and for most people, getting to those first 10 minutes is the toughest part.

The topic of exercise can get enormously complicated. There are so many types, so many muscles, so much gear, so much sweat, so much spandex, and so many excuses. We wish to boil this down to a few simple edicts.

- **There are no excuses.** Just get moving.
- **There are no rules.** Whatever gets you moving is fine by us. Whatever you wear is fine by us. Wherever you do it is fine by us.
- **There are no measurements.** You want to breathe a little hard, but not so hard that you can't talk. After that, just do it.

Your simple goal: Again, to move actively for at least 10 minutes a day. Out of that, an exercise habit or a hobby or even a passion could be born in time. When that time comes, we'll be cheering, and you'll need to get a good exercise book. Until then, don't complicate things.

Want some suggestions to get you started? Here are a few.

☐ **Take a walk.** There is no better choice than taking an energetic walk after lunch, for an afternoon break, or after dinner. For regular people who aren't interested in rigorous exercise programs, walking is perfect.

☐ **Do a stretching routine.** Find a health book with a thorough, full-body stretching routine and practice it until you have it memorized. Do it every morning, every night before bed, or right before dinner.

☐ **Work out with stretch bands.** A pair of exercise-grade stretch bands is out-standing for strengthening muscles, stretching your body, and burning calories—and they are so much more fun than weights.

☐ **Dance.** Most of us listen to music at home. Commit to dancing to at least two songs every day. Dancing alone is perfectly fine.

☐ **Do calisthenics in front of the TV.** Watch the evening news standing up. Do stretches, jumping jacks, simulated weight lifts, marching in place, or shadow boxing.

relax

Here's where the techniques we talked about in chapter 10 come in handy. Pick one technique from the list below, then find a class, practitioner, video, or book and commit to doing it at least once a week.

- Yoga
- Tai chi
- Professional massage
- Biofeedback
- Meditation
- Progressive relaxation
- Hypnosis

If none of the above appeal to you, make a concerted effort to do lots more of the following each day. Although there are no studies directly linking them to a reduction in allergy or asthma symptoms, they have been shown to reduce stress hormones.

☐ **Sing.** Studies have found that singing, particularly choral singing, results in lower levels of the stress hormone cortisol.

☐ **Laugh.** It costs nothing, and it really works. When researchers divided 33 healthy adult women into two groups and had one watch a humorous video while the other viewed a tourism video, not only did those who laughed experience a drop in their stress levels, but their immune function increased when compared with that of the women watching the tourism video.

☐ **Enjoy your pet.** Numerous studies attest to the stress-relieving benefits of pets. In one, researchers evaluated the heart health of 240 couples, half of whom owned a pet. People with pets had significantly lower heart rates and blood pressure levels when exposed to stressors than those who were petless. In fact, pets worked even better than spouses at buffering stress. If you're allergic to dogs or cats, try a turtle or even a bird. Whatever pet you decide on, test it out on a trial basis first to make sure it doesn't aggravate your allergies or asthma.

☐ **Pray.** Studies suggest that people who attend church regularly have stronger immune systems. This is one reason, researchers suggest, that other studies have found regular churchgoers to have better physical health overall. It makes sense when you think about it: Sitting in a church or temple is like meditating. It's quiet and peaceful.

☐ **Love.** We're not talking sex, but love. Hugs, holding hands, giving compliments, playing with kids, looking at the stars together, eating out together, forgiving, teasing, pillow fighting, sharing. Isn't this what really matters most? If you can find it within yourself to share your love with your family and friends, then you will have made a major step toward conquering stress.

keep a journal

You wouldn't think the simple act of writing down your thoughts for 10 minutes a day or so could affect your health, but it does. A 1999 study published in the *Journal of the American Medical Association* found that people with asthma who wrote about their most stressful life event showed a 19 percent improvement on a lung function test, an improvement that lasted up to four months after the experiment ended.

You don't have to be a Hemingway to write in your journal. You just have to find a quiet spot, uncap your pen (or fire up your computer), and begin. Write about your day, listing not only what you did but also how you felt about what you did. Write about your dream last night. Write about your plans for the weekend, your fears about work, and your hopes for your children. If you're blocked, try the following phrases to get started.

I am eager to _____
_____

I doubt myself when _____
_____

I feel powerful when _____
_____

I'm proud of myself because _____
_____

My 10 favorite things are _____
_____

I am most grateful for _____
_____

I can simplify my life by living without _____
_____

I feel my mission in life is to _____
_____

In my wildest dreams, I _____
_____

I believe in myself because _____
_____

I wish I could _____
_____

I am happiest when _____
_____

I hope to _____
_____

develop a positive attitude

Are you a glass-half-full or a glass-half-empty kind of person? If you're the latter, it's likely that you're exposing your body to far greater levels of stress hormones than if you're the former. In this final phase of the Breathe Easy stress-busting plan, we offer advice for turning your view of the world around or, if you'd rather, right side up.

The whole idea of positive psychology (a fancy name for optimism and personal resilience) is a relatively new concept in the mental health field, but it's one with a growing body of evidence to support it. In a nutshell, researchers find that people with inner resilience—that is, a good ability to cope with and overcome the many challenges that life throws at us—can form a shield against the harmful effects of stress.

Developing resilience is an extremely personal matter; it's not something that lends itself to a formal program. All we can ask is that you work at it—constantly. After all, being happy is better than being sad, isn't it? Not only does resliience help your life become more important, more hallowed, more uplifting, but indirectly, it…umm…helps your allergies and asthma. Which is where we started.

Here then are some opening thoughts on developing your personal resilience *before* a crisis hits.

- **Appreciate all you do** instead of worrying about all that remains to be done.
- **Foster your sense of humor.** If you can laugh at a situation rather than getting angry, you'll automatically lower your stress hormones.
- **Realize that you have choices** in your life and that there are always second chances. You don't have to handle everything perfectly the first time.
- **Remind yourself** that even the very worst situation, event, or feeling eventually passes.
- **Reframe reality, don't ignore it.** That means considering yourself to be a capable person, even if you've made mistakes or have constraints. The vision of yourself as strong empowers you, enabling you to feel less stressed and overwhelmed when crises or problems do hit and thus protecting your health. One study found that how women *perceive* stress can affect health as much as major stressors such as poverty. The researchers had women rank themselves on a picture of a ladder representing where people stood in society economically, with those who were best off at the top and those who were worst off at the bottom. Women who perceived themselves as being lower on the ladder, regardless of their actual socioeconomic status, had more stress hormones than women at the same socioeconomic level who perceived themselves as being higher. Call it the power of perception.

So there you have it: a plan to not only reduce the stress *in* your life but also to modify how you react to that stress and arm yourself against its negative health effects. All of this will greatly help your allergies and asthma, but we hope that's only the beginning of the benefits.

STEP SIX

live to beat allergies & asthma

We've covered a lot of ground so far in the Breathe Easy Plan, from medications and diet to home cleaning and stress relief. But you cover a lot of ground in your life as well, so in this step, we move beyond your home and provide easy-to-follow advice to help you cope with your allergies and asthma 365 days a year, 24 hours a day, no matter where you are or what time of year it is. We even point you toward allergy-related products we've tried ourselves, recommended to others, and found to be worth your money.

What you will be doing

This step is similar to step 3, in which we asked you to go room by room and make the changes needed to help your condition. This time, though, we'll focus on six scenarios or locations beyond your everyday life at home. They are your garden, your car, your workplace, travel, the holidays, and the seasons. For each of these areas, we offer the best tips we know for managing your allergies or asthma. Find the ones that are most appropriate for your situation, then act on them.

How you should prepare

Rethink where you spend your time and where allergies and asthma tend to flare up most. You may wish to review some of the forms you filled out in part 1 to help you focus on the most problematic areas. Then, be prepared to do some cleaning and purging and perhaps buy some new products to help manage your condition.

What to have on hand

No special gear is needed. Each of the following sections is independent, so unlike previous steps in the plan, you may be able to skip a section or sections if they are not relevant to your condition or lifestyle.

make your world safe from allergens

And here we go: dozens of tips, hints, and clever bits of advice for managing allergies and asthma outside your home. Remember: Take action! Only you can do what's needed to manage your allergies and asthma effectively.

In the garden

If you're allergic to pollens, it's impossible, regardless of what any book says, to plant an entirely "allergy-free" garden. Pollens can drift hundreds of miles from their original sources as well as a few hundred feet from the perennial garden next door. Still, there are some steps you can take so you can continue gardening in relative comfort.

☐ **Take the right medication.** That means a second-generation, nonsedating antihistamine such as fexofenadine (Allegra). During gardening season, take it daily even if you aren't having symptoms. That way, you'll be protected from pollen every day as well as when the urge to weed hits. You might also talk to your doctor about whether you're a good candidate for immunotherapy.

☐ **Wear the right equipment.** That means a face mask to filter pollen grains from the air before they hit your nose and mouth. You may feel silly, but wear it anyhow (consider it like wearing a bike helmet—unflattering, perhaps, but a mandatory safety practice). These days, you can find a variety of comfortable and effective face masks online and from the manufacturers listed on page 278. If your eyes bother you, don goggles or wraparound sunglasses. And try smearing petroleum jelly inside your nose. Yes, it sounds disgusting, but it can help stop pollen and mold spores from settling on the lining of your nose.

☐ **Watch the clock.** Pollens are at their worst in the afternoon during the spring and in the morning during the fall. Do your gardening when they're at their lowest levels.

☐ **Check the map.** Before you plan a day in the garden, check the updated pollen map at www.accuweather.com/adcbin/airpollen_maps?nav=health&type=over to see what's in store for your area.

☐ **Keep an eye on the weather.** If it's windy and dry, stay inside. You're better off gardening on still, even sultry days, when there's less airborne pollen. The best days? Misty, with just a bit of drizzle to keep down the dust and pollen.

☐ **Clean up properly.** When you finish gardening, leave your shoes by the back door, immediately strip off your clothing, and shower. Don't forget to wash your hair; otherwise, you could transfer pollens to your pillow when you go to bed. Toss your dirty clothes into the wash right away to avoid spreading pollens and other airborne allergens around the house.

☐ **Reduce molds.** Substitute gravel, other rocks, or black plastic mulch for wood and leaf mulch to cut down on the number of mold spores you come in contact with while you are gardening.

☐ **Keep it airy.** Heavy hedges can trap dust, pollen, and mold. Opt for a fence.

continued »

☐ **Opt for low-allergy plants.** Thomas Leo Ogren, author of *Allergy-Free Gardening* (the gardening bible for people with allergies), created the Ogren Plant-Allergy Scale (OPALS), which ranks plants according to their allergen potential.

Although there is no way to avoid pollens entirely, Ogren makes some suggestions for planting a garden that he says should reduce sneezing and itching. One of his main theories—although not everyone agrees with it—is that the dominance of "male" plants in landscapes and gardens is causing an overabundance of pollen in yards and public spaces. "Female" plants produce more seeds, flowers, and/or fruit and thus are messier to care for, but they are receivers of pollen rather than generators. Among his suggestions:

• **Stick with plants that have both male and female parts** (such as apple trees and roses). These pollens don't have to travel far (since both sexes are right *there*, get it?), so they are less likely to invade your nose and eyes. The same theory is at work with what are called monoecious-flowered plants, such as corn, which have separate male and female flowers on the same plant.

• **Go for female only.** Ogren recommends creating a "female-only" landscape, focusing on cleaner trees such as ash, willow, mulberry, juniper, and maple. As he notes, "such a garden would not release a single grain of pollen, ever!" The problem is that without any males around for pollination, you can forget about having any fruit from your trees.

☐ **Emphasize flowers, not bushes**, in your landscape. As we made clear in chapter 3, the pollen in flowers rarely causes allergies, thanks to its large size. It's the microscopic pollens from many bushes and trees that are the culprits, so build a fence if you need privacy, and get those bulbs planted!

While traveling

Having asthma or allergies shouldn't confine you to your home, but they can pose some unique challenges when you're traveling. To ensure a healthy, sneeze-free vacation or business trip, try these tips.

On the plane

☐ **Ask the nonobvious questions.** Call the airline and ask about its "pets on board" travel policy. If it allows passengers to bring small dogs and cats into the cabin, insist that you be seated as far away as possible from anyone carrying an animal. Some airlines also have a peanut-free policy.

☐ **Leave early.** Book the first flight of the day; you'll travel on a freshly cleaned plane.

☐ **Consider an upgrade.** The fabric seats in economy class are perfect havens for dust mites and other allergens. Often, seats in business class are leather, making them much less hospitable to allergens.

☐ **Consider a filtering face mask.** If the highly processed and recycled air on an airplane has triggered responses before, forget about what people may think and wear a mask. This can greatly cut down on the allergens you breathe.

☐ **Have your medications with you.** There's simply no more important advice we can give you, particularly in this day of airline delays, changes, and long waits. And premedicate: Take antihistamines the morning of your flight and a puff of your inhaler before boarding the plane.

- **Pack properly.** Add your own pillow and blanket to your carry-on bag for long flights, and carry an emergency phone number for your doctor.
- **Carry extra drinking water.** Having a large bottle of water on an airplane trip is always useful. Even when the flight attendants are diligent about serving water, they give you small cups, so you may end up feeling dehydrated.

At your destination

- **Consider the season.** Just as weather varies widely around the globe, so do regional allergy seasons. Check the average pollen counts for your destination before booking your trip.
- **See the medical sights.** Make sure you know where the closest emergency medical facility is located—just in case.
- **Pick the right lodging.** You're probably better off at a modern, albeit sterile, hotel than at a cozy (and probably allergen heavy) bed-and-breakfast or inn. It's also much better to stay in a hotel than in a friend or relative's home.

Some hotels even have special allergy-free rooms or provide allergy packs, including face masks, special pillows, and mattress covers. See if you can find a room without carpeting in a hotel that forbids pets.

- **Pick the right destination.** How about the beach or the mountains, where the air is clearer? In other words, exploring damp, musty caves or touring old, historic houses probably isn't the best vacation for you. However, a cruise on the pollen-free open seas could be a good alternative.
- **Use housekeeping services.** To save water and energy, many hotels today ask if they can change the sheets every other day or when you leave instead of daily. That's fine for most people, but someone with allergies needs clean sheets daily.
- **Pack your own.** If you're wary of your hotel's cleaning practices, pack a queen- or king-size sheet to throw over the bedspread so you're not exposed to the dust mites and other allergens lurking in the cover.

In the car

Americans spend an average of 75 minutes daily in their cars. These days, we often treat them like extensions of our homes and offices. We chat on the phone in our cars, check our e-mail from them, dine in them, and even take naps in them (preferably with the engine off).

Since most cars spend their lives exposed to the elements, they can quickly become minefields when it comes to allergies and asthma. Here's how to keep your moving living room as allergen-free as possible.

- **Sniff the air.** If your car smells like dirty socks, you've probably got mold. Check the air-conditioning coil, which may harbor mold; the carpet in the interior and trunk; and that wet blanket you threw in the backseat after your son's soccer game last weekend.
- **Avoid air fresheners.** The scent can exacerbate your asthma.

- **Clean your car regularly.** That means more than running it through the car wash. It means steam-cleaning the carpet and upholstery (unless you have leather seats), wiping down the interior with a damp cloth every couple of weeks, and throwing out trash daily.
- **Time your commute.** If at all possible, avoid congested streets and rush-hour traffic that

continued »

can emit high levels of fuel exhaust, possibly making your asthma worse.

☐ **Keep the inside dry.** Wet feet, spilled drinks, and a window left open over a rainy night can all be catalysts for some serious mold, thanks to the absorbent fabrics found on so many car seats and floors. If your car's interior does get wet, do what you can to dry it quickly. Use towels to sop up all the moisture you can and consider using a fan to dry up any remaining dampness. Remember to lift the mats.

☐ **Avoid eating in your car.** A car that's full of crumbs, shriveled French fries, lettuce leaves from a burger, and apple cores in the ashtray is a car full of mold and bacteria.

☐ **Use the AC.** Turn it on even on cool days, and set the airflow switch to "recirculate." This combination minimizes the amount of external pollen and dust that comes into the car.

At work

As you'll learn in chapter 15, there are numerous chemicals and odors in office buildings that can trigger allergy or asthma attacks, particularly given today's sealed-tight office environments. Additionally, some office equipment, such as photocopiers, computers, fax machines, and printers, gives off ozone and other irritants that can exacerbate asthma. Yet a British Allergy Foundation survey found that 94 percent of office workers don't even know that the equipment that surrounds them gives off ozone.

Overall, the Occupational Safety and Health Administration estimates that 11 million workers are exposed to some 200 substances associated with occupational asthma, and about 15 percent of "disabling" cases of asthma are related to the workplace. If you fall into this category, you have two options: Change jobs or change your environment. As part of the Breathe Easy Plan, we want you to do what you can to make your work environment healthier, using the following tips as a start. If you feel your company is not taking health-related factors in your building seriously enough, you'll find more pointed advice in chapter 15.

☐ **Treat your work space like your home.** Go back to step 3 of the Breathe Easy Plan and apply the same worksheets and advice you used for improving your living room or den to your work space. Identify the most likely sources of allergens and irritants and make as many improvements as your boss will allow.

☐ **Keep it clean.** Piles of paper, books, tools, and product samples cause two problems: First, they attract dust and allergens, and second, they prevent the cleaning staff from doing their job. If you can't manage to keep yourself organized and neat for professional reasons, do it for health reasons.

☐ **Develop a green thumb.** Live plants around the office can help absorb chemical emissions. A study conducted by researchers from NASA and the Associated Landscape Contractors of America found that philodendron, spider plant, and golden pothos were the plants most effective at removing formaldehyde molecules, while flowering plants such as gerbera daisy and chrysanthemum were best at removing benzene. Just be sure to water them properly and keep the leaves dust-free. Plants and their soil can generate their own host of allergens and molds if you aren't careful. Also be aware of any insects your plant may carry.

- **Pick the right spot.** Ask if you can sit in a part of the building that has solid-surface flooring near a window that opens. If your allergies or asthma are serious, make your case stronger by enlisting your doctor to either write a note or call your manager.

- **Minimize food and drink in your work space.** Unwashed coffee cups, bagel crumbs on the floor, a half-eaten sandwich left overnight on your desk: All of these contribute to dirt, mold, and a generally unhealthy atmosphere. Turn over your computer keyboard and give it a gentle shake. If crumbs fall out, you need to change your snacking and meal habits.

- **Speak up.** Don't be afraid to talk to your boss if a change in office policy suddenly lets employees bring their pets to work or if a coworker's perfume or office environment makes you wheeze. The Americans with Disabilities Act (ADA) of 1990, which requires employers to take reasonable measures to accommodate employees with special health issues and disabilities, covers asthma.

- **Track it.** Use the symptom tracking log on page 86 to track your asthma/allergy symptoms in the workplace and identify specific triggers. This will provide valuable information that you can share with both your boss and your doctor.

- **Work in the right section.** If you work in a retail business, such as a department store, arrange to cover a section of the store that doesn't include perfumes, scented candles, and potpourri. The appliance or housewares department would be just right for someone like you.

- **Get your orders straight.** If you work in a restaurant and have allergies or asthma, you're facing a double whammy. For one, cigarette smoke can trigger an asthma attack. For another, if you're allergic to certain foods, just touching them or even breathing in their vapors can trigger an allergic reaction. If wait service is your forte, be sure you're assigned to the nonsmoking section. And, if you have allergies to certain foods your guests order, turn your table over to another server.

During the holidays

'Tis the season...for major asthma and allergy attacks, if you're not careful. With live evergreens heading indoors to deck the halls amid potpourri-scented air, the Christmas holidays can turn the most cheerful allergy/asthma sufferer into a growling Grinch. But preparing ahead can guarantee a jolly time for all.

- **Get the right tree.** That would be artificial. Today, these trees are so realistic that you have to pinch the needles between your fingers to realize they're not alive. The artificial rule also goes for wreaths and mantel decorations. Even if you're not allergic to pine or other types of evergreens, fresh trees have to be kept damp for weeks between the time they're cut and when they're sold, so they can harbor mold.

- **Clean the decorations.** They've been down in your basement or up in your attic all year. Make sure you wipe them off thoroughly with a damp cloth to remove any dust, and throw away any that show signs of mold.

- **Handle the stress.** Now is when you need to make sure you're following the advice in step 5 of the Breathe Easy Plan. Christmas, with its parties, family tensions, travel, decorating, and financial woes, can send your stress levels

continued »

skyrocketing. Take extra time away from of the bustle just for you. Have a quiet lunch in an out-of-the-way inn, a night at the symphony, or a walk in the snowy woods. Take a day off from work to shop in the middle of the week when stores are less crowded and salespeople less surly. Hire some help. For instance, at www.Hallmark.com, you can arrange to have personalized Christmas cards mailed to people on a list that you supply. Housekeeping services come in real handy at this time of year, and most supermarkets these days stock an enticing array of prepared foods that work quite well as part or all of a company meal.

☐ **Scent your home naturally.** Instead of scented candles and potpourri or scented sprays, simmer a couple of cinnamon sticks and some orange peel in water on low heat on the back of your stove. Or put out small bowls of vanilla-soaked cotton balls to absorb odors.

☐ **Decorate the fireplace.** No, not the mantel, the *fireplace*. No matter how cozy, a blazing fire won't help your asthma or allergies, so you're better off using it to display a dried flower arrangement or covering it with a decorative screen.

☐ **Watch what you eat.** If you have food allergies, you should be especially vigilant during the holidays. Watch out for eggnog, Christmas cookies that may contain nuts, and candies that may harbor peanut butter.

Through the seasons

As you probably know all too well, weather conditions can mean the difference between a productive, energetic day and one in which you can do little more than reach for your inhaler and swallow antihistamines. You also know that many forms of allergies and asthma are seasonal—that is, they occur at around the same time each year.

We've already given you lots of advice about managing particular allergens and environmental issues, but there's more to be said on the topic. In this part of the Breathe Easy Plan, we ask that you be mindful of seasonal weather issues that might affect your condition—and then take action.

General guidelines

☐ **Monitor the weather.** If you have allergies or asthma, the Weather Channel should be the first thing you watch in the morning, and www.weather.gov should be set as your home page on your computer. Knowing the temperature, the humidity, and the chance of rain or snow ahead of time gives you the information necessary to take medication preemptively and prepare yourself for a potential onslaught of symptoms.

☐ **Manage your coats—and pockets.** People with allergies or asthma should have a year-round plan for their outerwear. For example, you may wish to keep four primary coats in your wardrobe: a winter coat for work and evenings out, a winter jacket for casual wear and outdoor fun, a cool-weather jacket for spring and fall, and a windbreaker or raincoat for warm but wet or windy days. Once you have implemented your coat strategy, stock the pockets of each with the items you need to manage your condition during that season: tissues, rescue medications, scarves, sunglasses, throat lozenges, and so on.

Winter

☐ **Bundle up your face.** Wear a scarf or face mask over your nose and mouth on very cold days to warm the air you breathe. And wrap your face *before* you head outside. All it takes is a few full breaths of raw, cold air to bring on an attack. If cold air is a trigger for your asthma, try taking a dose of your inhaler 10 minutes before heading outside.

☐ **Take it slowly.** If you live in a snowy locale, you know that the mere act of walking outside in winter can be tough exercise. If you're susceptible to exercise-induced asthma attacks, be particularly careful as you walk, shovel snow, or play. Start slowly and increase exertion only if your body has responded without any sign of stress after at least 15 minutes of activity.

Spring

☐ **Watch for lightning.** If thunderstorms are predicted, try to stay indoors in air conditioning. At the very least, keep all your windows closed. As we discussed in chapter 4, studies have found that airborne fungal spores nearly double during thunderstorms, significantly aggravating asthma.

☐ **Clear out the rot.** No matter how well you cleaned up four months earlier, spring—particularly in snowy areas—reveals the remains of the past autumn in all its allergy-inducing glory: rotted leaves, crumpled flower remains, broken branches, fallen pine cones, and so on. Rain and warmer weather can turn all that organic waste into a haven for mold and mildew. While a good garden needs compost, clear out the waste that isn't going to contribute to your prize-winning roses and tomatoes come summer.

Summer

☐ **Pay attention to ozone.** Ozone tends to be worst during the May-to-October "smog season," so try to limit outdoor activities on bad ozone days. Most municipalities now issue smog or ozone alerts during the summer when the air is particularly bad. On those days, stay inside in air conditioning as much as possible. If you don't have air conditioning, go to a library or mall during the afternoon, which is the worst part of the day for ozone.

☐ **Wear black.** Or at least stick to solid colors in neutral tones. Bright colors that mimic the colors of flowers entice stinging insects.

☐ **Beware the hot air.** For some people, hot, dry air can be as irritating to the lungs as icy air. If the temperature exceeds 85°F, be cautious as you go about your outdoor business. If your lungs start aching, go back inside.

Fall

☐ **Hands off the leaves.** Ideally, have someone else rake and pick up your leaves, which harbor mold and other allergens. If no one volunteers, buy a leaf blower so you have less contact with the mold. And while you're at it, wear a face mask to filter the air.

☐ **Clean out the garden.** Cut down old perennials and rake out dead leaves and plants. The more air circulates, the less mold will grow.

☐ **Do a fall cleaning inside.** The days are shorter, the weather's less inviting—autumn begins the "indoors" season. Why wait until spring to do a thorough housecleaning? Instead, do a preemptive top-to-bottom cleaning of your home each October. Get the house in the best shape possible for several months of comfortable, allergen-free nesting.

STEP SEVEN

breathe to beat allergies & asthma

We normally don't think much about breathing. After all, it's a reflex, something we perform as unconsciously as sleeping. If you have asthma or allergies, however, chances are you stopped taking breathing for granted long ago. In this final step of the Breathe Easy Plan, you'll learn how to focus on the way you breathe and strengthen your diaphragm to improve your breathing.

This may seem like a stretch, but it's not. As any athlete knows, lung power can be developed. After all, breathing is controlled by muscles that—like your biceps or thigh muscles—can be exercised, strengthened, and conditioned.

We'll show you an easy way to do that, using a method called Breathing Coordination. It's based on the fact that with asthma, the problem isn't so much getting air into your lungs as it is getting air completely *out*. As airways narrow and fill with mucus, your body struggles to exhale all the air you've inhaled. Thus, carbon dioxide–laden air builds up in your lungs as you take in less oxygen with each breath.

To help people move more carbon dioxide out of their lungs, researcher Carl Stough created the Breathing Coordination process. The goal is to strengthen your diaphragm muscle so you can move air out of and into your lungs more efficiently. Also, by teaching you to extend your exhale, the exercise can reduce the panic that often occurs with an asthma attack, helping you to self-limit the attack and its severity.

"The most common problem I see among people with asthma is that they're overinhaling," says Lynn Martin, a Breathing Coordination instructor in New York City who also lectures to anatomy students at New York University. "They're working too hard to try to pull more air into the lungs, using musculature that isn't appropriate for this use," she says. This could be one reason that people with asthma often complain of a sore back after an attack.

By systematically developing the diaphragm using the following exercise, Martin says, you will be able to more easily exhale air from your lungs, preventing the shortness of breath and shallow breathing so common in those with asthma.

What you will be doing	**How you should prepare**	**What to have on hand**
Learning the Breathing Coordination technique to strengthen your diaphragm and improve your breathing.	Pick a time when you will have no interruptions, choose a quiet place, and wear comfortable, loose clothing.	Two pillows, plus whatever else you need to lie comfortably on the floor.

TASK 1

the breathing coordination exercise

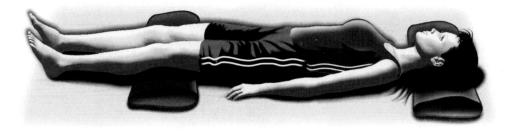

1. Although you can do this exercise while sitting or standing, the most relaxing position is **lying on your back with a pillow under your knees and another under your head.** In this position, your diaphragm doesn't work against gravity, and you don't need to bring any voluntary muscles into play just to balance and support your body. Remember: You're not supposed to work at inhaling or exhaling.

2. Make sure your **jaw is loose and your mouth** is open when you inhale. This doesn't mean that you do all mouth breathing, but at this point, it helps to keep your throat open.

3. Inhale, and then on the exhale, **count without sound**, with easy jaw and tongue movements. Build the silent count in **continuous rounds of the numbers** from 1 to 10 (1-2-3-4-5-6-7-8-9-10-1-2-3-4-5-6-7-8-9-10). You have to speak the numbers, but you can do it very softly, below the level of an audible whisper. This tricks the space between the vocal folds to stay open and extends the exhale without any pressure.

4. Continue the relaxed exhale **as long as possible** in order to cause a reflex inhale. Make sure your jaw is still loose and your mouth is open on the inhale. Repeat the process of exhaling with extended silent counting for a few minutes.

5. Next, continue the process, but **start making audible sound** in your larynx. This challenges the diaphragm a bit more by providing a progressive resistance exercise for the diaphragm to work against on the exhale. Start the audible counting very simply, with only five digits at a time (1-2-3-4-5). Once you start, remember that you want to be heard. Don't make a special effort to be loud, but think of projecting the sound so the air will continue to flow out freely while you count.

6. **Repeat the process** of exhaling with extended audible counting for a few minutes.

continued »

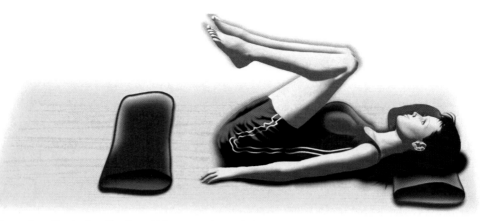

7. Occasionally during the breathing exercise, while lying down and continuing to count during exhales, **bring your knees up** toward your chest and, with your feet off the floor, **gently swing your legs** from side to side.

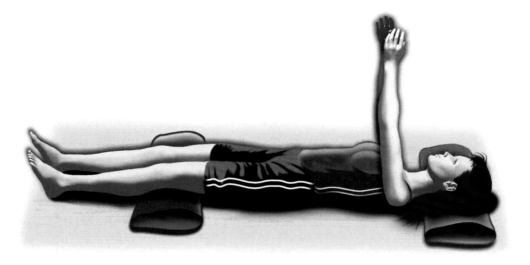

8. After swinging your legs, and while still continuing the breathing exercise, **raise your arms** toward the ceiling and **let them swing** from side to side to loosen your shoulders. These leg and arm movements reduce tension in the lower back and shoulder girdle, which is important because these muscles often interfere with the diaphragm's freedom of movement and with the freedom of the ribs to move in response to the diaphragm. Be sure that the swinging motions **occur on an exhale**, and keep counting quietly to keep the exhale going.

9. Do this exercise for **10 minutes a day,** either in one steady effort or in smaller increments.

Extra tips

- Once you feel comfortable with the Breathing Coordination exercise, you can **practice wherever you like**—maybe while driving your car or taking a shower or cooking dinner. In particular, you can do the silent portion of the breathing exercise anywhere, anytime. If you do the exercise daily for the prescribed time, Martin says you should feel an improvement in your breathing strength in about two weeks.

- **Never force either inhaling or exhaling.** You may be able to get to an exhale count of 40 or 50 without rushing, but keep your diaphragm moving by doing it in a sing-song. If your count is too precise, your diaphragm may not move as smoothly.

- While counting, **make sure your diaphragm rises.** If the count goes too long and your diaphragm begins to tense, you will feel pressure in your lower abdomen between your hip bones. This means that your abdomen isn't contracting but is dropping inward when your diaphragm rises. Don't push past that. When your diaphragm rises, everything above it and below it releases, so you can feel your chest and lower abdomen drop toward your spine. That's what you want to feel.

- As this exercise becomes easier, you should be able to accomplish the same thing **sitting or standing,** with a similar sensation.

- The best times to practice are **first thing in the morning** and **last thing at night.** You should also prime your breathing before you start making physical demands on your body, such as a little walking or some calisthenics. If you do it right before bed, it should be very relaxing and provide you with a better night's sleep.

- The more you practice, the faster your muscles will develop. Just make sure all practice is **done in a relaxed way.** The length of the practice depends on your success. If it's going very well and you have the time, continue. If it's not going well, let it go and try again later.

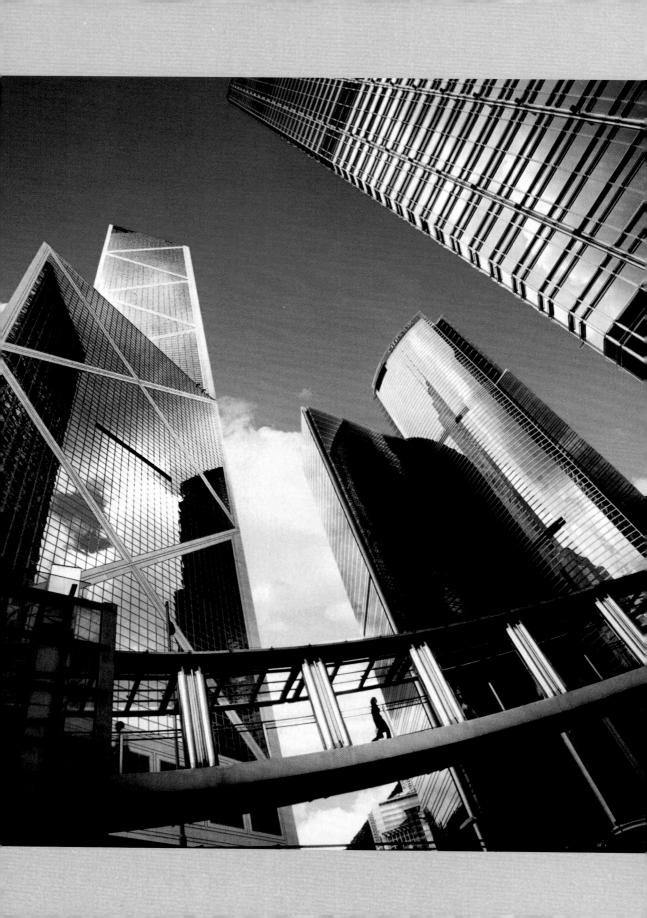

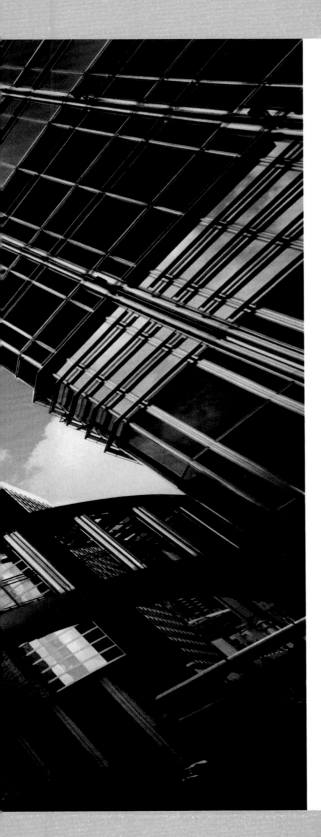

PART FOUR

special
situations

The Breathe Easy Plan was built
to be effective for most types of
allergies and asthma, but some
forms of these conditions require
unique advice. In the pages ahead,
we offer customized advice for
skin and insect allergies, "sick buildings," and exercise-induced asthma.
Most important, we provide guidance for parents of children with
allergies or asthma.

chapter twelve

allergies & asthma in
children

In the opening pages of this book, we talked about the allergy and asthma epidemic that is increasing in this country. It's a problem for people of all ages, of all backgrounds, and in all locations. That said, the epicenter of the epidemic truly lies with our children. Just consider:

■ Between 1980 and 1994, the number of asthma cases in children under 5 increased by more than 160 percent and rose by 74 percent among children ages 5 through 14.

■ Asthma is the most common chronic childhood illness; in 1998 (the latest year for which statistics are available), it affected an estimated 8.65 million American children—more than 12 percent of the entire under-18 population. In 1994, that figure was just 5 percent. Allergic rhinitis is even more prevalent, affecting an estimated 20 to 40 percent of children.

■ Asthma accounts for an estimated 11.8 million missed school days nationally and costs more than $1 billion per year in lost productivity in the United States due to parents staying home to care for their children.

In chapter 1, we discussed many of the reasons for the dramatic increase in asthma and allergies, including a "too-clean" environment, diet, actions a woman takes during her pregnancy, and environmental exposure. In this chapter, we focus on how allergies and asthma differ between children and adults, tell you how to recognize these conditions in your child and possibly prevent allergies from advancing to asthma, show you ways to handle the everyday issues of having a child with allergies or asthma, and provide easy-to-use charts on medications for children.

signs to watch for

See that scaly red patch on your baby's arm or chest? Watch it closely. It could be atopic dermatitis, better known as eczema, a chronic itch that develops into a rash. It can be quite uncomfortable, making your baby fussy and irritable.

Don't dismiss the problem as merely the sensitive skin of a child. Eczema is a sign—a canary-in-the-mineshaft kind of sign—that your child may soon develop allergies and/or asthma. Roughly 40 percent of infants with eczema develop asthma by age 4, and about 30 percent of all eczema cases in toddlers are linked to an allergy, of which a third are food related. So, if you see red, dry patches on your child's skin, talk to your doctor about allergy testing. The

Recognizing Asthma and Allergies in Children

From 50 to 80 percent of children with asthma develop symptoms before age 5. The vast majority of their asthma symptoms, however, are triggered by viral infections, not allergies. That's one reason symptoms of early asthma often mimic those of other childhood diseases, such as respiratory infections or stomach flu, and are often ignored by physicians. If you find that your child has periodic or persistent coughing, wheezing, shortness of breath, rapid breathing, or chest tightness, and if these symptoms get worse during the evening or early morning or are associated with triggers such as exercise or allergen exposure, ask your doctor to evaluate your child for asthma.

Keep in mind that just because your child isn't wheezing doesn't mean that he doesn't have asthma; not all children with asthma wheeze. Conversely, not all children who wheeze have asthma. Respiratory infections, rhinitis, sinusitis, and vocal cord dysfunction can all cause wheezing.

Allergic rhinitis hits a bit later, usually at about 9 or 10, so if your child has already been diagnosed with asthma and then develops nasal symptoms that suggest allergies, you should be concerned. Expect the first two or three years of coping with childhood allergies to be the worst; after that, symptoms generally level off and may even improve by the time your kid turns into an adult. In fact, about 20 percent of children with allergic rhinitis find that their symptoms disappear as they enter adulthood.

Like asthma, allergic rhinitis often goes undiagnosed and untreated in children. Signs to be on the lookout for include "allergic shiners" under your child's eyes, an "allergic crease" on his nose from constant rubbing, a nasal voice, constant mouth breathing and chapped lips, frequent snoring, coughing from postnasal drainage, frequent sneezing, and gaping of the mouth. Other possible symptoms include weakness, fatigue, irritability, and poor appetite.

earlier allergies are identified and treated, the less likely they are to become more severe or even develop into asthma. Identifying and treating asthma early on can prevent the kind of long-term lung damage that can make the condition worse.

Another clue that your child may be prone to allergies is gastrointestinal upset. Food sensitivities—although not necessarily full-blown allergies—can cause the symptoms. Children who have early and long-lasting food sensitivities

Beyond a Spoonful of Sugar

It's not always easy to get a recalcitrant preschooler to take medicine, especially if that medicine involves putting on a mask, as with a nebulizer. Even older children can be loath to swallow pills or use their inhalers. So what's a parent to do?

Nebulizers

Children age 5 and under are more likely to use a nebulizer with a face mask, particularly during an asthma emergency. Unfortunately, toddlers and infants hate the "trapped" feeling they get when the mask is pulled over their face, so parents often simply hold the mask up to the child's face in the hope that some medicine gets in. Studies have found, however, that this technique, called "blow by," is useless. If you don't have a closed seal when you use a nebulizer mask, virtually none of the medicine gets into the child's lungs, and the treatment is ineffective (except maybe for the nearby houseplants). Even a tiny space between the mask and the face allows most of the medicine to dissipate into the air. Given, then, that you must make your child wear the mask properly, concentrate on ways to divert and entertain her during the session.

Make it a game. If you have a very young child, try giving nebulizer treatments to her favorite doll or stuffed animal first, so she becomes comfortable with the procedure.

Make it special. Keep a special video that your child can watch only during nebulizer treatments. Also have a special treat on hand that she may have only after treatments or medication.

Inhalers and medications

Studies have found that even when children succeed in mastering metered dose inhalers (MDI), just 10 to 15 percent of the medication reaches the lungs. If your child has to take medicine with an MDI, ask your doctor to prescribe a spacer, which holds the "puff" of medicine between the patient and the MDI so it can be inhaled slowly and more completely. Spacers are effective at delivering medicine to the lungs more easily and successfully.

Another possibility for older kids (5 and up) is a dry-powder inhaler, which gets more medicine to the lungs. Be sure you and your child know how to use it, however, or again, the medicine will be wasted. Here are some other ideas for getting your child to take medication.

Use a sticker program. Each time the child takes the medicine without complaining, award a sticker. When he earns 10 stickers, give him a nice reward.

Make it taste good. If your child's medicine tastes bad, check into pharmacies that add appealing flavors to liquid medicines.

Make it easier to swallow. Wetting a gelatin capsule can soften it and make it easier to take. You can also ask your doctor if you can put oral medication in a cup of juice or mash it into applesauce or ice cream.

Ask about giving it less frequently. Ask your doctor if there are longer-acting dosages your child can take or if it's okay to take a twice-a-day medicine all at once. Both will reduce the stress of "medicine time."

are three times more likely to develop allergic rhinitis than children who don't have them, and they're more than five times more likely to develop asthma.

Eczema and gastric upsets are the first steps in what researchers call the allergic march, a constellation of clues in early life that signal a child's increased risk for allergies and asthma.

The allergic march begins with a genetic predisposition, i.e., parents, siblings, or other close relatives who have allergies or asthma. It continues with the skin rashes and stomach upsets described above and progresses to recurrent ear infections (as many as 79 percent of children with chronic ear infections have confirmed allergic rhinitis), nasal congestion, and asthma.

Most primary care physicians are not trained to recognize the signs of the allergic march. If you're aware of the clues, however, they can give you an early heads-up about your child's health, enabling you to avoid treatments that won't work and allowing you to start on treatments that will—and possibly even prevent the ultimate destination of the march, asthma.

For instance, some research suggests that early use of inhaled corticosteroids may prevent the early development of asthma in at-risk children. A large national study sponsored by the National Institutes of Health called Prevention of Early Asthma in Kids (PEAK) hopes to have more definitive information on that in a few years.

Another study gave one- and two-year-olds who already had atopic dermatitis the antihistamine cetirizine (Zyrtec). Eighteen months after treatment, researchers found, the children who received Zyrtec who were allergic to grass and/or dust mites were significantly less likely to develop asthma than those who didn't receive the drug. The benefit continued for up to 18 months after the children stopped taking the medication.

Early treatment also helps your child avoid the psychosocial effects of allergies and asthma. Children with allergic rhinitis, for instance, are more likely to be shy, depressed, anxious, and fearful than other children. Sleep problems and missed school days can interfere with their academic development and their self-esteem.

Don't start medicating your child on your own, however. Before you do anything, have her tested. If your doctor finds evidence of allergies or asthma, discuss steps you can take to minimize their effects on her health. They may include environmental changes, starting the proper medications, or removing any allergy-causing foods from her diet. In fact, the Breathe Easy Plan is every bit as appropriate and effective for a child as it is for an adult. Make following the plan a family affair, and everyone's health will benefit.

Finally, you might consider allergy shots for your child. Studies suggest that an early course of immunotherapy in children with allergic rhinitis significantly reduces their risk of developing asthma. It's a rigorous, difficult treatment for a child, but the payoff may last for many years.

it's different for children

Researchers are beginning to suspect that asthma in children is actually a different disease than asthma in adults. "Kids clearly seem different," says Joseph Spahn, M.D., associate professor of pediatrics at the National Jewish Medical and Research Center in Denver. Children and adults from around the country come to the center for treatment for severe asthma, the type that isn't easily controlled by medicine.

When Dr. Spahn and his colleagues evaluated 260 people with severe asthma, ranging in age from 2 to 74 years, they found significant differences between the kids and the grownups. For one, even though the children were classified as having severe asthma, their lung function tests put them in the mild to moderate category. This could have been because the children hadn't had the disease as long as the adults and thus had better lung function overall. But what concerns Dr. Spahn is that national guidelines for evaluating asthma severity don't distinguish between adults and children. In other words, even though a child has a lung function test that suggests mild to moderate asthma, that child may in fact have severe asthma and require more aggressive treatment.

Dr. Spahn's study also found that lung function in children with severe asthma deteriorated much more rapidly than in adults, suggesting that the disease progresses more quickly. Thus, he says, pediatricians should measure a child's lung function just as they measure a child's growth over time, looking for early signs of decline.

These may seem like esoteric facts, but if your child is constantly sick, can't seem to get his asthma under control, and yet is classified as having only mild to moderate asthma—and treated accordingly—you may want to talk to your doctor about taking a more aggressive approach.

asthma and gender differences

Another difference between adults and children when it comes to asthma is that males are more likely to have asthma in childhood, but females are more likely to have it in adolescence and adulthood. In fact, about 65 percent of young children with asthma are boys. That number flips in adolescence and beyond, however, and 65 percent of adults with asthma are women.

One theory about the gender difference is that boys may be born with smaller airways in relation to their lung size, says Dr. Spahn, so they're more prone to airflow obstruction. Once they hit adolescence and its growth spurts, however, their airways also grow. This sends their asthma into remission, he says, but still puts them at risk for later recurrences.

With girls, researchers suspect that the hormones of puberty—estrogen and progesterone—play some role in the increased rates of asthma, but girls, unlike boys, are unlikely to go into remission. In fact, simply being female increases a girl's risk of having persistent asthma into adulthood by nearly twofold.

explaining asthma to your child

So you've just learned that your 7-year-old's chronic cough and wheezing are due not to a viral infection but to asthma. He now has to take medicine every day, learn to use a peak flow meter, and remain hypersensitive to things most kids never think about, such as weather changes and whether his friends have pets in their homes. How do you explain all this?

■ **Use simple language.** You don't want to get into areas such as the immune system and mucus and airway constriction. Instead, first explain what the lungs do—"They're where the air goes when you breathe in"—and then explain what happens when you have asthma—"Your lungs just don't work as well. It's kind of like a clogged sink."

■ **Use visual aids.** There are numerous children's books that explain how our bodies work, as well as several specifically targeted toward children that explain asthma. You can also ask your doctor for any pamphlets or coloring books intended for kids. Finally, one of the best resources for parents is a group called Allergy and Asthma Network Mothers of Asthmatics (www.aanma.org).

■ **Be honest.** Don't pretend the medicine is candy or a "cure." Instead, tell your child that she is very lucky, because today there is medicine to help her lungs work better, but it's important that she take it every day. And don't minimize the seriousness of the condition. Make sure your child understands what to do if she can't breathe.

■ **Involve your child.** Depending on your child's age, she can help participate in managing the condition.

parents **ask**

Are Allergy Shots Safe for Kids?

Definitely. A collaborative committee of the three major allergy and immunology medical societies found that immunotherapy for children is effective and often well tolerated. The committee recommends allergy shots for children with allergic rhinitis, allergic asthma, and allergies to stinging insects. Most exciting: Studies suggest that allergy shots in children with allergic rhinitis may *prevent* them from ever developing asthma (about 20 percent of children who have hay fever develop asthma within 8 to 10 years). Generally, children don't start immunotherapy until they're about 5, both because it's difficult to get young children to submit to the shots and because children generally don't develop pollen sensitivity until at least that age.

Does your child scream at the sight of needles? One 10-year European study on the use of oral immunotherapy (the SLIT technique discussed on page 107) found that it provides long-term relief for children as young as 4.

For instance, she can fill in the peak flow meter chart every day or keep a journal to track how she feels. If your child is too young to write, set aside a few minutes each day during which she tells you how she's feeling and *you* write it in the journal.

■ **Explain the warning signs.** Make sure your child knows what to do if she feels "funny" or "weird." Be sure she understands that this is a sign that an asthma or allergy attack may be imminent, and she should tell you, her teacher, or another adult.

building a support team

You love your pediatrician, who has answered every late-night phone call about fevers and rashes and fussiness and that weird mark on your toddler's back you were sure signaled Lyme disease. Still, a pediatrician may not be the best doctor to treat your child's asthma or allergies.

Too often, general pediatricians and family practitioners simply aren't as aware of the latest treatments and recommendations as allergy specialists are. For instance, initial data from a large study of children found that many who wind up in the emergency room are not using controlling medications or are using them inappropriately. The vast majority did not have asthma action plans or use a peak flow meters, suggesting that they were being undertreated.

If your child has mild asthma or allergies that are easily controlled, you probably don't need to see a specialist. But if your child's condition results in missed school days, emergency room visits, hospitalizations, and a noticeable effect on his quality of life, ask your pediatrician for a referral to a specialist. Chances are, you'll find that your child's condition will be better managed.

No matter which doctor you settle on, remember that managing your child's condition is a team effort. You need to enlist all of the following to make sure your child is getting the best support possible.

■ **Your child's doctor and all of the medical office staff.** Not only is the doctor crucial, but so are the nurses, the receptionist who makes the appointments, and the asthma educators in the doctor's practice. Even printed material is important: The doctor should be a major source of information on the medicines and treatments he provides.

■ **Your child's school.** Remember that school is to children as work is to you—that is, the place where they spend a lot of time and focus and where they have a unique set of people with whom they interact daily. Your child's teacher is at the forefront, but there are also the school nurse, coaches, bus drivers, and administrators who oversee your child's school days. In a moment, we'll give you lots of advice on the best ways to work with your child's school.

■ **Other adults in your child's life.** From the parents of your child's friends to the piano teachers, swimming instructors, and church leaders with whom your child interacts, each adult should be aware of his unique health needs. Sometimes a mere 1-minute conversation is enough to let them know the essentials of your child's condition.

■ **Your family.** The golden rule of health care today is to take responsibility. Managing the condition is a family commitment for you, your spouse, and your child; it's not your doctor's or anyone else's job. Reading this book is a great start. Exploring the resources provided on page 277 is also key. Most of all, talking extensively with each other is crucial. If there are other children in the family who don't have allergies or asthma, they need to be told about their sibling's health and how they can help. Encourage them to ask questions and explain any special equipment.

asthma-friendly schools

You've torn up your carpets, thrown out your 6-year-old's stuffed animals, encased his bed in mattress and pillow covers, and invested in HEPA filters for your entire house and heating system. But have you thought about what awaits him at school?

Studies have shown that children in half the nation's 115,000 schools have health problems linked to poor indoor air quality. Overall, pollutant levels inside classrooms and other indoor school facilities are often two to five times higher than outdoor levels and can trigger asthma attacks, notes the Environmental Protection Agency (EPA).

If you have a child with asthma or allergies, no matter how carefully you've modified your home environment, sending him to school can be like sending him into a war zone. No wonder children with asthma miss an estimated 10 million days of school a year.

The implication is that you have two broad responsibilities when it comes to your child's school: first, enlisting the partnership of the teachers and coaches in monitoring and helping your child; and second, making sure that the environment is as healthy as possible. The truth is, the latter is much harder than the former. After

You can succeed at improving the indoor *air quality at your child's school,* but it will take time and effort.

all, what teachers don't want to help the kids in their classes? Getting a school district to agree to better cleaning and maintenance techniques, though, takes some persuasion.

Let's start with the environmental issues. To determine how "health-friendly" your child's school is, answer the following questions from the National Heart, Lung, and Blood Institute. To help get accurate answers, consider asking the principal for an honest assessment of the school's health, environmental, and cleaning policies. Plus, get permission to do your own walkthrough of the school while it's in session to check out the situation.

1. Is the school free of tobacco smoke at all times, including during school-sponsored events?   yes ☐   no ☐

2. Does the school maintain good indoor air quality? Does it actively seek to reduce or eliminate allergens and irritants that can make asthma worse, such as:

✓ Cockroaches   yes ☐   no ☐

✓ Dust mites (commonly found in humid climates in pillows, carpets, upholstery, and stuffed toys)   yes ☐   no ☐

✓ Mold   yes ☐   no ☐

✓ Animals in cages, particularly those with fur or feathers   yes ☐   no ☐

✓ Strong odors or fumes from arts and crafts supplies, pesticides, paint, perfumes, air fresheners, or cleaning chemicals   yes ☐   no ☐

3. Is there a nurse at the school all day, every day? If not, is a nurse regularly available to help the school write plans and give guidance on medicines, physical education, and field trips for students with allergies or asthma?   yes ☐   no ☐

4. Can children take medicines at school as recommended by their doctors and parents? May they carry their own asthma or allergy medications?   yes ☐   no ☐

5. Does someone teach school staff about allergies and asthma and their treatments? Does someone teach students about allergies and asthma and how to help a classmate who has one or both?   yes ☐   no ☐

6. Do students with allergies or asthma have good options for fully and safely participating in physical education classes and recess? For example, do students have access to their medicine before exercise? Can they choose modified or alternative activities when medically necessary?   yes ☐   no ☐

If the answer to any of these questions is *no*, your child may be facing obstacles to controlling his condition once he enters the classroom. Don't despair, though. There are numerous things you can do to improve the indoor air quality at your child's school. It will take some effort and time, but it's worth it—for your child and probably for others with allergies or asthma as well.

The school principal is in charge and is the person to deal with. If your questions or concerns seem to catch the principal by surprise, let him know about the Indoor Air Quality Tools for Schools kit from the EPA, available online at www.epa.gov/iaq/schools/-tools4s2.html. The free kit includes easy-to-follow checklists, videos, sample memos and policies, and a recommended management plan to help schools identify, correct, and prevent indoor air-quality problems. Then lobby the principal to follow these steps, which are recommended by the American Academy of Allergy, Asthma, and Immunology.

- Use HEPA vacuum cleaners and filters to clean the school.
- Remove pets (guinea pigs, gerbils, and mice) from everyday classrooms.
- Remove any newspaper piles in classrooms. They can harbor mold, not to mention dust mites.
- Check books and shelves frequently for mold growth and dust accumulation.
- Check that classroom closets are free of dust-accumulating items, old clothes, and moisture sources.
- Provide adequate fresh air ventilation in classrooms. One way to do that is to trim trees, shrubs, hedges, and flowers away from classroom windows.
- Prohibit smoking on school premises, both indoors and out.
- Make sure vacuuming and cleaning with chemical solutions are done after school hours.
- Check that the school is well ventilated and that systems/filters are cleaned or replaced regularly.

While it's not in your power to make sure these measures are taken, it is fair and legitimate for you to inquire regularly and to have access to your child's classroom to see if the environment is healthy. If you're not getting an appropriate response, you're also within your rights to make your dissatisfaction clear

parents ask

Should My Child Stay Home Today?

If your child is in the midst of a major asthma or allergy attack, this question is a no-brainer. But what if he just has a cold or was coughing more than usual last night? These guidelines from the Center for Interdisciplinary Research on Immunologic Diseases at Georgetown University in Washington, D.C., can provide some guidance.

Your child can go to school with:
- A stuffy nose but no wheezing
- Mild wheezing that clears after medication
- The ability to do usual daily activities
- No difficulty breathing

Keep your child home with:
- Evidence of infection, sore throat, or swollen, painful neck glands
- A fever over 100°F, measured orally; a hot, flushed face
- Wheezing that continues to be labored 1 hour after medicine is given
- Weakness or tiredness that makes it hard to take part in usual daily activities
- Difficulty breathing

Also keep a close watch on your child's peak flow meter readings. If they are lower than normal, and your child has signs of infection or simply isn't acting like himself, you may want to keep him home for a day just in case an attack is imminent.

at the next board of education meeting. If the board members take your concerns seriously, rest assured that the school will take them more seriously as well.

While it may take some time and effort to effect change in a school's environmental policies, enlisting people to help monitor and care for your child should take just a few conversations. Make an appointment with your child's teacher and, if possible, the school nurse, prior to the start of the school year to introduce them to your child and make them aware of her condition. Offer to visit the classroom and talk about asthma so other children understand why your daughter sometimes needs her inhaler or gets out of breath quickly.

Also talk to school officials about allowing your child to carry her medication with her at all times rather than having to go the nurse's office every time she needs her inhaler. Added up throughout the year, these little side visits could cost your child a lot of valuable school time. She can carry her medicine in a fanny pack, in a pocket of her backpack, or in a purse. But warn your child that the medicine is not a toy; she shouldn't take it out and show it to friends or "play" with it when she's bored.

Are you the activist type? Then consider starting an asthma club for the kids in your child's school with the disease. Given the high numbers of children with asthma these days, it's a sure bet you'd get a good turnout. Not only will the children learn "kid-specific" tips for managing their asthma, they won't feel that they're alone. And there's a bonus: You'll meet other parents who can provide support when things get tough, and if any legal issues arise with the school, you'll have a larger voice.

You also need to make a special effort with your child's coaches and gym teachers. Be sure they have a typed list of emergency phone numbers and actions, and list step-by-step instructions for what to do in an emergency. If exercise tends to act as a trigger (as it does for most kids with asthma), be sure they know that your child needs to use an inhaler before activities. Stress that asthma is not a reason to cut out exercise or keep a child off a team.

safe drugs for children

National guidelines on the treatment of asthma in children call for doctors to start with the most aggressive therapy necessary to achieve control, then gradually "step down" medication dosages and types to the minimal therapy that will maintain control. Choosing the right medication is a bit more complicated for children than for adults, because not all medications have been officially approved for use in children. Don't worry, though, if your doctor prescribes a medication for your 6-year-old that is approved only for children 12 and over.

Many medications, particularly older drugs, have never been tested in children and so have never received formal FDA approval. Through long years of use, doctors have found what works in children and what doesn't.

For Allergic Rhinitis

You and your doctor should avoid giving your child any first-generation antihistamines, since they cause drowsiness and mental fuzziness that affects schoolwork, mood, and personality. Instead, ask your doctor for a prescription for one of the newer second-generation, nonsedating antihistamines. As for steroids, nasal versions carry lower risks than inhaled versions, but both are considered safe.

Antihistamines (prescription)

Brand/generic name	FDA-approved for ages	Comments
Astelin (azelastine HCl)	5 and up	unique antihistamine nasal spray
Allegra (fexofenadine)	6 and up	comes in 3 strengths (30, 60, and 180mg)
Allegra -D (fexofenadine+pseudoephedrine)	12 and up	antihistamine/decongestant
Clarinex (desloratadine)	12 and up	
Zyrtec tablets (cetirizine)	6 and up	comes in 2 strengths (5 and 10mg)
Zyrtec syrup (cetirizine)	6 months and up	only prescription nonsedating antihistamine in syrup form
Zyrtec-D (cetirizine+pseudoephedrine)	12 and up	antihistamine/decongestant

Antihistamines (over-the-counter)

Brand/generic name	FDA-approved for ages	Comments
Alavert (generic loratadine)	6 and up	quick dissolving tablet
Claritin tablets (loratadine)	6 and up	available in traditional tablet and quick dissolving forms
Claritin syrup (loratadine)	2 and up	
Claritin-D (loratadine+pseudoephedrine)	12 and up	antihistamine/decongestant (12- and 24-hour tablets)

Nasal Corticosteroids

Brand/generic name	FDA-approved for ages	Comments
Beconase AQ (beclomethasone)	6 and up	dose recommendation by age
Flonase (fluticasone propionate)	4 and up	dose recommendation by age
Nasacort AQ (triamcinolone acetonide)	6 and up	dose recommendation by age
Nasarel (flunisolide)	6 and up	dose recommendation by age
Nasonex (mometasone furoate monhydrate)	2 and up	dose recommendation by age
Rhinocort AQ (budesonide)	6 and up	dose recommendation by age
Vancenase AQ	6 and up	dose recommendation by age

For Asthma

Mast cell stabilizer drugs are generally effective for children, but if your child needs stronger anti-inflammatory medicine, do not hesitate to use inhaled corticosteroids. Studies show they can safely be used even in infants and young children, and evidence is strong that they improve the long-term condition of children of all ages with mild to moderate persistent asthma better than using beta2-agonists alone during attacks. Although corticosteroids may cause some temporary growth delay, children taking oral versions still reach their normal predicted adult height.

Mast Cell Stabilizers

Brand/generic name	FDA-approved for ages	Comments
Intal MDI (cromolyn sodium)	5 and up	
Intal Inhalation Solution (cromolyn sodium)	2 and up	inhalation solution only available in generic
Tilade MDI (nedocromil)	6 and up	

Leukotriene Modifiers

Brand/generic name	FDA-approved for ages	Comments
Accolate Tablets (zafirlukast)	5 and up	available in 2 strengths (10 and 20mg)
Singulair Tablets (montelukast sodium)	12 months and up	available in 3 strengths of chewable tablets (4, 5, and 10mg) and dissolvable granules (4mg); dose recommendation by age

Inhaled Corticosteroids

Brand/generic name	FDA-approved for ages	Comments
Aerobid (flunisolide)	6 and up	available in mint flavoring
Advair (fluticasone & salmeterol)	12 and up	available in 3 strengths (100/50, 250/50, and 500/50); combination of long-acting bronchodialator and inhaled corticosteroid
Azmacort (triamcinolone)	6 and up	dose recommendation by age
Flovent MDI (fluticasone propionate)	12 and up	available in 3 strengths (44, 110, and 220mcg)
Flovent Rotadisk (fluticasone propionate)	4 and up	available in 3 strengths (50, 100, and 250mcg)
Pulmicort (budesonide)	12 months and up	only inhaled corticosteroid available in both a nebulized solution (0.25 and 0.5mg) and dry powder inhaler; approved for use through pregnancy
QVAR (beclomethasone dipropionate)	5 and up	new propellant that can deliver smaller particles to the lungs

Short-Acting Bronchodialator

Brand/generic name	FDA-approved for ages	Comments
AccuNeb Inhalation (Albuterol)	2 and up	nebulizer solution; available in 2 strengths (0.63 and 1.25mg)
Alupent MDI (metaproterenol)	12 and up	
Generic Albuterol MDI	12 and up	
Brethine tablets (terbutaline)	12 and up	available in 2 strengths (2.5 and 5mg)
Proventil-HFA MDI (albuterol)	4 and up	CFC-free propellant
Proventil Inhalation Solution (albuterol)	12 and up	nebulizer solution

Long-Acting Bronchodialator

Brand/generic name	FDA-approved for ages	Comments
Foradil Aerolizer (formoterol fumarate)	5 and up	unique delivery system; rapid onset of action
Serevent Diskus (salmeterol)	4 and up	

Oral Steroids

Brand/generic name	FDA-approved for ages	Comments
Prednisolone syrup	not established	dosage based on severity of symptoms
Orapred syrup	not established	dosage based on severity of symptoms
Pediapred syrup	not established	dosage based on severity of symptoms
Prelone syrup	not established	available in 2 strengths (15 and 5mg/1 tsp); dosage based on severity of symptoms
Prednisone tablets	not established	available in multiple strengths
Medrol (methylprednisolone)	not established	available in multiple strengths

exercise-induced
asthma

Watching children run and play outside—whether on a playground or a soccer field—is one of the great joys in life. They seem to move so effortlessly—running freely, stooping, and jumping, their bodies seemingly made for motion, activity, and energy. But for a child—or an adult—with asthma, exercise is all too often a foe, not a friend: It triggers attacks in 80 to 90 percent of people with asthma. Amateur and professional athletes have particularly high rates of exercise-induced asthma, with studies finding that between 11 and 50 percent are affected.

Make no mistake: Exercise-induced asthma, also called exercise-induced bronchospasm, is asthma. It's not a type of asthma, an "asthma-like" condition, or a separate disease. It's diagnosed when you have an asthma attack, or spasm of the bronchial airways, 5 to 15 minutes after beginning or ending physical exertion. The main cause isn't really known, but researchers suspect it's related to the loss of heat, water, or both from the lungs during exercise. This occurs because of the common tendency to breathe through your mouth when you're exercising, so you take in cooler, drier air that hasn't had a chance to pass through your nose (which warms and moistens it).

Unfortunately, if exercise is the *only* trigger for asthma, the condition may go undiagnosed, particularly in athletes. The breathlessness and wheezing you experience after exercise may be the only symptom of exercise-induced asthma, leading you to think that you just get out of breath easily. That could be why one study found unrecognized exercise-induced bronchospasm in as many as 29 percent of athletes studied.

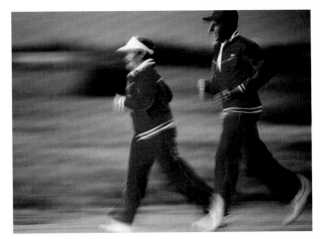

Researchers suspect exercise-induced asthma is related to *the loss of heat, water, or both from the lungs* during exercise.

Don't let this happen to you. As you learned in earlier chapters, asthma is often a chronic disease that requires treatment on a regular basis, not just when symptoms occur. When you exercise, watch out for shortness of breath or wheezing, decreased exercise endurance, chest pain or tightness, cough, upset stomach or stomachache, and sore throat. If you experience any of these symptoms, stop exercising and allow your breathing and heart rate to return to normal. Generally, the "attack" lasts only a few minutes, but it can be just as scary as any other asthma attack, often leading otherwise healthy people to avoid exercise altogether.

The only way to know for sure if your symptoms are related to asthma is to see a specialist, who may conduct an "exercise challenge" test to confirm a diagnosis. This usually involves evaluating your lung function before and after you've run on a treadmill or used an exercise bicycle for about 10 minutes.

preventive strategies

As with any form of asthma, medication plays a major role in controlling your symptoms, but there are also several nonmedical steps you can take to avoid exercise-induced asthma.

- Improve your overall physical condition. The better shape you're in, the stronger your lungs are. Thus, they'll be less sensitive to the cool, dry air you take in while exercising.
- Warm up for at least 10 minutes before you start exercising.
- Try not to exercise outside in cold weather. If you do (as with skiing), cover your mouth and nose with a scarf or face mask to warm and moisten the air.
- Exercise in warm, humidified environments. Swimming in a heated indoor

pool is often considered a good exercise for people with exercise-induced asthma.

- Try not to exercise outside in areas of high pollution or at times when the air quality is poor. For example, don't run alongside a busy road or bike on hot days when ozone levels are high.
- Wait at least 2 hours after eating before exercising. This ensures that your stomach has emptied and reduces the risk of gastric reflux, or heartburn, which could lead to aspirating bits of food into your lungs if you have an asthma attack.
- Try to breathe through your nose, not your mouth.

Also consider changing your sport. The American Academy of Allergy, Asthma, and Immunology recommends sports with intermittent periods of activity, such as swimming, baseball, wrestling, golf, walking, leisure biking, hiking, and downhill skiing, rather than sports such as jogging, tennis, basketball, or soccer. And monitor your condition with a peak flow meter. If your readings indicate that your asthma is getting worse, it's a signal to put off strenuous exercise.

medications

Most asthma medications control exercise-induced asthma quite well. What you'll need and how much you'll need depend on a variety of factors, such as whether exercise is the only trigger for your asthma, how often you exercise,

When Exercise Becomes Dangerous

Exercise-induced anaphylaxis is a rare condition in which intense exercise actually leads to a life-threatening systemic reaction. Symptoms range from relatively mild, such as hives, to severe, such as a sudden drop in blood pressure, loss of consciousness, and even death. However, since the condition was first identified in the 1970s, just one death has been reported. Either most people have mild symptoms, or doctors fail to recognize it as a cause of death. If you have ever had a dramatic reaction to exercise, such as breaking out in hives or becoming dizzy (a sign of low blood pressure), you should talk to your doctor about it, and from now on, never exercise alone. Make sure you always have an EpiPen with you and that you're with someone who knows how to administer the epinephrine. At the first sign of flushing or hives, stop exercising and use the EpiPen.

To help avoid anaphylaxis, wait 4 to 6 hours after eating before exercising; don't use aspirin or other nonsteroidal anti-inflammatory medications, such as ibuprofen, before exercising; and, if you're female, don't exercise just before or during menstruation. Studies have found that taking an antihistamine before exercising can also help prevent problems.

and your fitness level. For instance, if you work out only a couple of times a week and have a reaction once in a while, you may be able to get by with just a short-acting bronchodilator (rescue medication), which can prevent symptoms if you take it 15 minutes before exercising. It lasts 4 to 6 hours—more than enough time for a good workout. Other preworkout medications include the mast cell stabilizers cromolyn sodium and nedocromil sodium.

If, however, you're an athlete—say, a competitive runner or bicyclist—your doctor may put you on a more aggressive regimen that includes long-acting bronchodilators and inhaled corticosteroids.

asthma **sufferers ask**

Can I Exercise if I Have Asthma?

Absolutely. In fact, it's a myth that you can't or shouldn't exercise if you have asthma. Unfortunately, too many children with asthma are still kept from recess at school and forbidden to participate on sports teams. Just consider that several studies have found that children with asthma are "unfit" not as a result of their disease but because of their lack of physical activity. Given today's growing epidemic of obesity among children, that thinking is not only wrong, it's dangerous, since numerous studies have found that physical conditioning improves asthma.

As you can see throughout this chapter, proper treatment of asthma, along with taking certain precautions before you head out to the playing field, will enable you to run, jump, and roll with the best of them, with no negative effects.

the bottom line

You need a healthy body to cope with asthma, even if exercise triggers attacks. The trick is to identify the types of exercise and other physical activities you can participate in without triggering symptoms, pretreat your asthma before exercise according to your doctor's instructions, and follow the guidelines outlined above. Don't let your asthma stand in the way of a healthy body or a good workout. Done correctly, exercise will greatly help your condition.

skin
and **insect**
allergies

No one wants to get stung by a bee. It hurts. But if you knew that the potential result of a bee sting was widespread swelling, cardiac arrest, and even death, you'd be justifiably terrified—and that's how serious an insect allergy can be.

Skin allergies, on the other hand, are generally more benign, but that doesn't make them easy or insubstantial. Just ask the thousands of people who wear long-sleeved shirts in summer solely to keep scaly patches on their arms hidden from sight. With their incessant itchiness and high visibility, skin allergies can be as frustrating and debilitating as any other form of allergy.

In this chapter, we explore both of these issues—skin allergies first, then insect allergies—and tell you how to minimize their interference with your life by avoiding the causes or recognizing and treating reactions if you're not able to prevent them.

skin allergies

Hear that scratching sound? The sound of fingernails on skin? That's the sound of allergies and asthma. It often turns out that one of the first signs of both conditions isn't sneezing, coughing, or wheezing but a skin rash called atopic dermatitis, or eczema. It affects more than 15 million Americans and accounts for 10 to 20 percent of all visits to dermatologists.

The name *atopic dermatitis* actually defines the condition. *Dermatitis* means "inflammation of the skin," and *atopic* refers to an inherited tendency to develop allergic conditions. Put it together, and it means that your skin reacts when you eat or inhale a substance to which your body is allergic.

This is an important point. A common misconception is that an allergic reaction on the skin has to be caused by something touching that skin. And indeed, there is a type of eczema, called allergic contact dermatitis, in which your skin has an immune system reaction to direct contact with an allergen, such as poison ivy or certain preservatives in creams and lotions. But that's not true in the majority of cases of skin allergy. Rather, atopic dermatitis is usually an external reaction to an internal trigger, such as food.

In either case, skin allergies aren't life-threatening, but they can seriously affect your quality of life. In fact, one study found that people with eczema reported worse quality of life than those with heart disease or high blood pressure.

It makes sense when you think about it. After all, no one needs to know that you have high blood pressure, and certainly no one can tell by looking at you. But with eczema—or any skin condition, for that matter—your situation is highlighted for the world to see. That can lead to embarrassment, shame,

Eczema Defined

Although the terms *atopic dermatitis* and *eczema* are often used interchangeably, atopic dermatitis is actually just one of several types of eczema, albeit the most common one. Here are the other forms.

Contact eczema. A localized reaction that includes redness, itching, and burning where the skin has come into contact with an irritant such as an acid, a cleaning agent, or other chemical.

Dyshidrotic eczema. Irritation of the skin on the palms of the hands and soles of the feet characterized by clear, deep blisters that itch and burn. Doctors aren't sure of the causes, but stress and ingestion of certain minerals (such as nickel, chromium, or cobalt) may be a factor. It's most common in adolescents and young adults.

Neurodermatitis. Chronic, itchy inflammation of the top layer of the skin, usually caused by chronic scratching. Sometimes the itch has no apparent cause, while at other times, an insect bite or other irritant can launch the itch-scratch-itch cycle.

Nummular eczema. Coin-shaped patches of irritated skin that may be crusted, scaly, and extremely itchy. They are most common on the arms, back, buttocks, and lower legs. The coin shape of the spots makes this eczema distinct, but its causes are unknown.

Seborrheic eczema. Yellowish, oily, scaly patches on the scalp, face, and occasionally other parts of the body. Its cause is unknown.

Stasis dermatitis. Irritated skin on the lower legs that's generally related to circulatory problems, such as pooling of blood or other fluids in the leg veins.

Skin Allergy Glossary

If you're coping with any form of dermatitis, you may hear and read some pretty confusing words. Here's a simple glossary to help you better understand what your doctor says and what you may be reading about your condition.

Atopic pleat (Dennie-Morgan fold). An extra fold of skin that develops under the eyes and points to a tendency toward asthma and allergies.

Cheilitis. Inflammation of the skin on and around the lips.

Hyperlinear palms. Increased skin creases on the palms.

Hyperpigmented eyelids. Eyelids that have darkened in color due to inflammation or hay fever.

Ichthyosis. Dry, rectangular scales on the skin.

Keratosis pilaris. Small, rough bumps, generally on the face, upper arms, and thighs.

Lichenification. Thick, leathery skin due to constant scratching and rubbing.

Papules. Small bumps that may open when scratched and become crusty and infected.

Urticaria. Hives (red bumps) that may occur after exposure to an allergen, at the beginning of flare-ups, or after exercise or a hot bath.

shyness, and general withdrawal from public life. Children with eczema, for instance, often refuse to wear shorts or short-sleeved shirts for fear someone will see their reddened, scaly skin. Then there's the constant itching and scratching, which can lead to redness, swelling, cracking, "weeping" of clear fluid, and finally, crusting and scaling of the skin.

The disease itself tends to ebb and flow, sometimes getting worse (often due to stress) and sometimes disappearing altogether. It generally appears before age 5 and in some instances may disappear with age; in other cases, it's a lifelong condition.

There is no single test to diagnose atopic dermatitis. Even allergy tests aren't always accurate, because people with eczema generally have skin sensitivities to a variety of substances. However, food allergies can play an important role in this condition. To find out if your eczema stems from food allergies, try eliminating one of the seven most common food allergens—eggs, milk, peanuts, wheat, tree nuts, soybeans, and seafood—one at a time and see if your skin improves.

Treating Atopic Dermatitis

Traditionally, eczema has been treated with corticosteroid creams and ointments that help by keeping the immune response that causes it in check. But steroids bring with them their own problems, including thinning of the skin, dilated blood vessels, stretch marks, and infection.

In recent years, however, two new nonsteroidal drugs known as topical immunomodulators have come on the market: tacrolimus (Protopic) ointment and pimecrolimus (Elidel) cream. Although researchers don't know exactly how they work, it's thought that they block immune cells from creating the chemical messages that lead to eczema. Both drugs have been approved for use in children 2 and older, as well as adults. The main side effect of both is that they increase your skin's sensitivity to sunlight and other UV light, so keep the part of your body on which you're using either product covered up when you're outside.

If neither of these treatments works, you may need systemic steroids to suppress your immune system and prevent flare-ups. These drugs are given only in very serious cases, however, and then only for a short time. Other immune-suppressing drugs, such as methotrexate and cyclosporine, may be prescribed, again for a short time. Your doctor may also recommend antibiotics to prevent infection if your skin is in bad shape from all the scratching, along with first-generation antihistamines to reduce itching at night and help you sleep.

Phototherapy, or the use of ultraviolet A or B light waves, alone or combined, is also used to treat atopic dermatitis. Since it can increase your risk of skin cancer down the road, however, your doctor needs to monitor this treatment carefully. *Don't* self-treat by going to a tanning salon!

There's also some evidence that St. John's wort, best known as an herbal treatment for depression, can treat atopic dermatitis when used as a cream.

Meanwhile, there are things you can do to reduce the incidence and severity of flare-ups.

■ **Treat your skin kindly.** In particular, avoid irritants that can make your condition worse, such as perfumes and dyes in laundry detergents, soaps and body creams, scratchy fabrics, and exposure to chemicals and smoke.

■ **Dress in light, loose layers.** Natural fibers such as cotton are most gentle on the skin. In fact, 100 percent cotton is the best fabric for those with eczema. Wash new clothes before wearing them so they're softer, and cut out any labels that may further irritate your skin. Also stick to 100 percent cotton sheets and blankets.

revealing **research**

Piercing and Metal Allergies

The trend toward piercing numerous parts of the body—ears, nose, tongue, navel, breasts, and genitalia—is behind dramatically increasing rates of metal allergies as well as an increase in latex allergies, with studies finding that the more piercings you have, the more likely you are to be allergic to metal, generally nickel. Overall, nickel allergies increased by 40 percent in the five years between 1995 and 2000, says the American Academy of Dermatology. The allergy may cause redness, watery blisters, hives, or eczema. Often the symptoms are only at the site of contact, but in some cases, they spread over the entire body.

Just getting rid of the body jewelry won't help; once you have a metal allergy, you've got it for life. And nickel is everywhere, including in many coins and everyday alloys. In Europe, for instance, Euro coins have such high levels of nickel that some people develop reactions just from handling their money!

If you think you're safe sticking with gold or silver studs, you should be aware that many still contain nickel. A European study that tested 66 earrings found that 25 exceeded European Union limits on the amount of nickel they could safely contain. Other studies have found even worse results with jewelry intended for other parts of the body. The safest jewelry? Titanium and surgical-grade stainless steel, the kind used for implants.

■ **Stay cool.** Sweating, as well as sudden changes in temperature, can aggravate atopic dermatitis. If you're in the midst of an outbreak, take a day off from the gym or limit your workout to light stretching. Also maintain a cool temperature in your home and office.

■ **Try cool baths to help the itching.** Avoid water that's warmer than room temperature, as heat dilates the blood vessels in your skin, which results in even worse itching. After your bath, gently pat your skin with a soft towel and apply a nonscented cream or lotion to seal in moisture. Use emollient lotions, which are thick and thus provide a stronger barrier between your skin and bacteria.

■ **Divert your hands.** If you can't seem to stop scratching the itch, try to keep your hands busy with activities such as knitting or crossword puzzles. Also, keep your nails short to avoid tearing the skin when you do scratch. If possible, "scratch" with a flat hand, rubbing the itchy spot rather than raking it with your nails.

■ **Reduce stress in your life.** Or at least moderate how you react to it. Stress, while not a cause of atopic dermatitis as once thought, can definitely make it worse. Follow the stress-relieving guidelines in step 5 of the Breathe Easy Plan.

■ **Dip into the yogurt.** If you have an infant with eczema, try adding probiotics to her diet with either yogurt or supplements. A Finnish study found that consumption of the probiotic *Lactobacillus acidophilus* (safe to use at an early age) halved the incidence of infant eczema, compared with infants receiving a placebo. Go ahead and add one container of live-culture yogurt to your daily diet, too, as long as you're not allergic to dairy foods. Although studies have not been done yet, it may work just as well for adults as for babies.

Latex Allergies

In 1985, as a direct result of the AIDS epidemic, health authorities implemented the use of universal health precautions to protect against transmission of HIV and hepatitis C. Basically, that meant that all health care and emergency workers—anyone who could conceivably come into contact with blood or other body fluids—began wearing protective gear, including surgical gloves, which are typically made from natural rubber, or latex. Today, it's estimated that more than 5.6 million American health care workers use more than 7 billion pairs of gloves each year. That has resulted in a significant increase in latex allergies, with an estimated 1 to 6 percent of the general population affected, and 5 to 10 percent of health care workers.

The occurrence of the allergy is directly proportional to the frequency and degree of exposure to latex. That wouldn't be so bad, except that latex is everywhere. It's found not only in surgical gloves but also in condoms and diaphragms, surgical masks, adhesive strips, balloons, diapers, incontinence pads, feeding nipples, rubber bands, sports equipment and athletic shoes, water toys and equipment, and even zipper-seal plastic storage bags.

One major problem for those allergic to latex is that latex proteins can become fastened to the lubricant powder used in some gloves to make them easier to put on and take off. When workers change gloves, the protein/powder particles become airborne and can be inhaled.

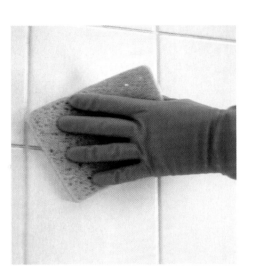

Symptoms of latex allergy include relatively mild reactions, such as itchy, red, watery eyes; sneezing or runny nose; coughing; and a rash or hives. It can also lead to severe reactions, up to and including anaphylactic shock. Unlike most allergic reactions, however, it doesn't cause immediate symptoms such as itchy eyes and a runny nose. Instead, you may not notice any symptoms for 24 to 48 hours after your exposure, when the part of your body that came in contact with the latex breaks out in an itchy rash.

*The occurrence of a latex allergy is determined by the frequency and degree of exposure. The problem is that **latex is everywhere**.*

If you suspect you're allergic or sensitive to latex, you must try to avoid any products that contain natural rubber latex, or NRL. Read labels carefully, ask questions, and, if you're in doubt, don't touch it. Also, if you need to be examined by health care professionals, tell them about your allergy so they don't use latex gloves and masks. You should also wear a medical alert bracelet in case you're injured and unable to communicate.

If you work in an industry that uses latex products, the Occupational Safety and Health Administration (OSHA) recommends the following precautions to reduce your risk of developing an allergy.

■ **Switch gloves.** Use nonlatex gloves for activities that aren't likely to involve contact with infectious materials, such as food preparation, routine housekeeping, and general maintenance.

■ **Go powder-free.** If you use latex gloves when handling infectious material, choose powder-free gloves with reduced protein content, which lessen exposure to latex protein and reduce the risk of latex allergy.

■ **Be wary of marketing claims.** So-called hypoallergenic latex gloves do not reduce the risk of latex allergy, but they may reduce allergic reactions to chemical additives in the latex.

■ **Skip the lotion.** When wearing latex gloves, don't use oil-based hand creams or lotions, which can cause glove deterioration.

■ **Wash after use.** After removing latex gloves, wash your hands with mild soap and dry them thoroughly.

■ **Practice good housekeeping.** Frequently clean areas and equipment contaminated with latex-containing dust.

■ **Be watchful.** Learn to recognize the symptoms of latex allergy: skin rash; hives; flushing; itching; nasal, eye, or sinus symptoms; asthma; and (rarely) shock.

insect allergies

If you're allergic to the stings or bites of insects, navigating your way through the summer can be more dangerous than bicycling through New York City. An estimated 2 million Americans have insect allergies, which send more than 500,000 of them to the hospital and cause at least 50 deaths each year. That figure may actually be higher, since some insect-allergy–related deaths may not be recognized as such. Almost half of fatal reactions occur in people who have no history of insect allergies. If you suspect that you may be allergic, ask your doctor to do a skin test.

The culprits include stinging insects, such as bees, hornets, yellow jackets, wasps, and fire ants, and biting insects, such as mosquitoes and bedbugs—most of which are most plentiful in late July, August, and early September. You'll know you're allergic to one of them if, after you've been bitten, you develop

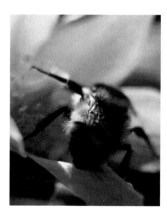

Almost half of fatal reactions occur in people who have *no history of insect allergies*.

hives, itchiness, swelling in areas other than the sting site, difficulty breathing, dizziness, a hoarse voice, and/or swelling of the tongue. In severe reactions, you may lose consciousness and go into cardiac arrest as your body becomes overwhelmed and goes into anaphylactic shock. If it's any consolation, the more severe reactions usually occur only with insect stings. Don't be surprised if the symptoms hit several hours after your encounter with the insect and gradually worsen before dissipating.

Once you've had a systemic reaction to an insect sting, such as hives or swelling, you have a 50 percent chance of experiencing anaphylactic shock if you're stung again. That's why people who know they're allergic should *never* be without an emergency kit containing epinephrine (adrenaline). The good news is that your risk of a severe reaction tends to drop with time, down to 25 percent 10 or more years after the initial reaction. Also, reactions generally don't become more severe with successive stings.

There's really no way to know if you're allergic to an insect until you've been stung, since this is one of the few allergies in which there is no clear family

Hiring a Pest-Control Specialist

These recommendations for choosing a pest-control service come from the Massachusetts Department of Agricultural Resources.

Shop around. Ask friends, neighbors, or business associates for names of firms with which they have had positive experiences. Get estimates from several companies, but make your selection based on the value of their service, not the price.

Choose the right company. That means one that employs knowledgeable and competent professionals who take the time to explain your problems and options and the best way to achieve control of pests.

Be wary of special deals and high-pressure sales tactics. The lowest price may not be the best value if the company cuts corners on safety.

Choose a company that meets your needs. Competent pest-management companies will outline a program that identifies the pests to be controlled, the extent of the infestation, the specific pesticides they intend to use, and the steps you can take to minimize the chance of future infestation. The initial inspection may even indicate that pesticides are not necessary.

Choose the right treatment. If the company claims that its treatments include "secret" chemicals or offers to provide you with a special discount if you have the work done immediately, say you'll pass.

Ask the company to discuss Integrated Pest Management (IPM) options. IPM techniques involve the use of monitoring devices, formulations, insect growth regulators (IGRP), sanitation, cultural practices, and other physical steps to avoid or reduce problems. The company should be able to help you understand your pest problem and what to do about it.

Check licensing and references. Most states license those who work as pest-control specialists. Also check with the Better Business Bureau (www.bbb.com) and the local chamber of commerce. A reputable company will belong to both.

Check affiliations. Membership in a professional organization reflects a commitment to integrity and responsibility, offering opportunities for training in the latest developments in technology, safety, research, and regulations.

history. Just because your mother is allergic to bee stings doesn't mean you will be; conversely, just because no one in your family dating back three generations has had an insect allergy doesn't mean you're off the hook.

If you are stung, try applying cold compresses and/or an over-the-counter hydrocortisone cream to reduce the stinging and swelling, but even if that first reaction is mild, make sure you see an allergist. Not only do you need a doctor's prescription for the epinephrine kit, you should also ask if you're a candidate for venom immunotherapy, or allergy shots, which can desensitize you to most insect stings. Studies have found that immunotherapy is more than 97 percent effective in protecting allergic people from potentially life-threatening reactions to insect stings. The downside? The injections may carry a higher risk of adverse reactions than allergy shots given for airborne allergens.

The other critical step you need to take is avoiding contact with these insects in the first place. Forget insect repellents, though; they don't work against stinging insects such as bees and yellow jackets. Instead:

■ **Avoid the beeline.** When honey bees are foraging for pollen, they fly a direct route (the fabled "beeline") from the food source to the hive. So, if you can, try to figure out their beeline and make sure you're not caught in the middle.

■ **If you're stung, don't slap!** Fast hand motions combined with the scent released from a stinging bee can bring more bees. Remove the stinger as soon as possible after a sting by scraping and pulling it out with your fingernails. Don't grab and pull, because squeezing the little sac at the end of the stinger can force more venom into the wound, making the sting worse. Try meat tenderizer or ice to alleviate the pain.

■ **Wear a hat.** Furry animals steal honey from bees, so if bees see anything that looks like fur, they get nervous and generally stay away.

■ **Hold still.** The worst thing you can do if you see bees approaching is to wave your arms and run away. It's the rapid movement that startles the bee and encourages stinging. Instead, be as still as a statue.

■ **Blow gently.** Try this if a bee lands on you; it can encourage the bee to move on while not startling it.

■ **Wear shoes.** It's much easier to step on and crush a bee when you're wearing a pair of Nikes than when you're barefoot or in flip-flops.

■ **Pinch tightly.** If a bee gets caught in your hair or tangled in your clothing, quickly and calmly pinch it to kill it.

■ **Avoid scented soaps and loud clothing.** If you smell or even look like a flower (by dressing in bright colors and floral prints), you'll attract bees.

■ **Picnic properly.** That means keeping food covered when you're eating outdoors, and never drinking from soft drink or juice cans. Stinging insects are attracted to the sweetness and may crawl inside a can. Even if you use a cup, always check the contents before sipping.

■ **Maintain your home.** Store garbage cans outside and covered with tight-fitting lids, and keep window and door screens in good repair.

■ **Drive safely.** That means with the car windows closed. Also check for any stinging insects before you climb in.

■ **Hire a gardener.** If you have an insect allergy, you're obviously putting yourself at risk any time you garden. If it's not a beloved hobby, cross gardening off your list of chores and hire someone to do it. If gardening *is* a passion, hire someone anyhow—to do the less creative or pleasing maintenance work, such as cutting grass or weeding. Save your time outdoors for the most rewarding work, such as planting new flowers and harvesting herbs and vegetables.

■ **Hire an exterminator.** Just as the first roses begin blooming, hire a professional pest-control service to check your property for beehives and wasp nests. If the service person finds any, give very specific instructions, i.e., *get rid of them!* If you hire a pest-control contractor, quarterly inspections are generally all you need. Be wary of any contractor who gives you a quote over the telephone to use pesticides without first thoroughly inspecting your home.

Fire Ants: A Growing Menace

If you live in the southeastern portion of the United States, you have to worry about more than bees and yellow jackets. You also have to be concerned with red and black fire ants, which can be found in 11 states so far: Texas, Louisiana, Mississippi, Alabama, Florida, Georgia, South Carolina and adjacent regions in North Carolina, Arkansas, Tennessee, and Oklahoma.

Once the ants invade an area, half of the people living there can expect to be stung. In a troubling development, studies suggest that up to 17 percent or more of a population may be allergic to the annoying pests. If you have a reaction, you can expect an immediate burning sensation due to toxic oily alkaloids in the venom. Within 18 to 24 hours of the sting, pustules develop, which may persist for a week and may cause scarring. Fire ant stings can be serious; the American Academy of Allergy, Asthma, and Immunology notes that about 1 to 16 percent of fire ant stings result in anaphylaxis.

Chances are you'll be stung more than once, since unlike bees, which die after stinging, fire ants can sting repeatedly. They're also very difficult to eradicate because you can't destroy the colony unless you kill the queen ant. Your best bet is exterminating all ants you find with liquid pesticides, including pouring some down any anthills you see. One product touted for fire ant destruction is called EXXANT, available online and in hardware stores. Bait containing an insect growth regulator can also help, although it takes longer to work and often requires several applications. It's best to hire a professional to deal with fire ants, since they're like phoenixes—they keep coming back. Here's how to avoid the fiery creatures in the first place.

■ **Protect your feet and hands.** Wear shoes with closed toes, socks, and gloves, when gardening, and tuck your pant legs into your socks.

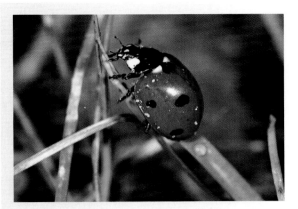

Beware the Gentle Ladybugs

As more gardeners turn to nontoxic methods of controlling pests, the ladybug, star of the children's rhyme exhorting it to "fly away home," has become a predator of choice to vanquish aphids from the garden. As the numbers of ladybugs proliferate in some areas, doctors have begun noticing that some patients are allergic to the red-and-black bugs. If your allergy symptoms worsen (or appear for the first time) soon after introducing a load of ladybugs to your garden, consider another aphid-control approach.

■ **Take fast action.** If you see any fire ant mounds, pour several pots of boiling water directly into them (wear protective clothing, and be careful to stay away from the ants). You can also place shallow bowls of ant poison throughout your garden and across your lawn. Report any suspected mounds near your home to your local agricultural extension service.

■ **Warn others.** Let your children and any visitors know if you have fire ants on your property and what to do if they find any crawling in the yard or house or on their skin.

■ **Stock up on insect bite remedies.** Treat stings with an approved product that deadens pain and provides protection against secondary infection, such as Sting-Kill External Anesthetic, which contains benzocaine.

■ **Keep your hands away.** If you are stung, don't scratch. You run the risk of the blisters becoming infected.

■ **Be cautious.** If you have a severe reaction, see a doctor immediately.

Mosquitoes: Beyond West Nile

It's not enough that mosquitoes carry the potentially deadly West Nile virus; they can also cause an allergic reaction in susceptible people. If you have a mosquito allergy, you'll experience far worse than the typical itchy reactions that last for a few hours. Because of your increased antibody reaction to mosquito saliva, you can expect a large red swelling, skin blisters, bruises, or even hives, all lasting a week or more. The good news? Systemic reactions (anaphylactic shock) are relatively rare with mosquito allergies.

Even if you're not allergic, you should take the following steps to reduce your exposure to mosquitoes.

■ **Drain all standing water on your property.** Get in the habit of walking around your property after each summer rain to find any watering cans, upside-down Frisbees, flower pots, garbage can lids, and other receptacles that need to be dumped. The reason? Mosquitoes lay their eggs in standing water.

■ **Use insect repellent.** In particular, use repellent containing DEET when you're outside during mosquito season. The U.S. government has declared DEET safe for kids and adults of all ages when used as instructed on the package.

■ **Avoid sitting outside at dusk.** Mosquitoes are at their most active when the sun sets and in the first half-hour or so of darkness.

■ **Wear protective clothing when outdoors.** That means long-sleeved shirts, long pants, socks, and closed shoes (no sandals or clogs). Add a hat and gardening gloves when doing yard work. The reason is obvious: You offer less skin for mosquitoes to bite.

■ **Nix the perfumes.** You don't want anything that could draw the blood-sucking bugs to you.

Bedbugs: They're Still Biting

The bed bug—now there's a name that says it all. Bed bugs, or *Cimex Lectularius*, often live inside mattresses, or between mattresses and box springs. These tiny bugs come out at night to feed on human blood. About the only good thing you can say about bedbugs is that they don't carry disease, so a bite probably won't make you sick. And they are so small that a bite won't hurt. However, they are terribly dangerous if you're allergic to them: Their bite has been known to cause anaphylaxis.

Newsflash: Bedbugs are staging a resurgence in many parts of the country, even turning up in the beds of some of the finest hotels. Pest-control companies are reporting a surge in calls about them and expect the numbers to keep rising.

With no immunotherapy treatment available for bedbug bites, your best bet is avoidance (and no, repeating the old childhood bedtime saying "don't let the bedbugs bite" as your personal mantra simply isn't enough). Here's what to do.

■ **Check your luggage at the door.** Bedbugs typically enter a home via clothing or luggage. If you've been on a trip, vacuum your luggage upon your return, then immediately wash all your travel clothes in the hottest water available, whether you wore them or not.

■ **Manage your laundry smartly.** Be diligent about washing all your clothes soon after wearing, and don't leave dirty clothes hanging out near your bed. This applies to everyone in your family, particularly children, who can pick up bedbugs from contact with other kids at school.

■ **Be watchful.** Bedbugs look like tiny lentils: flat, oval, brown, and about ¼ inch long. They come out only at night and congregate where people sleep, since their only food is blood. Typically, they can be found in the seams of a mattress (they spend their days resting inside). An infested area tends to have a faint cucumber smell.

■ **React fast.** If you spot bedbugs, get rid of your mattress (purging the critters from a mattress is nearly impossible), wash your bedding and clothes in hot, soapy water, and call a pest-control expert. Bedbugs are virtually impossible to get rid of on your own; you really do need an expert.

■ **Don't act as if you're dealing with ants, cockroaches, or dust mites.** Unlike many other insects, bedbugs are not drawn to dirt or repelled by cleanliness, so maintaining a pristine house is no deterrent. What they seek is blood and blood alone.

■ **Remove clutter from your bedroom.** This reduces the number of places where they can hide.

■ **Sleep in long-legged, long-sleeved pajamas and socks.** Since the bugs bite only bare skin, the less you have exposed, the less likely you are to be bitten.

sick
buildings
the truth and
the response

How could something that we have peacefully coexisted with for thousands of years, that led us to the most important medicine of our time (penicillin), and that is the foundation of one of our tastiest foods (cheese) now be responsible for sending us fleeing from our homes?

That's the rap mold has gotten. According to recent media reports, families have been rendered nearly insensible by its toxic effects, and multimillion-dollar homes have had to be stripped down to the foundation to eradicate it. Mold, according to the reports, has single-handedly sparked a crisis in the home insurance industry. Add it up, and mold has taken on an evil persona topped only by that of a bomb-toting terrorist. In fact, you might even call mold "the homeowner's terrorist."

Mold is the biggest culprit we think of when we hear about something called sick building syndrome (SBS), but that isn't quite fair. Far more headaches and dry coughs can be linked to poor ventilation, toxic fumes from building materials, and poorly managed heating and air-conditioning systems than to mold.

Before we even get into examining how to deal with these villains, we need to talk about the realities—and the falsehoods—regarding the health risks posed by buildings and the role of mold. What is the problem, exactly? Where does it come from? And, perhaps the most controversial and confusing question: Is sick building syndrome even real?

SBS defined

The term *sick building syndrome* refers to situations in which specific health complaints appear to be linked to the building in which you work or live but for which no specific illness or cause can be identified. It shouldn't be confused with a building-related illness, in which symptoms of diagnosable illnesses such as asthma and allergies can be directly attributed to airborne contaminants in a building, such as dust mites, animal dander, and pollen.

Whether or not SBS is real, complaints about sick buildings are certainly on the rise. A recent American Lung Association survey of office workers found that one in four believed their workplaces had air-quality problems, and one in five believed those problems interfered with their work.

No surprise there. As we've discussed in earlier chapters, energy-saving construction methods, begun in the 1970s, led to levels of air pollution that were higher inside many buildings than outside. Less fresh air filters into buildings these days, as we become more reliant on complex automated heating and cooling systems. At the same time, buildings have fewer humidification systems, and rarely can you find a window you can open if you need a breath of fresh air.

Sick building syndrome remains controversial in medical circles, however. Some researchers dismiss SBS complaints as psychosomatic, attributing them to stress, worker fatigue, and boredom. Others, however, point to a growing body of evidence that links a building's environment to an array of individual symptoms, such as headaches, fatigue, cough, dizziness and nausea, difficulty concentrating, and sensitivity to odors.

But does it truly matter if the syndrome is real? In other words, if you *think* something in the building is causing your symptoms, and you *know* these symptoms are interfering with your ability to work or live your normal life, does it matter if the building is really "sick"? The bottom line is that you want the problem solved and your symptoms relieved.

pinning the blame

No one is saying that the air in your office building is crystal clear. Suspected offenders when it comes to SBS include:

■ **Volatile organic compounds.** These are chemical irritants released by sources inside the building, such as adhesives, carpeting, upholstery,

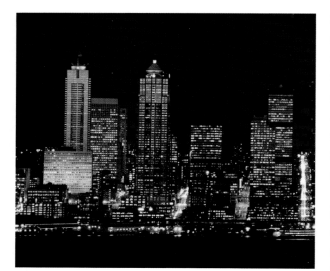

manufactured wood products such as drywall, copy machines, pesticides, and cleaning agents. They also include formaldehyde, which, according to the American Lung Association, can cause headaches, sore throats, and fatigue, as well as rashes, nausea, dizziness, and eye and respiratory tract irritation.

■ **Carbon monoxide.** This odorless gas is regulated in the outside environment but not the inside environment, where it can cause significant health problems. The

Less fresh air filters into buildings these days, as we have become more reliant on complex automated heating and cooling systems.

American Lung Association reports that in some office buildings, afternoon levels of carbon monoxide can be 10 to 20 times greater than the daily standard for outdoor air quality, as set by the Environmental Protection Agency (EPA). Major sources include improperly vented garages and loading docks and leaks in ductwork that enable the gas to seep into offices. It causes a variety of health effects, including fatigue, confusion, headache, dizziness, and nausea.

■ **Inadequate ventilation.** This is probably one of the major causes of SBS symptoms. For this, you can blame OPEC. Before the 1973 oil embargo, building ventilation standards called for approximately 15 cubic feet per minute (CFM) of outside air for each building occupant. After the embargo and the resulting spike in energy costs, that requirement was reduced to 5 CFM per person, a rate that's often inadequate to maintain the health and comfort of building occupants, the EPA notes. Fortunately, in the early 1990s, the American Society of Heating, Refrigerating, and Air-Conditioning Engineers revised its standards back to the minimum 15 CFM (20 CFM in office spaces). If you're in an older building, though, the feeling that you can't breathe may be very real indeed. And, for the record, there is *no* standard requirement for indoor air quality in this country.

■ **Outdoor chemical contaminants.** Although many buildings today are well sealed (perhaps too well sealed), outdoor contaminants from motor vehicle and building exhausts can still enter through poorly located intake vents, windows, and other openings, says the EPA. If your office is located over the parking garage, take note.

■ **Biological contaminants.** These include mold, bacteria, pollen, and viruses. For instance, the bacterium *Legionella pneumophila* causes both

Legionnaire's disease and Pontiac fever. But, as we discuss in the next section, the issue of whether mold is really responsible for the havoc attributed to it is still largely unknown and, for the most part, unlikely.

■ **Climate control.** Simple temperature problems—whether too warm or too cold—can often be blamed for common complaints such as headache, fatigue, and dryness.

mold: uncovering the truth

There's no question that mold can be a potent trigger for allergies and asthma, but contrary to popular perception, there has been no increase in the number of allergies to mold, and mold is not getting worse in this country. Also, regardless of what you may read in *People* magazine, there's no evidence that mold, even the much-maligned *Stachybotrys chartarum*, is responsible for the neurological problems and other health effects often attributed to it. In fact, a special article on the health effects of residential mold published in the September 2003 issue of the journal *Annals of Allergy, Asthma & Immunology* was headlined "Toxic Mold: Phantom Risk vs. Science."

A Healthy Home

Whether you have allergies, asthma, or multiple chemical sensitivities, one way to improve your symptoms is to live in the right place. That means building a "healthy home" or renovating your current one, using nontoxic materials. Today, you can find builders and architects who specialize in this type of work, creating homes and offices designed to both conserve resources and reduce indoor air pollutants. If you're undertaking new construction or renovation, consider incorporating the following tips into your building plans.

• Avoid wall-to-wall carpeting and synthetic flooring and choose natural, hard-surfaced materials such as tile and wood.

• Choose low-odor paints, caulking, and sealants specially designed to reduce exposure for people with chemical sensitivities.

• Use natural, colored plaster instead of paint.

• Choose a foundation that lifts the home off the ground to separate it from both radon and moisture.

• Choose nontoxic, nonallergenic insulation materials such as cork, cotton, and even "cementitious foam" insulation made from magnesium silicate.

• Stick to low-formaldehyde products for furniture, cabinets, and finishes.

• Use metal pipes for plumbing instead of plastic pipes, which allow organic matter to seep into the water.

• Consider using steel or other modern construction materials rather than the standard particleboard.

• Insist on a quality ventilation system.

For more tips and resources, check out the Healthy Home Coalition (www.herc.org/hhc), the Healthy House Institute (www.hhinst.com), and MCS Housing Resources (http://world.std.com/~habib/thegarden//mcs).

"At this point," concluded the five physicians who wrote the article, "there is little science to support the public concern and to justify the prodigious number of lawsuits [over mold-infested homes]. In many respects, this area remains a 'black box' in which there is little science to support the public reaction."

Here's what we do know about mold and its health effects.

- Mold is a fungus, of which there are thought to be more than 1.5 million species. Less than 100 are known to be infectious in humans or animals.

- You probably have at least six different types of mold spores in your house right now, regardless of how well you clean and how dry the air is. They come in from the outside on your clothing or your pets or subsist on houseplants. Contaminated air conditioners and humidifiers can also circulate indoor spores.

- There's no way to know if the amount of mold you have in your home is healthy or unhealthy. That's because there's no standardized method for accurately collecting, measuring, and identifying mold spores in a home. Even if you do have good measurements of the mold in your home, there's no consensus on how to interpret the data; more than 20 suggested guidelines exist for indoor airborne or surface mold. Thus, if you hire some air-quality inspector who tells you that you have high levels of mold, he's really not telling you anything.

- The mold you can't see (the mold growing inside your walls) is no more dangerous than the mold on your bathroom shower curtain. Finding mold in your walls doesn't mean that your house has to be ripped apart; it's been estimated that 70 percent of homes have mold growing there.

- When it comes to the much-feared *Stachybotrys* and other molds, the concern is not so much the fungus itself but the toxins the organism normally produces as a by-product of living. However, there has been no conclusive proof linking *Stachybotrys* to any specific health conditions.

So what does all this mean?

Well, no one is claiming that mold is benign. Not only does it exacerbate allergies and asthma, but people with compromised immune systems or underlying lung disease are particularly susceptible to infection. In fact, 9 percent of all hospital-acquired infections are related to fungi, including mold. Foods contaminated with certain toxins that mold and other fungal products can cause have been linked to liver and kidney cancer. Many respiratory illnesses among workers are attributed to mold exposure, such as hypersensitivity pneumonitis (also called farmer's lung, woodworker's lung, and malt worker's lung).

Whether residential molds cause bleeding in the lungs (pulmonary hemorrhage), memory loss, or lethargy—all symptoms attributed to the fungi in recent lawsuits and media reports—is still unproven and unknown.

Hopefully, we'll have more answers soon. The Institute of Medicine of the National Academies of Science was expected to release a report on the relationship between damp or moldy indoor environments and health effects in early 2004. And the Centers for Disease Control and Prevention is continuing to investigate and evaluate the health effects and risks associated with mold and poor indoor air quality.

breathing better at work

If the stale air in your office is getting to you, there are steps you can take to, ahem, clear the air. Back in step 6 of the Breathe Easy Plan, we provided a host of things you can do to improve your personal work space. But what if you lack control over your work environment? Here's what you can do.

■ **Be proactive.** You can't set policies, but you certainly have a right to know what they are. If you suspect that something in your workplace is triggering your asthma or allergies, politely ask questions. Your boss probably doesn't know the answers, so get his permission to talk to the building maintenance supervisor on behalf of yourself and your fellow workers. Find out when the heating and ventilation systems were last cleaned and repaired. Ask if the systems meet, at a minimum, local building codes for ventilation standards. Ask if all systems use HEPA filters. If storage areas have been turned into office space, ask if appropriate ventilation changes were made.

■ **Make a list.** See any water-stained ceiling tiles or damp patches on the carpet? How about volatile compounds (such as copy machine toner, pesticides, and cleaning supplies) stored in unventilated areas? Make a list of such problems and send a memo (politely worded) to the maintenance chief.

■ **Walk around outside.** Are outtake vents blocked by dirt or weeds? Are intake vents located too close to the parking lot? If so, add these problems to your list for the maintenance supervisor.

■ **Consider space planning.** Are furniture and/or boxes blocking supply or return air registers? Is heat-generating equipment placed close to thermostats? Are too many desks crammed into too small a space? These are all contributors to poor air quality that can be easily corrected. Again, notify the maintenance supervisor if you see problems.

If you take all these steps and find that your supervisor or building maintenance chief is unresponsive, you can contact the Occupational Safety and Health Administration (OSHA), which has regional offices throughout the United States. To find the address and phone number of the one nearest you, go to www.osha.gov, find the U.S. map, and click on your region.

glossary

ACTION PLAN A written set of directions or a chart that tells you what to do when asthma symptoms occur as well as preventive steps to take when you're not having symptoms.

ALLERGEN A substance that triggers an allergic reaction. Many allergens, including dust mites, animal dander, mold, and cockroaches, also trigger asthma.

ALLERGIC RHINITIS A condition that occurs when an allergen binds with IgE antibodies linked to cells that line the mucous membranes in the nose, causing the release of chemicals that lead to classic allergy symptoms: scratchy, runny nose; watery eyes; sneezing; and so on. Also known as hay fever.

ALLERGIST A doctor with additional specialty training in the care of asthma, allergies, and related conditions.

ALLERGY An inappropriate or exaggerated reaction of the immune system to substances that cause no symptoms in the majority of people.

ALVEOLI Tiny air sacs in the lungs where oxygen is transferred into the bloodstream and carbon dioxide waste enters the airways, from which it is exhaled.

ANAPHYLAXIS A severe, sudden, and life-threatening allergic reaction. Although rare, it can occur after an insect sting or as a reaction to an injected drug, such as penicillin or anti-tetanus (horse) serum. Less commonly, it occurs after consumption of a particular food or drug. Also known as anaphylactic shock.

ANTIBODY A specialized defender protein that latches onto invaders and marks them so other immune system cells can destroy them. Antibodies also send out chemical signals calling white blood cells into action.

ANTIGEN A substance, usually a protein, that the body perceives as foreign.

ANTIHISTAMINE A medication that prevents symptoms such as congestion, sneezing, and itchy, runny nose by blocking histamine receptors.

ANTI-INFLAMMATORY A medication that reduces inflammation; used to reduce airway inflammation in asthma. See also *Inflammation*.

ASTHMA A chronic inflammatory disorder of the airways of the lungs.

ASTHMA ATTACK A period of coughing, wheezing, breathlessness, and chest tightness. Also known as asthma episode.

ASTHMA MANAGEMENT A comprehensive approach to controlling asthma.

ATOPIC DERMATITIS An eczema-type rash triggered by exposure to an allergen.

ATOPY The propensity, usually genetic, to develop IgE-mediated responses to common environmental allergens.

B LYMPHOCYTE An immune cell that produces antibodies.

BASOPHIL A white blood cell filled with granules of toxic chemicals that can digest microorganisms. Also known as granular leukocyte.

BETA-AGONIST An asthma drug (bronchodilator) that relaxes the muscles around the bronchial tubes, thus opening the airways or helping to keep them open. There are two main types: long-acting, taken daily to prevent symptoms, often in combination with an inhaled steroid; and short-acting, used for quick relief of symptoms during an asthma attack.

BRONCHIAL TUBES Airways in the lungs. One major branch goes into each lung, then divides into many smaller branches.

BRONCHIOLES The smallest airways in the lungs.

BRONCHOCONSTRICTION Constriction of the airways that occurs when the muscles that wrap them tighten forcefully, pinching them closed.

BRONCHODILATOR A medication used to relax and open the airways. See also *Beta-agonist*.

CONJUNCTIVITIS Allergic inflammation of the inside of the eyelid, causing itchy, watery, red, swollen eyes.

CONTACT DERMATITIS An inflammatory skin rash caused by contact with various irritating substances.

CONTRIBUTING FACTOR A risk factor that either adds to the likelihood of a medical condition developing with exposure to it or may increase susceptibility to that condition. For asthma, contributing factors include smoking, viral infections, small size at birth, and environmental pollutants.

CORTICOSTEROID A type of medication used to reduce inflammation in people with asthma. The inhaled form is the most common and effective drug used for long-term daily control of asthma.

CROMOLYN SODIUM A medication used to prevent asthma and/or allergic rhinitis symptoms.

DANDER Tiny flakes of skin.

DECONGESTANT A medication that shrinks nasal tissues to relieve symptoms of swelling and congestion.

DERMATITIS Inflammation of the skin, due to either direct contact with an irritating substance or an allergic reaction. Symptoms include redness, itching, and a rash.

DRUG ALLERGY An allergic reaction to a specific medication. The most common cause of drug allergies is penicillin.

DRY-POWDER INHALER A small device similar to a metered-dose inhaler but in which the drug is in powder form and is breath activated instead of aerosol activated.

DUST MITES Microscopic creatures that survive on skin flakes and other dust components and are common triggers for allergies.

ECZEMA Inflammation of the skin, usually causing itching and sometimes accompanied by crusting, oozing, and scaling.

ELIMINATION DIET A diet in which certain foods are temporarily discontinued to rule them out as possible causes of allergy symptoms.

ELISA (enzyme-linked immunosorbent assay) A blood test used to identify substances that cause allergy symptoms and to estimate a relative sensitivity.

ENVIRONMENTAL CONTROL The removal of risk factors and allergy and asthma triggers from the environment.

EOSINOPHIL A white blood cell that secretes chemicals that trigger the inflammatory process and helps destroy foreign cells.

EPINEPHRINE A form of adrenaline medication used to treat severe allergic reactions, such as anaphylaxis.

EXACERBATION Any worsening of asthma or allergy symptoms.

EXERCISE-INDUCED ASTHMA Asthma triggered by physical activity.

EXTRINSIC ASTHMA Asthma triggered by an allergic reaction, usually to something that is inhaled.

FOOD ALLERGY An allergic reaction to proteins in certain foods. The most common foods involved in food allergy include milk, eggs, seafood, peanuts, tree nuts, and soy.

HAY FEVER See *Allergic rhinitis*.

HEPA FILTER (high-efficiency particulate air) A filter that removes particles from the air by forcing it through screens containing microscopic pores.

HISTAMINE A naturally occurring substance released by mast cells and basophils after exposure to an allergen. It attaches to receptors on blood vessels, causing them to dilate, and binds to other receptors in nasal tissues, causing redness, swelling, itching, and changes in secretions.

HIVES Itchy, swollen, red bumps or patches on the skin that appear suddenly as a result of the body's adverse reaction to the release of histamine and other chemicals. Also known as urticaria.

HYPOALLERGENIC Formulated to contain the fewest possible allergens.

IgE Immunoglobulin E, a type of immunoglobulin that triggers the release of histamine from mast cells, resulting in an allergic reaction.

IMMUNOGLOBULIN See *Antibody*.

IMMUNOTHERAPY A series of injections to help build the immune system's tolerance to an asthma or allergy trigger.

INFLAMMATION The body's response to a host of insults, including invasion by bacteria or viruses, injury, or reaction to your own tissues. When tissues are injured, they and the cells that flock to the injury release a barrage of chemicals, including histamine, bradykinin, serotonin, and others that cause blood vessels to leak fluid into the tissues, leading to swelling, redness, and heat.

INHALER A small plastic device used to deliver medication to the airways.

INTRINSIC ASTHMA Asthma with no apparent external cause.

IRRITANT A substance that irritates the lungs and sets off an allergy or asthma attack.

LATEX ALLERGY An allergy that develops after sensitizing contact with latex (natural rubber).

LEUKOTRIENE MODIFIER A type of oral medication used to treat mild to moderate asthma.

MACROPHAGE A large immune cell that engulfs and destroys large particles such as bacteria, yeast, and dying cells.

MAST CELL A type of cell present in most body tissues but particularly numerous in connective tissue lining the skin and airways. In an allergic response, an allergen stimulates the release of antibodies, which attach themselves to mast cells. Following subsequent allergen exposure, the mast cells release substances such as histamine into the tissue, triggering an allergic reaction.

METERED-DOSE INHALER The most common device used to deliver asthma medication, allowing inhalation of a specific amount of medicine (a metered dose).

MUCOUS MEMBRANE Moist tissue that lines body cavities with an external opening, such as the respiratory, digestive, and urinary tracts.

MUCUS The liquid secretions of the mucus glands, which can change according to allergic reactions.

NEBULIZER A device that creates a mist from an asthma drug, which can then be inhaled into the lungs.

NEUTROPHIL The most numerous type of white blood cell and the first to arrive on the scene after a body insult occurs, especially an infection.

PEAK FLOW A measurement of how well you can blow air out of your lungs. If your airways become narrow and blocked due to asthma, you can't blow air out as well, and your peak flow values drop.

PEAK FLOW METER A small, portable device that measures airflow from the lungs.

POLLEN AND MOLD COUNTS Measurements of the amount of allergens in the air.

PROSTAGLANDIN A chemical released during an allergic reaction that contributes to allergy symptoms.

RAST (radioallergosorbent test) A blood test used to identify substances that cause allergy symptoms and to estimate a relative sensitivity.

RESCUE MEDICATION A drug used as needed to relieve symptoms during an allergy or asthma attack.

SINUSITIS Inflammation or infection of one or more of the sinuses, the hollow air spaces located around the nose and between and over the eyes.

SKIN TEST Injection of a small quantity of an allergen into the skin to determine which allergens trigger an allergic response.

SPACER A device that works with a metered-dose inhaler to deliver medication more easily and effectively and reduce side effects. It holds the "puff" of medicine between you and the inhaler so you can inhale it slowly and more completely.

SPIROMETRY The most important test for diagnosing asthma. A spirometer measures the maximum volume of air you can exhale after breathing in as much as you can. The total volume you exhale is called forced vital capacity, or FVC. The spirometer also measures the volume of air you exhale in the first second, called forced expiratory volume in 1 second, or FEV1. In general, the more air you breathe out during the first second of a full exhalation, the better.

T LYMPHOCYTE An immune system cell that secretes potent substances to attract other immune system cells that destroy invaders. Some T lymphocytes also attack and destroy diseased cells. Also known as T cell.

THEOPHYLLINE A drug sometimes used to help control mild to moderate persistent asthma, especially to prevent nighttime symptoms.

TRIGGER Any substance that causes or worsens an allergy or asthma attack.

URTICARIA See *Hives*.

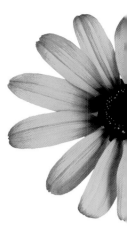

resources

This book should be a starting point in your search for information and understanding about allergies and asthma. In this section, we provide you with some of the best online and print resources for these two serious health conditions.

WebSites/Organizations

The amount of consumer health information on the Internet these days can be overwhelming, so we've carefully selected several of the best, most accurate, and most trustworthy sites for your research.

All Allergy Net (www.allallergy.net) Serves as a gateway to allergy sites on the Web.

Allergy & Asthma Network Mothers of Asthmatics (www.aanma.org) A national nonprofit network of families whose desire is to overcome, not just cope with, allergies and asthma.

American Lung Association (www.lungusa.org) Provides environmental and consumer health information about asthma and allergies.

Asthma and Allergy Foundation of America (www.aafa.org) Offers trustworthy information about asthma and allergies, educational programs for consumers and health professionals, advocacy to improve the quality of life for patients, and support for research to find a cure.

Asthma Research at the National Institute of Environmental Health Science (www.niehs.nih.gov/airborne/home.htm) Part of the National Institutes of Health; offers links to three major subjects—research studies, allergy prevention, and resources.

Centers for Disease Control and Prevention (www.cdc.gov/nceh/airpollution/asthma) Pro-vides information on the connection between air quality and asthma.

Childhood Asthma Research and Education Network (www.asthma-carenet.org) Centers funded by the National Institutes of Health that evaluate treatments for children with asthma.

Environmental Protection Agency (www.epa.gov/iaq/asthma) Offers a plethora of background and resources about asthma and environmental influences on the disease.

Food Allergy & Anaphylaxis Network (www.foodallergy.org) A leading organization for food allergy and anaphylaxis awareness and the issues surrounding the condition.

National Institute of Allergy and Infectious Diseases (www.niaid.nih.gov) Provides print and online consumer resources for allergies and asthma.

National Jewish Medical and Research Center (www.njc.org) The only medical and research center in the United States devoted entirely to respiratory, allergic, and immune system diseases, including asthma, tuberculosis, emphysema, severe allergies, AIDS, cancer, and autoimmune diseases such as lupus.

Books

In addition to this book, library and bookstore shelves are filled with asthma/allergy tomes. Here are a few we particularly like.

Asthma for Dummies by William E. Berger, M.D. (Wiley, 2004)

Allergy-Free Living: How to Create a Healthy, Allergy-Free Home and Lifestyle by Anita Reid, Dr. Peter Howarth, and Asa Briggs (Mitchell Beazley, 2000)

My House Is Killing Me: The Home Guide for Families with Allergies and Asthma by Jeffrey C. May and Jonathan M. Samet (Johns Hopkins University Press, 2001)

The Allergy Bible by Linda Gamlin (Reader's Digest, 2001)

Major Allergy Associations

Both of these organizations hold annual medical meetings during which the latest research in the field is presented. Check their websites for press releases, abstracts, and other information from the meetings, as well as extensive consumer/patient information on allergies and asthma.

American Academy of Allergy, Asthma, and Immunology (www.aaaai.org)

American College of Allergy, Asthma, and Immunology (www.acaai.org)

Major Asthma/Allergy Journals

You can view free abstracts from these journals at www.pubmed.gov or on their websites. Some also allow you to sign up for e-mail delivery of their tables of contents.

Chest (www.chestjournal.org) Published by the American College of Chest Physicians.

Journal of Asthma
(www.dekker.com/servlet/product/productid/JAS) The official journal of the Association for the Care of Asthma.

Lung
(www.springerlink.com/app/home/journal.asp?wasp=570cdglhwk0wtul3hjf3&referrer=parent&backto=browsepublicationsresults,318,509) Publishes original articles, reviews, and editorials on all aspects of healthy and diseased lungs, the airways, and breathing.

Thorax (http://thorax.bmjjournals.com) A leading respiratory medicine journal that publishes articles on clinical and experimental research in respiratory medicine, pediatrics, immunology, pharmacology, pathology, and surgery.

Products for Allergy Sufferers

Here are three major suppliers of allergy-related products that we recommend. They stock everything from vent filters and cleaners to "de-miting" laundry additives and mattress and pillow casings. There are numerous others out there, but we've found these three to have the best selections, prices, and quality. All have full-color brochures that they'll send you.

Allergy-Free

905 Gemini
Houston, TX 77058
Phone: 800-255-3749
Fax: 281-486-9317
www.800allergy.com

National Allergy

1620-D Satellite Blvd.
Duluth, GA 30097
Phone: 800-522-1448
Fax: 770-623-5568
www.nationalallergy.com

Vitaire for Allergy

Phone: 800-447-4344
Fax: 201-592-6612
P.O. Box 800088
Elmhurst, NY 11380
www.vitaire.com

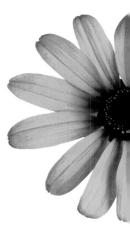

index